Integrated Women's Health: Holistic Approaches for Comprehensive Care

Edited by

Ellen Olshansky, DNSc, RNC

Associate Professor, Chair of the PhD in
Nursing Program, and Women's Health Care
Nurse Practitioner
Duquesne University School of Nursing
Pittsburgh, Pennsylvania

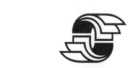

AN ASPEN PUBLICATION®
Aspen Publishers, Inc.
Gaithersburg, Maryland
2000

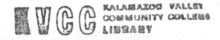

The author has made every effort to ensure the accuracy of the information herein. However, appropriate information sources should be consulted, especially for new or unfamiliar procedures. It is the responsibility of every practitioner to evaluate the appropriateness of a particular opinion in the context of actual clinical situations and with due considerations to new developments. The author, editors, and the publisher cannot be held responsible for any typographical or other errors found in this book.

Library of Congress Cataloging-in-Publication Data

Olshansky, Ellen Frances, 1949–
Integrated women's health: holistic approaches for comprehensive care/Ellen Olshansky.
p. ; cm.
Includes bibliographical references and index.
ISBN 0-8342-1219-6
1. Holistic nursing—United States.   2. Women—Health and hygiene—United States.
I. Title.
[DNLM: 1. Holistic Nursing—United States.   2. Women's Health—United States.
3. Health Promotion—United States.   WY 86.5 O52i 2000]
RT120.I5 O476 2000
613'.04244—dc21
00-020617

Orders: (800) 638-8437
Customer Service: (800) 234-1660

About Aspen Publishers • For more than 40 years, Aspen has been a leading professional publisher in a variety of disciplines. Aspen's vast information resources are available in both print and electronic formats. We are committed to providing the highest quality information available in the most appropriate format for our customers. Visit Aspen's Internet site for more information resources, directories, articles, and a searchable version of Aspen's full catalog, including the most recent publications: **www.aspenpublishers.com**
Aspen Publishers, Inc. • The hallmark of quality in publishing
Member of the worldwide Wolters Kluwer group.

Editorial Services: Kate Hawker
Library of Congress Catalog Card Number: 00-020617
ISBN: 0-8342-1219-6

Printed in the United States of America

1 2 3 4 5

*This book is dedicated to my family:
My parents, Jack and Lillian Olshansky;
my in-laws, David and Muriel Pattis;
my husband, Richard Pattis,
and my sons, Alexander and Mark Pattis*

Contents

Contributors

Gerri Adreon, BA
Assistant to the Dean
Duquesne University
School of Nursing
Pittsburgh, Pennsylvania

Brian Scott Austin, MS, CSCS
Head Strength and Conditioning
    Coach
Duquesne University
Pittsburgh, Pennsylvania

Joanne Banks-Wallace, PhD, RN
Assistant Professor
The University of Missouri
Sinclair School of Nursing
Columbia, Missouri

**Sister Donna Marie Beck, PhD,
    FAMI, MT-BC**
Associate Professor
School of Music
Department of Music Therapy
Duquesne University
Pittsburgh, Pennsylvania

Leslie Bonci, MPH, RD
Center for Sports Medicine
Pittsburgh, Pennsylvania

B. Jane Cornman, PhD, RN
Senior Lecturer
Department of Family and Child
    Nursing
University of Washington
School of Nursing
Seattle, Washington

**Leah Vota Cunningham, RN,
    MSN**
Assistant Professor and Vice
    Chair, BSN Program
School of Nursing
Duquesne University
Pittsburgh, Pennsylvania

Patricia Fedorka, RNC, PhD
Assistant Professor
Duquesne University
School of Nursing
Pittsburgh, Pennsylvania

Penny Lewis, PhD, ADTR, RDT-BCT
Executive Director and Co-Director
Alternative Route Training
Certificate in Transpersonal Drama Therapy
Institute for Healing and Wellness, Inc.
Depth Psychotherapist
Private Practice
Amesbury, Massachusetts
Senior Faculty
Antioch-New England Graduate School
Keene, New Hampshire

Joan Such Lockhart, PhD, RN, CORLN
Associate Professor and Chair, BSN Program
Duquesne University
School of Nursing
Pittsburgh, Pennsylvania

Michele Maloy, MSN, RN, CNRN, CRNP
Nurse Practitioner
Allegheny General Hospital
Department of Psychiatry
Pittsburgh, Pennsylvania

Christine D. Meyer, MSN, RN, FACCE
PhD Candidate
Duquesne University
School of Nursing
Pittsburgh, Pennsylvania

Ellen Olshansky, DNSc, RNC
Associate Professor,
Chair of the PhD in Nursing Program, Women's Health Care Nurse Practitioner
Duquesne University School of Nursing
Pittsburgh, Pennsylvania

Carol Patton, DrPH, RN, CRNP
Assistant Professor
Director of Family Nurse Practitioner Program
Duquesne University
School of Nursing
Pittsburgh, Pennsylvania

Natalie Pavlovich, PhD, RN, DiHt
Professor
Duquesne University
School of Nursing
Pittsburgh, Pennsylvania

Nicole Rawson, RN, ND, CNM, MPH
Interim Director
Center for International Nursing
Duquesne University
School of Nursing
Pittsburgh, Pennsylvania

Lenore K. Resick, MSN, RN, CS, CRNP
Assistant Professor
Director, Nurse-Managed Wellness Clinics
Duquesne University
School of Nursing
Pittsburgh, Pennsylvania

Melinda Kai Smith, PhD, RN
Associate Professor
Duquesne University
School of Nursing
Pittsburgh, Pennsylvania

**Shirley Powe Smith, MNEd,
   RN, CRNP**
Assistant Professor
Duquesne University
School of Nursing
Pittsburgh, Pennsylvania

Foreword

Integrated Women's Health: Holistic Approaches for Comprehensive Care
is a timely contribution to the literature on women's health. Indeed, it
is a book to lead practice into the twenty-first century. As the U.S.
population becomes increasingly diverse in its ethnic and cultural
makeup, new ideas about health and health care have permeated
American thinking. Not surprisingly, this new influence on our frame
of reference for health care is evident among women. Since the beginning of recorded history, women have assumed responsibility for the
health of their families, as well as their own health. Women have been
the keepers of the traditions, passing down the home remedies from
one generation to the next and seeking out new remedies to promote
health and treat disease.

Contemporary studies show that women engage in health-seeking
behavior for themselves and for their families. Women are often first
to notice a health problem, seek an explanation for that problem, investigate its significance and severity, and posit solutions, evaluating
which treatments seem to be effective. Likewise, women seem particularly motivated to engage in health-promoting behaviors and preventive and screening activities to reduce the chances of developing more
serious disease. In times of illness, women are often the first to attempt
to manage their own symptoms and those of their family member(s)
before seeking help from a professional. Women's social networks often have been the source of advice about self-care activities as well as
referral sources for professional care. In times of illness, particularly

chronic illness, or when family members need long-term or palliative care, women are likely to be the caretakers.

Integrated Women's Health offers a unique focus on women's health, one that reflects that health is not merely a matter of the body, but also psychological-emotional, social-cultural, and spiritual. In seeking health, women have been attracted to complementary therapies, those that often have been part of the culture for centuries. Only recently have scientists attempted to study these therapies in an attempt to evaluate their efficacy. As these complementary, yet traditional, therapies are evaluated, it is important to remember that they need to be viewed in the context of their administration to truly assess their efficacy. If only the herbal preparation is evaluated without reference to the interpersonal relationship in which it is administered, there may be little understanding of the true therapeutic value. This appreciation is clearly evident in *Integrated Women's Health*. Careful examination of the growing number of complementary therapies is a significant contribution to women's health. *Integrated Women's Health* provides women and health professionals with an important set of understandings about ways to enhance women's health.

Nancy Fugate Woods, PhD, RN, FAAN
Dean and Professor, University of Washington School of Nursing
Founding Director, Center for Women's Health Research
Seattle, Washington

Preface

WHY FOCUS ON WOMEN'S HOLISTIC HEALTH AND WELLNESS?

This book began originally as a comprehensive overview of health promotion for women. As the ideas for the book evolved, however, the concept of holistic health and women's wellness became clearly evident. In addressing health promotion for women in a comprehensive way, it seemed only natural to focus on a holistic approach, which encompasses a convergence of various methods of achieving and maintaining health; and health promotion naturally lent itself to a focus on wellness. This book, therefore, became centered around comprehensive, holistic approaches to achieving optimum wellness for women.

The foundation for the book is based on a bio-psycho-social-cultural-spiritual framework for understanding women's health and wellness (Figure 1–1 in Chapter 1). Women's health is described from this framework and then various "interventions" or approaches to optimizing women's health are described. These approaches include both traditional and alternative therapies with the intent of conceptualizing all of the therapies as "complementary" to one another. The intent of the book is to present these various approaches in the hopes that one, some, or a combination of a few may be useful for health care professionals who provide care for women. While the majority of the chapters present an overview of each approach with a review of the research to support our current knowledge, a few chapters provide some unique aspects. The chapter on storytelling among women (Chapter 21) is actually a reprint of an article that originally appeared in *MCN: The American Journal of Maternal-Child Nursing,* based on the author's own experiences in working in this area. The chapter on art therapy (Chapter 20) is a "journalistic" report of an interview with a woman who quilts and organizes groups of women quilters and who views her work as a way of contributing to women's wellness. The chapter on a woman's own experience in "coming to wellness" after suffering a stroke (Chapter 22) is an example of this woman's own life story, providing an example of how one can make constructive changes to achieve a higher level of wellness.

As we approach the twenty-first century, we have witnessed an incredible upsurge in technology, allowing for the development of many intricate health care interventions. While these interventions have assisted in enhancing longevity and quality of life, some disadvantages exist also. In this age of technology there is simultaneously an increased interest in "natural" or "folk" remedies as well. While these "natural" remedies have also assisted in enhancing longevity and quality of life, some disadvantages exist with these remedies too. Thus, the intent of this book is to provide an overview of various remedies and interventions in an effort to present a truly holistic, comprehensive approach to women's wellness, incorporating a variety of approaches.

The book does not contain specific "prescriptions" for women's wellness. Rather, there is a strong recognition of individual differences among both women and their care providers. Decisions regarding specific treatments, then, are based on recognizing, appreciating, and valuing these individual differences. This book was written in the spirit of celebrating women's strengths and the strengths of those who provide care for women.

I thank each of the contributors to this book. They have truly helped to enhance our understanding of women and their health. I also thank the editors at Aspen Publishers, Inc., in particular Mary Anne Langdon, Senior Developmental Editor, Martha Sasser, Editorial Director, Kate Hawker, Associate Editor, and Jill Berry, Freelance Production Editor. In addition, I am very thankful to Carmen Warner for her inspiration and motivation, and to Bob Howard, former acquisitions manager at Aspen, for his encouragement. And finally, my love and gratitude go to my family: my husband, Richard Pattis, and my two sons, Alex and Mark Pattis, who have consistently supported and encouraged me.

Ellen Olshansky, DNSc, RNC

CHAPTER 1

Conceptual Framework for Approaching Women's Wellness

Ellen Olshansky

Fundamental to holistic healing is the idea that the body, mind, and spirit form an integrated whole and that the individual is deeply connected to herself, her environment, and her community.

—Boston Women's Health Collective, 1998, p. 102

Groundbreaking work in the area of understanding women's health from the perspective of women themselves was done in the early 1970s with the first publication of *Our Bodies, Our Selves* (Boston Women's Health Collective, 1970). That publication generated an openness among women to talk with one another about common and shared health concerns that, until that time, were often difficult for women to discuss. Much of what was addressed in that now classic book was not addressed adequately by the scientific and medical community. The Boston Women's Health Collective and the women's health movement paved the way for the scientific community to begin to focus attention on the health care needs and concerns of women. The last decade of the twentieth century has witnessed a surge of interest in women's health as comprising unique and important aspects, and, as we move into the twenty-first century, women's health issues continue to raise important questions for scientists, health care providers, and women and their families. One challenge as we gain more scientific understanding of women is to keep that understanding merged with the Boston Women's Health Collective's appreciation for women's own experiences and perspectives of those experiences as they influence their own health and wellness.

Historically, women's health has been equated with reproductive health, limiting the scientific concerns regarding women to their reproductive organs only (Cohen, Mitchell, Olesen, Olshansky, & Taylor, 1993). As a result, other systems in women's bodies, such as cardiac and respiratory, were understood only in terms of men as the norm against whom women were measured or assessed. Traditional views of women reflected the perspective that it was only women's reproductive capacity that distinguished women from men. Early biblical stories, such as the creation of woman (Eve) from man (Adam's rib), contributed to the notion that, other than reproductive capacity, women's bodies functioned similarly to men's. As scientific findings have begun to reveal that women's health conditions are often different from men's and that women often experience symptoms of conditions different from the way men do, women's health issues, as unique and different from men's health, have received increasing attention recently, both from the media and from health care and research institutions. Historically, women have often been omitted from health and medical research because of fears related to pregnancy and potential harm to the fetus, but also because of concerns that the fact that women menstruate introduces extraneous variables into the study findings. The very fact of menstruation and the hormonal differences between men and women, however, are now being found to be key explanatory variables in why women and men experience many health conditions differently (Institute of Medicine, 1993). Beginning in 1993, the National Institutes of Health has mandated that women be included in all research studies, unless there is obvious reason to exclude women. The National Institutes of Health (NIH) funding for the Women's Health Initiative and the recently developed Office of Women's Health Research reflect the acknowledgment on the part of the U.S. government that research in women's health has been sorely lacking, and this funding was one step in beginning to rectify this lack. This is only one step, however. More knowledge is needed to understand women's health in all of its complexities.

As we do begin to focus increased attention on women's health needs and issues, it is critical that these issues not be viewed in isolation as only physical concerns. Women's bodily concerns need to be viewed and understood in relation to their psychological-emotional, social-cultural, and spiritual concerns and needs as well. Therefore, while the close of the twentieth century is witnessing greater interest and concern for women's health, we continue to be challenged to view and appreciate women's health as a complex, dynamic process that is influenced by many simultaneously interacting factors. While nurses have traditionally always valued health from a bio-psycho-social-cultural-spiritual perspective, we are challenged to continue to take this perspective and it is hoped that all health care providers, regardless of discipline, will incorporate such a perspective into their practice.

An important trend that is apparent in looking back on the women's movement as well as the women's health movement is that initially issues of concern were centered on white, middle-class, heterosexual women. Women within the women's movement were criticized for taking a largely ethnocentric approach to women's issues. Important recent contributions from women of diverse backgrounds have contributed a richer and more complex understanding and appreciation of the myriad challenges to women and society as we seek higher-level wellness. Issues of gender, race, class, and sexual orientation cannot be viewed as separate and distinct variables, but, rather, they must be viewed as constantly interacting factors that influence the health and well-being of each individual woman as well as the understanding of women's health from the perspective of the community and society.

IMPORTANT CONCEPTS

A holistic and integrated approach, wherein women are viewed as bio-psycho-social-cultural-spiritual beings, will enhance both our understanding of women's health in a more profound way and will enable the development of comprehensive approaches to the care of women. The purpose of this book is to present a comprehensive overview of significant health care issues for women, based on a holistic approach to understanding these issues and to suggest ways of assisting or intervening with women in regard to these issues. The focus of the book is on health promotion and disease prevention, emphasizing wellness. Therefore, serious health conditions such as cancer or heart disease are discussed in terms of preventing such conditions in an effort to promote optimal wellness. The emphasis is not on treatment of such conditions, but rather on prevention and early detection. Several concepts are emphasized throughout this book: integrated, holistic, complementary, and comprehensive approaches to care; dynamic and interacting factors that influence health; wellness and well-being; and health promotion and illness prevention. These concepts are represented in Figure 1–1 and they are described in the following section.

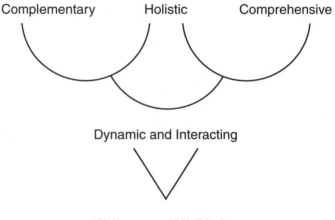

Figure 1–1 Conceptual Framework for Holistic Approach to Women's Health and Health Care.

Integrated

By *integrated*, this approach emphasizes the interrelationship of biological, psychological, emotional, social/cultural, and spiritual aspects that contribute to an individual's level of wellness or illness. Each one of these aspects, by itself, represents an aspect of a woman's level of wellness. Taken together, however, these aspects are more than the sum of their parts; they represent the woman's wellness in its entirety. This perspective of an integrated approach to understanding a woman's individual makeup is contrary to the widely accepted philosophy of Descartes (1960), who purported that mind and body are two distinctly separate entities. His philosophy undergirded Western medicine's philosophy of searching for the one cause of a particular disease in the hopes that that cause can be eliminated through medical procedures. While miraculous advances have been achieved in Western medicine and many infectious organisms have been wiped out, an integrated approach embodies the belief that illnesses are explained by more than one offending organism and that complex and dynamic interactions are occurring within one's self and one's social context that influence and contribute to one's overall sense of health and wellness. These interactions highlight the concept of integration, as various aspects of one's self are integrated with one another as they interact with one another.

Holistic

The term *holistic* has many connotations, which is why it is important to clarify its meaning as it is used in this book. *Holism,* from which holistic is derived, refers to a philosophy in which the belief is that whole entities are greater than the sum of their parts and that the parts can only be understood in relation to the whole entity (Random House Dictionary, 2nd edition, 1997). A holistic approach to health and health care, then, reflects a philosophical belief that optimal health care is comprehensive; complementary; balanced; multidisciplinary; and encompasses a biobehavioral, mental, emotional, and spiritual approach to wellness and well-being, as well as a health promotion and disease prevention approach. Dossey, Keegan, Guzzetta, and Kolkmeier (1995) described holism as meaning an integrated whole that is greater than the sum of its parts and that has a separate reality from each individual part. These authors focus on the importance of personal meaning as a key component in one's integrated and whole self. While we know that physiological changes affect women's lives, it is also important to understand how social and family changes directly affect women's lives, particularly in the many and varied concurrent roles that women must fulfill. The socioeconomic context has a major influence not only on access to health care, but also on the feasibility and ease with which women can make certain lifestyle changes to enhance their well-being. Psychological and spiritual factors also influence women's well-being. A holistic approach to women's health care takes into account these multiple factors that affect women's health and women's lives.

Often the term *holistic* connotes only alternative treatment or alternative approaches to care. For the purposes of this book, holistic means a comprehensive and integrated approach to health care. We are witnessing a surge of interest in naturalist health care approaches, including the use of herbs, nutrition, therapeutic touch, and acupuncture. The Office of Alternative Medicine (OAM), created within the National Institutes of Health, is evidence of this interest (Dossey,

1998). Dossey (1998) reported that 10 centers have been funded through OAM to study several holistic health therapies, and that the budget of the OAM is now $20 million annually, which was recently increased from $12 million. Dossey emphasized that the intent of these various studies is to enable integration of valid complementary therapies into the mainstream traditional health care system. In addition, several professional organizations have been developed, such as the American Holistic Nurses' Association, to focus on these "alternative" health care approaches. Many of these newly supported health care practices are directly relevant to women. At the same time, many of the traditional practices and interventions in health care have specific relevance to women. By including both traditional and nontraditional approaches to the health care of women, a truly holistic approach can be achieved, which is the intent of this book.

Comprehensive and Complementary

By *comprehensive*, this approach includes both traditional and alternative modalities of care. The book is not espousing a particular modality, but, instead is espousing a wide array of health care approaches that complement one another when used correctly and appropriately. For example, in our highly technological world we are fortunate to have many advanced and complex medical treatments, while at the same time human touch in the form of massage, therapeutic touch, or other modalities will complement this technology. Another term for comprehensive could be *complementary*, in which various health care modalities are recognized and used to provide maximum benefits to individuals. When these various health care modalities together provide optimum health care, the whole of these modalities is clearly greater than the sum of the individual parts. Thus, the concepts of comprehensive and complementary are closely related to the concept of holistic and are integral aspects of a holistic approach to care.

Dynamic and Interacting Factors Influencing Health

An essential aspect of taking and embracing a holistic approach to women's wellness is to understand and appreciate the depth of complexity of the constantly *interacting* and *dynamic* factors that influence women's health. The larger social and political issues cannot be separated out from this approach. Understanding how racism, sexism, and

heterosexism affect health is of central importance in truly comprehending the extent of factors involved in a holistic approach. The
larger social context of violence, particularly against women, also
must be included in understanding the multiple factors that influence
women's lives and women's health. These factors are also dynamic in
that their emphasis may change depending on changes within the
larger context.

Wellness and Well-being

Wellness and *well-being* are other terms that need to be defined for
the purposes of this book. Wellness is a state of health as experienced
by the person herself. Well-being refers to a sense of wellness or health,
wherein a woman experiences a balance of the various aspects of
health noted above. A key concept here is to recognize that wellness
and well-being have personal meaning for individual women.

Well-being is something that is subjective and may be measured differently by individual women. A woman with a chronic illness will
likely define well-being differently from a woman with no illnesses.
For example, a woman with severe arthritis may feel that she has made
good progress in an exercise routine if she can do sustained walking on
a treadmill for 15 minutes. A woman without arthritis, however, may
perceive good progress if she runs 3 miles. A woman in an abusive
relationship with a man may view well-being as an ability to seek help
from a women's shelter. Therefore, in understanding the concept of
well-being it is important to note that this is a concept that has different meanings and perceptions based on individual differences and
contexts of health. These various contexts cannot be separated out
from understanding well-being from the perspective of individual
women themselves.

Health Promotion and Illness Prevention

Health promotion and *illness prevention* are yet additional important
terms used in this book. Health promotion refers to the goal of maxi-
mizing one's state of health based on that particular individual. Similar to the concepts of wellness and well-being, health promotion has
different meanings for different persons based on their own particular
contexts. Illness prevention means engaging in activities to lessen the
chance of becoming ill. Prevention includes becoming involved in
healthy lifestyle habits in order to maximize one's potential for good

health. Prevention also includes undergoing routine assessments in an effort to detect any abnormalities at an early stage when they are most amenable to treatment, a situation known as secondary prevention. In order for women to benefit from secondary prevention, however, all women must have good access to health care. The American Nurses' Association is currently developing a set of guidelines for health care providers working in a managed care system, in which they emphasize the importance of access to care for all (Trossman, 1998). Understanding and improving the context of health care is important as we strive to achieve health promotion and illness prevention. Therefore, understanding and appreciating social and cultural aspects, as well as economic aspects of health care, are essential in this endeavor.

Perceptions of Health and Self

A key concept that transcends all of the concepts described above is the perception of the woman herself. That is, we, as health care providers, must be cognizant of the woman's own perception of her health and herself. Asking questions such as "what does wellness and well-being mean to her?" or "what does she perceive as important in treating or managing any of her particular health conditions?" are essential in allowing us to understand better her perceptions of her own health.

RATIONALE FOR TAKING A HOLISTIC APPROACH TO WOMEN'S WELLNESS

Current statistics on the status of women's health provide strong rationale for the need to develop more comprehensive approaches to the care of women. Woods (1995) described what she terms the "paradox" (p. 1) that is seen in the relationship between morbidity and mortality when viewed in terms of gender differences. Women experience lower mortality rates than do men for most causes of death in the United States, but the women tend to suffer a higher morbidity, or degree of illness, than do men. Women tend to suffer illnesses more often than men, but men tend to experience a higher mortality from illnesses than do women. Women make more visits to health care providers, although part of that may be due to taking children in for health care. While women experience a greater number of episodes of illness, women live longer than men. The fact that statistics do reveal a longer life span for women than for men is sometimes used as an argument for directing most health research toward men. Living longer, however, does not necessarily mean living a higher quality of life. Older women experience loneliness and depression as well as poverty and social isolation, and these factors must be taken into account when providing health care to these women.

The leading cause of cancer death in women is lung cancer, which is considered to be a largely preventable disease if people would not smoke. The fact that women are contracting lung cancer in greater numbers may be a reflection of a social or cultural issue related to why women smoke, whether it is due to stress, to being seduced by the media, or for other reasons. The fact that young women experience eating disorders, such as anorexia and bulimia, may also be a reflection of a social or cultural issue related to women's perceptions of the meaning of being thin. The fact that women suffer depression to a greater extent than do men may be a reflection of a combination of unique stressors that women experience as well as a biological makeup that is specific to women.

Women's physical health issues, other than reproductive health, have been largely ignored by the scientific and medical communities. Furthermore, the complexities of women's lives as reflected in their health have not been well understood, if at all. By taking a holistic perspective and approach to women's health, physical health will be better understood as a complex process that encompasses women's bodies beyond their reproductive system and that interacts with psychological, social-cultural, and spiritual aspects as well.

ORGANIZATION OF THE BOOK

This book is organized in three parts. Each part contains a short introduction, followed by several chapters.

Part I addresses important health issues and goals for women. The purpose of Part I is to present an overview of the major issues of importance for women as they seek to improve or maintain their level of wellness. This part contains descriptions of the major health issues for women, information on the implications or controversial aspects of these issues, and ways of approaching these issues from a health promotion and illness prevention perspective. This overview serves as the basis for describing the major goals regarding the promotion and maintenance of women's wellness. This part includes a general approach for women as they seek to maintain optimal wellness or improve their level of wellness. The goals reflect a holistic philosophy of seeking to achieve a maximum level of well-being based on each individual woman's perceptions and meanings of her own life context. The purpose of Part I is to provide direction for particular remedies or interventions that optimally can assist in achieving high level wellness for women.

Part II addresses various strategies for achieving the stated goals in Part I, based on a holistic approach to health and health care. Each chapter in Part II includes a summary and synthesis of the current research conducted on each strategy presented, with examples of the relevance of each strategy for women's wellness. The purpose of Part II is to provide guidance in developing holistic and complementary health care programs for women with the goal of achieving high-level wellness. Part II is not organized according to specific women's health issues (e.g., chapters are not organized according to approaches to cardiovascular health, approaches to psychological health), but rather according to particular strategies that are part of a larger holistic approach to women's wellness. Certain strategies will likely be helpful for some women in some situations, while other strategies will be less helpful. The intent is to provide an array of approaches to care, which can then be individualized for each woman based on her particular needs and situation.

Part III addresses several personal perspectives of women's experiences of health and illness. Some are cultural and some are personal vignettes.

While the book is not organized according to age-specific women's health issues and concerns, each part includes discussion of women's health issues across the life span. Focus is on particular age-related issues based on the relevance of those particular issues at specific ages.

It is hoped that this book will enable health care providers and health care educators to understand and communicate to others a comprehensive approach to women's wellness. Each reader may have certain beliefs about how to practice and intervene with women, and some of the approaches may be controversial, particularly due to their newness within the mainstream health care community. Some of the approaches clearly need more research to provide enough evidence for their efficacy and safety. Such research, if conducted in a scientifically rigorous manner, would yield much-welcomed information for women and their families. The newer approaches are not necessarily intended to replace traditional approaches, but instead to complement them in an effort to provide women with more options and better chances to live healthy, productive, and high-quality lives. As women are living longer, it certainly follows that high-quality, productive lives should be a goal for all women.

REFERENCES

Boston Women's Health Collective. (1998). *Our bodies, ourselves for the new century.* New York: Touchstone.

Boston Women's Health Collective. (1970). *Our bodies, ourselves.* New York: Touchstone.

Cohen, S., Mitchell, E., Olesen, V., Olshansky, E., & Taylor, D. (1994). From female disease to women's health. In A. Dan (Ed.), *Reframing women's health.* Thousand Oaks, CA: Sage.

Descartes, R. (1960). Meditations on first philosophy. In M.C. Beardsley (Ed.), *The European philosophers from Descartes to Nietzche* (pp. 25–96). New York: Random House. [Descartes' original work was published in 1644].

Dossey, B.M. (1998). Holistic modalities and healing moments. *American Journal of Nursing, 98*(6), 44–47.

Dossey, B.M., Keegan, L., Guzzetta, C., & Kolkmeier, L.G. (1995). *Holistic nursing.* Gaithersburg, MD: Aspen Publishers, Inc.

Institute of Medicine. (1993). *Report of a workshop: Women and drug development.* Washington, DC: National Academy Press.

Random House Dictionary (1997). 2nd edition. New York: Random House.

Taylor, D.L., & Woods, N.F. (1991). *Menstruation, health, and illness.* New York: Hemisphere Publishing Corporation.

Trossman, S. (1998). Issues update: Quality managed care: A nursing perspective. *American Journal of Nursing, 98*(6), 56, 58.

Woods, N.F. (1995). Women and their health. In C.I. Fogel & N.F. Woods (Eds.), *Women's health care: A comprehensive handbook.* Thousand Oaks, CA: Sage.

PART I

Health Issues and Goals for Women

Ellen Olshansky

Part I provides an overview of the major health care issues of current concern to women. In keeping with a holistic approach as well as with an expanded view of women's health, this overview is, by necessity, broad. Rather than presenting women's health as consisting mainly of reproductive and sexual issues, a more comprehensive overview of women's health concerns and issues is provided.

These issues are presented as a basis for a description of goals for women's wellness. These goals seek to reframe traditional views of women's wellness, which are usually limited to physical concerns. Four specific goals are presented which, together, comprise a holistic understanding of what is meant by holistic and integrated women's health. These goals provide the foundation for Part II, in which various health care approaches, both traditional and alternative, are presented. A major caveat for the reader is to study these goals with the understanding that they vary with each individual woman and that they occur on a continuum, based on the individual context within which each individual woman lives and experiences her life.

Because Part I is an overview, the reader is advised to seek more detailed texts for additional specific information related to each issue presented. It is hoped, however, that Part I will continue to give a comprehensive and holistic view of what is meant by the much-used term *women's health.*

CHAPTER 2

Physical Health

Ellen Olshansky

Women and their health care professionals are beginning to assess health along a continuum of wellness. Instead of asking, "Am I sick?" more women are now asking, "How well am I?" and "How well can I be?"

—Judelson & Dell, 1998, p. 2

While a main underlying concept of holistic approaches to health and health care is the notion of integrating mind and body, a separate chapter devoted to physical health is necessary in order to present clearly and emphasize strongly important aspects of women's physical health. Consistent with the philosophical stance of this book, however, physical health is not viewed as separate from emotional, psychological, social, cultural, and spiritual factors. It is believed that the physical health of women is affected by and affects all of these other aspects of women's lives. In addition, women's physical health problems will be more effectively prevented or ameliorated by a comprehensive, holistic approach to care that embraces all of these factors.

Another important point regarding women's physical health is that traditionally women's health was considered to be only that limited to women's reproductive health. This traditional focus reflected a larger societal view of women as primarily reproductive beings whose main goal was to conceive, bear, and raise children. With evolving social views of women as encompassing other important aspects of their lives in addition to reproduction, and with the recent focus on primary care and disease prevention, the conceptualization of women's physical health has broadened to comprise all bodily systems and functions, which includes, but is not limited to, women's reproductive function. Because women's reproductive health, however, includes much detailed and complex information, this book includes a separate chapter that is devoted solely to women's reproductive health issues. This current chapter addresses aspects of women's physical health other than reproductive health.

Thus, the reader is asked to keep in mind two caveats while reading this chapter. First, physical health is not, in actuality, separate from all other aspects of a person's health. Second, women's physical health includes but is much more than, reproductive and sexual health. For purposes of clarity and emphasis, this chapter is devoted solely to a description of women's physical health issues and concerns. Many of the physical conditions addressed in this chapter are also relevant to men. In many instances, the issues are similar for both men and women, but in some cases certain specific issues are of particular concern to women and these issues are highlighted (see box "Physical Health Issues with Specific Concerns for Women").

Each portion of this chapter addresses a broad topic related to women's physical health, including an overview of the particular topic and its relevance to women, assessment of the condition, symptoms, controversies, and recommendations. The focus of each portion is directed toward health promotion and disease prevention. Because this chapter provides an overview of the most common physical health

---

Physical Health Issues with Specific Concerns for Women

Cardiovascular health
Respiratory health
Diabetes
Hypertension
Fibromyalgia
Arthritis
Chronic fatigue syndrome
Lung cancer
Breast cancer
Colorectal cancer
Endometrial cancer
Ovarian cancer

Lymphoma
Skin cancer
Bladder cancer
Pancreatic cancer
Cervical cancer
Multiple sclerosis
Human immunodeficiency virus/acquired immune deficiency syndrome (HIV/AIDS)
Systemic lupus erythematosus
Urinary tract infection

issues for women, each condition cannot be addressed in depth. The purpose of this chapter is to familiarize the reader with these most common physical health issues with a view toward promoting optimal wellness for individual women within their own physical constraints. Where relevant, psychosocial/cultural issues are highlighted as they affect women's experience of particular physical conditions. In other chapters, certain physical conditions of women are also discussed, when these conditions are relevant to particular treatment modalities being presented.

CARDIOVASCULAR HEALTH

Women's cardiovascular health is currently receiving increased attention from health care researchers. In the past, the knowledge that existed regarding cardiovascular health in men was simply applied to women, without specific research conducted on women's cardiovascular functioning (Beery, 1995). In fact, women were often told that they were not at risk for cardiovascular disease until after they had reached menopause, negating any emphasis on cardiac health promotion for women prior to menopause. We now know that cardiac disease is the number one killer of women after menopause (National Center for Health Statistics, 1988). In fact, more women than men die from cardiac disease (Arnstein, Buselli, & Rankin, 1996). There is a 46% chance over a woman's lifetime that she will develop coronary artery disease (LaCharity, 1997). The number one cause of death among women 65 years and older is cardiovascular disease (Woods, 1995). Even if the majority of women with cardiac disease are of menopausal age, from a health promotion standpoint we can begin encouraging healthy lifestyles well before menopause. Murdaugh (1990) strongly admonishes health care providers to encourage women of all ages to develop healthy lifestyles in an effort to promote cardiac health. Therefore, attention to cardiac health in women is warranted even before women reach menopause.

Current research is finding that women experience symptoms of cardiovascular disease differently from the way men experience such symptoms, and there are differences in risk factors between men and women (Jensen & King, 1997). In addition, research indicates that women may be at greater risk of death, cardiac distress, and cardiac reinfarction during the first post-myocardial infarction (MI) year as compared with men (Young & Kahana, 1993). Assessments of cardiovascular status also are sometimes different for women as opposed to men, for example, in the assessment of laboratory values related to hyperlipidemia and in the assessment of findings on angiograms. Despite some marked differences between men and women, there are also many similarities, but the focus of cardiovascular health has traditionally been directed toward men, under the belief that women do not suffer from cardiovascular disease as much as do men. Attention to maintenance of cardiovascular health and prevention of disease is a priority in attempts to achieve high-level wellness for women. This section presents an overview of the important aspects of assessment of cardiovascular status, symptoms of cardiac disease, and issues and controversies related to maintenance of cardiovascular health and prevention of cardiovascular disease.

Assessment/Risk Factors of Women for Cardiac Disease

The major risk factors for women for cardiac disease include obesity, hypertension, hyperlipidemia (in particular as evidenced by the ratio of total cholesterol to high-density lipoproteins [HDL]), smoking, high-fat diet, sedentary lifestyle, and family history of cardiac disease. While these are risk factors for both men and women, there are some important distinctions based on gender. For hyperlipidemia, total cholesterol levels are less important than HDL levels for women, and triglyceride levels appear to be more important as indicators of cardiac disease in women as opposed to men.

Signs/Symptoms of Cardiac Disease among Women

Symptoms of cardiac disease may be experienced differently for women as compared with men. Studies have indicated that fewer women experience an MI after angina than do men, but when women do experience an MI the mortality rate is greater than it is for men because symptoms of angina in women are different as compared with men and the symptoms in women are more likely to be attributed to conditions other than cardiac (Ferrary & Parker-Falzoi, 1998), often precluding appropriate treatment.

Current Issues/Controversies

Encouraging certain lifestyle changes is not controversial in terms of the scientific rationale for doing so, particularly those changes that include increasing exercise, stopping smoking, and eating a low-fat and high-fiber diet. The issues that are raised surrounding these suggested lifestyle changes have to do with the social context in which women struggle to make such changes. When women are bombarded with advertisements that reflect sophisticated, sexy women who smoke, their understanding of the importance of not smoking becomes quite complicated. Women in very poor socioeconomic conditions who struggle to have food on the plates of their children may not consider developing a routine exercise program to be important. A woman living in a homeless shelter for women will likely not analyze labels on food to make sure that she is eating a low-fat, high-fiber diet. Thus, while these recommendations are not controversial, they are not without very serious issues and implications for individual women in particular situations/contexts.

Other recommendations are controversial. The use of hormone replacement therapy (HRT) remains controversial even though studies have demonstrated that estrogen replacement lowers the risk of cardiac disease (Smith & Judd, 1994). The controversy is related to other potential negative effects of HRT. The risk of uterine cancer has been greatly diminished due to the use of opposed estrogen, wherein estrogen is given along with progesterone. The risk of breast cancer, however, continues to be a concern in relation to HRT. Recent research is beginning to reveal an association between social support and lower morbidity and mortality from cardiovascular disease. The work by Ornish (1997) cites numerous research studies that strongly suggest a positive correlation between social intimacy and better outcomes with and even prevention of cardiovascular disease.

Current Recommendations for Women Related to Promotion of Cardiac Health and Prevention of Cardiac Disease

The major recommendations for women in the area of preventing cardiac disease and promoting cardiovascular health involve managing any risk factors that are present and preventing the occurrence of additional risk factors. Therefore, maintaining a healthy body weight through a low-fat and high-fiber diet, exercising regularly, managing stress, ceasing smoking or continuing to not smoke, and taking alcohol in moderation only are important behaviors. In addition, depending on the woman's unique situation, following certain suggestions for intervention is important. In Part II of this book, several approaches to care are useful for promotion of cardiac health, in particular, good nutrition, exercise, and development of healthy interpersonal relationships.

RESPIRATORY HEALTH

Respiratory health includes common acute and chronic ailments such as bronchitis, other upper respiratory infections, and asthma, as well as lung cancer. Lung cancer is addressed under "Cancer" later in this chapter. From a health-promotion perspective, it is essential to address preventable risk factors and management of some of the chronic conditions with the goal of improving one's quality of life. Of particular concern for women in relation to respiratory health is the importance of smoking cessation. Because much of the advertising for smoking is targeted to women (with the ads of sexy, youthful-looking women making an autonomous choice to smoke in a manner portrayed as achieving a certain social status), women have become more vulnerable to certain respiratory conditions, especially lung cancer. In this regard, then, aspects of respiratory health reflect important women's issues concerning health promotion and illness prevention.

Asthma

Asthma is a common respiratory condition, which is more common in women than it is in men (Verdon, 1997). This condition could be addressed under "Chronic Conditions," but since it is a major respiratory disorder it is addressed in this section instead.

Ringsberg, Segesten, and Akerlind (1997) conducted a grounded theory study of 14 women who had asthmalike symptoms even though they were never diagnosed with asthma. The women in this study described themselves as "walking around in circles" in which they felt socially isolated and frustrated by the fact that no specific treatment was offered to them because no specific diagnosis was made. This study emphasizes the chronic nature of such respiratory symptoms and how these symptoms affected the women's daily lives. Asthma is a reversible condition in which the airway is obstructed and inflamed. Asthma often occurs in response to external stimuli such as pollen, ragweed, grass, animals, house dust, mites, mold, and smoke from tobacco and wood stoves (Verdon, 1997).

Assessment/Risk Factors for Asthma

Asthma is assessed based on specific pulmonary tests, which include assessing pulmonary function tests (PFTs) that show reversibility of the obstruction when a bronchodilator is used, or hyperresponsiveness of the airways when histamine or methacholine challenge is given in the presence of PFTs. Verdon (1997) noted, however, that it is often necessary to include the patient's history and response of the patient's symptoms to the use of a bronchodilator in order to make a more accurate diagnosis.

Signs/Symptoms of Asthma

The major symptoms of asthma include cough, dyspnea, chest tightness, and wheezing, with wheezing being a classic symptom. Symptoms particularly occur directly after exercise and also during the night (Verdon, 1997).

Current Issues/Controversies

One important issue related to the condition of asthma is the effect this chronic illness has on families, particularly mothers of young children with asthma. Palmer (1999) addressed this issue, emphasizing the stressful effect on daily lives of families. The diagnosis of asthma can be challenging at times, particularly when a person does not experience wheezing, but does have a cough, when asthma may be confused with bronchitis or congestive heart failure (Verdon, 1997).

Current Recommendations for Women Related to Asthma

The major concern in living with the chronic condition of asthma is to ensure that a woman with asthma is oxygenated well and that even during pregnancy, she makes sure that she continues her treatment/management regimen for asthma. From a wellness and health-promotion perspective, encouraging women not to smoke or to stop smoking if they already have started, is very important. It is also important to help women learn to live with their asthma or to learn to live with having a family member (especially a child) with asthma. Learning to manage stress in their daily lives is part of how they can learn to live with their asthma and still lead healthy, productive lives.

Respiratory Infections

Respiratory infections include such conditions as bronchitis, pneumonia, and tuberculosis. Bronchitis is usually a self-limiting condition that resolves in about 7 to 11 days. Pneumonia is more severe than bronchitis, and tuberculosis, which used to be a common cause of death, is now a treatable respiratory infection.

CHRONIC CONDITIONS

Chronic diseases or conditions include diabetes, hypertension, fibromyalgia, and arthritis. Sometimes, from a wellness perspective, it is preferable to refer to these circumstances as conditions rather than diseases, as many people work hard at living "healthy" lives despite the presence of a chronic condition. Here is an example of "health" being determined from the perspective of the person experiencing it. In the case of a person with a chronic condition, it may be that that person can live to his or her highest potential within that limitation.

The specific chronic conditions discussed here are diabetes, hypertension, fibromyalgia, and arthritis. While other chronic conditions exist, such as chronic fatigue syndrome (discussed briefly here), these four are common and many of the concepts described regarding these conditions can be applied to an understanding of other chronic conditions.

Diabetes

Diabetes is a dysfunction of the insulin-producing blood glucose factors. Different categories of diabetes diagnoses include insulin-dependent diabetes mellitus, non–insulin dependent diabetes mellitus (NIDDM), gestational diabetes, and impaired glucose tolerance. Diabetes is controlled by diet alone, diet in combination with oral hypoglycemic medication, or diet in combination with insulin injections. The goal in living with diabetes is to control the blood glucose levels as much as possible. A unique aspect of diabetes for women is the situation of gestational diabetes, which is diabetes that is induced specifically by pregnancy as a result of an insulin-resistant state induced by pregnancy (Brown, 1997). Gestational diabetes occurs in approximately 3% of pregnant women, and approximately 60% of those women will develop NIDDM over the subsequent 20 years. In addition, there is a 90% chance that a woman who has developed gestational diabetes with one pregnancy will develop it in a subsequent pregnancy. Women of childbearing age, therefore, deserve attention regarding prevention of diabetes. Another factor unique to women is the presence of polycystic ovarian syndrome, which is a condition in which multiple benign cysts grow on the ovaries with attendant anovulation and hirsutism. Associated with this syndrome is insulin resistance and diabetes (Brown, 1997). These women, then, represent another group that deserves attention regarding prevention of diabetes or, at least, regulation of diabetes to achieve the highest potential for their individual health.

Assessment/Risk Factors for Diabetes

Risk factors for the development of diabetes include a family history, obesity, high-carbohydrate and high-fat diet, and for women with a history of gestational diabetes and presence of polycystic ovarian disease. Screening for diabetes is through fasting plasma glucose levels.

Signs/Symptoms of Diabetes

The classic symptoms of diabetes are polyuria, polydipsia, and polyphagia, with associated fatigue, weight loss, and possibly blurred vision. If diabetes is discovered and treated before the development of ketoacidosis (or ketosis), this is preferable. Once ketoacidosis occurs, the pancreas has become unable to produce any insulin at all. The condition resulting is referred to as diabetic ketoacidosis, with symptoms of nausea, vomiting, and abdominal pain in addition to the other symptoms of diabetes.

Current Issues/Controversies

Health care providers are focusing more attention on health promotion specifically related to diabetes prevention and control during pregnancy. Advances in scientific understanding of diabetes have contributed to the ability of individuals to control their blood sugar levels to a much higher degree than was possible previously. Women are now able to have healthy pregnancies despite diabetes, although the image of a pregnant woman with diabetes as being like the character portrayed in the movie *Steel Magnolias* persists and, to an extent, has validity. The presence of diabetes concurrent with pregnancy continues to pose challenges to scientists, health care providers, and women and their families.

Current Recommendations To Prevent Diabetes in Women or To Promote the Health of Women with Diabetes

Maintaining a healthy diet is paramount in managing diabetes, as well as is following any particular treatment regimen that has been prescribed. Certain social constraints, however, may impede successful management of diabetes, as some persons may not have access to healthy foods; teenagers, in particular, may find it difficult to follow a healthy diet while their friends are eating French fries and drinking Cokes after school each day. It is important for health care providers to be empathic about the pressures on teenagers, while making sure to encourage healthy habits in an effort to attain high-level wellness despite the presence of diabetes.

Hypertension

Hypertension is a problem with the cardiovascular system and is commonly defined as a systolic blood pressure of 140 mm Hg or greater and a diastolic blood pressure of 90 mm Hg or greater (Gibbons, 1995). Hypertension is associated with heart disease, stroke, and kidney failure. It is believed that women can live with hypertension for a longer time than men can before cardiovascular changes become apparent. However, once these changes do occur, the process is accelerated in women (Gibbons, 1995). Few studies have been conducted of hypertension in women, making it difficult to understand the unique aspects of this condition for women (*Harvard Women's Health Watch*, September 1998).

Assessment/Risk Factors for Hypertension

Hypertension is often included as a risk factor for other illnesses, such as stroke or heart attack, but it is important to understand the risk factors for hypertension itself. Family history, obesity, a sedentary lifestyle, and a very stressful lifestyle are major risk factors. Epidemiological studies reveal that hypertension is more prevalent in older people and in blacks and in persons of lower socioeconomic status. It is also more common in men than in women during midlife, but during old age, more women than men are prone to developing hypertension. Of particular concern to women is that oral contraceptives are associated with hypertension in some women. Assessment is through periodic and regular blood pressure screenings, making sure that a diagnosis of hypertension is not made based on one blood pressure reading alone.

Signs/Symptoms of Hypertension

Hypertension is often referred to as the "silent killer," as there are frequently no apparent symptoms that alert a person to the fact that he or she may be hypertensive. Sometimes women do describe vague symptoms, such as headache, that they associate with hypertension.

Current Issues/Controversies Related to Hypertension

Health care providers tend to agree on the fact that hypertension must be controlled in women, as it is a major risk factor for cardiovascular disease, the number one killer in women. Some controversies exist over when to decide to treat hypertension and how to assess the presence of hypertension accurately. For example, many persons will have a slightly high blood pressure reading at one time and then a lower reading later. Making sure that several blood pressure readings are obtained is important in arriving at an accurate assessment.

Current Recommendations To Prevent Hypertension or To Promote the Health of Women with Hypertension

Preventive approaches to hypertension include dietary management, cessation of smoking, regular exercise routine, limiting alcohol intake, and maintaining a healthy body weight (*Harvard Women's Health Watch,* September 1998). For women already diagnosed with hypertension, the preventive approaches will help to manage their hypertension along with whatever treatment regimens are prescribed by their health care provider (often in the form of pharmacological treatment).

Fibromyalgia

Fibromyalgia is a muskuloskeletal disorder that tends to affect women proportionately more than it affects men, in fact, at a rate of 10 times more frequently in women (Williams & Kaul, 1995). There is no known specific cause for fibromyalgia, and it tends to be viewed as a syndrome that involves pain and tenderness in various and widespread areas of the body. While there is no known specific cause, many people do have what is often referred to as reactive fibromyalgia in which the condition occurs as a result of a catalytic event, such as an accident or perhaps a virus infection. Even these types of fibromyalgia are vague, however, in terms of causation.

Assessment/Risk Factors for Fibromyalgia

The main assessment technique for the presence of fibromyalgia is the detection of pain in 11 of 18 tender point sites that have been developed by the American College of Rheumatology (as cited in Williams & Kaul, 1995). In addition to these specific pain sites, the criterion of widespread pain is determined by several factors that include pain for more than 3 months, pain at sites both above and below the waist, pain on both the right and left sides of the body, and axial pain (cervical or anterior chest, thoracic spine, or lower back).

Signs/Symptoms of Fibromyalgia

Fibromyalgia includes widespread pain and tenderness as well as sleep disturbances, stiffness, and fatigue.

Current Issues and Controversies/Recommendations

The major issue that is raised in relation to fibromyalgia is the vagueness and chronicity of symptoms and often unknown etiology of symptoms. Treatment of fibromyalgia is directed at alleviating the symptoms. Pain management, education, exercise, and focusing on alleviating sleep disturbances all will help in the successful management of fibromyalgia. Smoking, because of its vasoconstrictive effects and consequent muscle ischemia, is believed to exacerbate symptoms of fibromyalgia. Alcohol, because of its propensity for contributing to sleep disturbances, is also believed possibly to exacerbate fibromyalgia. Therefore, tobacco and alcohol are substances that are considered harmful to persons with fibromyalgia and it is recommended that these substances be avoided.

Arthritis

Arthritis is a degenerative condition in which changes occur in the cartilage and inflammation occurs in the soft tissue, leading to pain in the joints. There are two major kinds of arthritis, osteoarthritis and rheumatoid arthritis, with both occurring more commonly in women than in men. Osteoarthritis, however, is the more common type of arthritis (Acheson & Abelson, 1997), affecting the joints of the hand, knee, hip, foot, spine, and other joints. Arthritis progressively worsens with age, affecting almost all people to some degree over age 80 (Acheson & Abelson, 1997) and can be very disabling.

Assessment/Risk Factors for Arthritis

Certain techniques for assessment of arthritis include examining the synovial fluid of the joints, which may reveal the presence of crystals, and radiological studies, which may indicate subchondral changes and narrowing of the joint spaces (Acheson & Abelson, 1997). Risk factors for the development of arthritis include age, female gender, repetitive joint stress, and obesity.

Signs/Symptoms of Arthritis

The major symptom of arthritis is pain, particularly an aching pain with morning stiffness. This pain is usually noted to occur in persons over age 45 and can be subtle initially, but can worsen over time.

Current Controversies

While it is not a major controversy, a major challenge in caring for a person with arthritis involves balancing the treatment with encouraging the person to maintain her activities of daily living. That is, health care providers must be sensitive to the patient's complaints of pain, but also encourage her to become active in self-help groups or other resources to learn to manage and live with the pain. While more treatments are being developed, such as improved hip replacement surgery, controversy often exists as to when such surgery is appropriate for an individual.

Current Recommendations

At this point, pharmacological treatment seems to be a major approach in the management of persons with arthritis. Several different pharmacological approaches can be employed (see Chapter 10). Other approaches include developing an exercise program, resting and protecting the joints, possibly applications of heat and/or cold; psychological approaches such as support groups; and, for more severe cases, arthroscopy or surgery. Certain lifestyle changes can assist women also. A study reported in the *University of California at Berkeley Wellness Letter* (September 1998) revealed that women who consistently wear high heels are at a greater risk of developing a condition called "torque," a rotational force applied around a joint, such as the knee, which, over time, can lead to arthritis.

Chronic Fatigue Syndrome

Chronic Fatigue Syndrome is a vague, although not uncommon, condition that appears to be more prevalent in women than it is in men (Buchwald, 1995). Many of the classic symptoms of this condition are also symptoms of underlying psychiatric disorders. It is interesting to note that in the attempts to distinguish the essential features of this condition, the difficulty in doing so stems from the overlap of such features with other conditions. This fact may, ironically, represent the need for a holistic approach to diagnosis of many conditions and, subsequently, the need for a holistic approach to treatment of such conditions.

CANCER

The major cancers of women, in order of incidence, are lung, breast, colorectal, endometrial, ovarian, lymphoma, skin, urinary bladder, pancreas, and cervix (American Cancer Society, 1997). Some cancers may be preventable, although much more research is needed in this area. Prevention includes lifestyle changes, early detection, and some specific factors related to specific cancers. For example, lung cancer is linked to smoking (U.S. Public Health Service, 1998), and some cancers are linked to high-fat diets (American Dietetic Association and Canadian Dietetic Association, 1995). Because the etiology of the various cancers is so complex, it would be quite misleading to assume that simply eliminating these suspect elements will eliminate the risk for a particular cancer. Much more research is needed and it is likely that a complex interaction of factors is responsible for particular cancers.

Lung Cancer

While breast cancer occurs more frequently in women than does lung cancer, lung cancer is the number one cause of cancer death for women (Beckett, 1995), making prevention of lung cancer a critical issue for women.

Assessment/Risk Factors for Lung Cancer

While some lung cancer is caused by exposure to radon, asbestos, and "secondary" smoke, research tells us that about 90% of lung cancers are a result of cigarette smoking (Risser, 1996). Cigarette smoking among women has increased over the past several decades (Beckett, 1995) and some research suggests that women have a greater susceptibility than men to smoking's carcinogenic effects.

Signs/Symptoms of Lung Cancer

The most common symptom of lung cancer is a chronic and persistent cough. In addition, a person may experience pain in her chest and increased sputum production that is occasionally bloody (Snyderman, 1996).

Current Issues/Controversies

Many cigarette advertisements target women, particularly younger women. Controversies center around the ethics of allowing such advertisements. Some estimates indicate that by the year 2000, more women than men will suffer mortality that is directly related to smoking (Moore, 1995). From a health-promotion perspective, the majority of lung cancer can be prevented by lifestyle changes that include cessation of smoking.

Current Recommendations

The most important recommendation in terms of primary prevention of lung cancer is to educate women about the importance of avoiding smoking. For women who do smoke, emphasizing smoking cessation programs is crucial.

Breast Cancer

Breast cancer is the most common form of cancer in women. While the majority of masses found in the breast are benign, any mass deserves further attention. Recent research has led to promising advances for the prevention and treatment of breast cancer (*Harvard Women's Health Watch*, July 1998). Two new approaches to prevention of breast cancer involve two drugs: Nolvadex (tamoxifen) and Evista (raloxifene). Two new approaches to treatment of breast cancer involve two other drugs: Taxol (paclitaxel) and herceptin.

Assessment/Risk Factors for Breast Cancer

Risk factors for breast cancer include a family history (particularly mother, grandmother, sister), and possibly a history of mammary dysplasia. It is important to note, however, that most women diagnosed with breast cancer do not have any known risk factors (Thirlby, 1995). Thirlby (1995), in fact, emphasized that all women, regardless of identified risk factors, should be evaluated routinely for breast cancer. Breast cancer itself is usually detected through one of the following or a combination of each: monthly breast-self examination, clinical breast examination, mammography, and possibly ultrasound, with biopsy of any suspicious lesions.

Signs/Symptoms of Breast Cancer

A benign condition, referred to as fibrocystic breasts, is prevalent in younger women. This condition consists of cyclic breast tenderness related to the menstrual period and the presence of symmetrical, palpable, mobile, incapsulated cysts. Benign masses are usually mobile with obvious margins and they are often tender. The usual first sign of breast cancer is a single, nontender, firm, immobile mass that is unilateral. Occasionally a woman may experience nipple discharge, but unless the discharge is bloody, it is usually not a sign of cancer. Rarely a woman may notice thickening of the skin of the breast, dimpling, or eczematoid nipple changes (Thirlby, 1995).

Current Issues/Controversies

Breast cancer has received heightened attention recently, leading both to greater understanding and improved detection and treatment techniques. Additionally, however, many controversies have risen to the forefront related to management of breast health, prevention of and screening for breast cancer, and treatment of breast cancer. Genetic research has led to the discovery of certain genetic factors that predispose a woman to breast cancer, leading to ethical questions regarding the implications of such information without assurance of what, in fact, this information means for an individual woman. The possibility of discrimination by health insurance companies against women with a known genetic predisposition to breast cancer cannot be ignored. Controversies over whether diet or exercise may help in preventing breast cancer continue, with further research needed in these areas. Issues related to appropriate guidelines for screening mammograms center around the degree of risk versus benefit of using screening, particularly related to the frequency with which women between the ages of 40 and 50 should be screened. The treatment for breast cancer continues to have some controversies surrounding it. For example, when is a simple lumpectomy just as effective as a radical mastectomy? While much progress has been made in this area, individual women continue to struggle with various treatment options. As with many health conditions, access to care raises issues of equal access. For example, Ashing-Giwa and Ganz (1997) found that most African-American women in their study received inadequate information and support as they went through the initial diagnosis and treatment phases of breast cancer. They also found that women with lower socioeconomic status and less education often received lower-quality health care, reflected in lack of coordinated care and poor patient-provider relationship.

Current Recommendations

Currently, women are advised to maintain a regular exercise program, a low-fat diet, and to perform breast self-examination monthly. It has been suggested that for menstruating women, it is best to examine the breasts approximately 1 week to 10 days after beginning the menses, when the breasts are least tender. For nonmenstruating women, it is important that they simply stay on a monthly schedule, whether it be every fourth Sunday, or whatever monthly schedule works for them. In addition to monthly breast self-exam, it is recommended that all women have a yearly clinical breast exam by a qualified health care provider. Mammograms are recommended yearly for all women from age 50 and up. For women ages 40 to 50, there is controversy around the frequency of recommended mammography. Some believe that women should have the procedure every 2 years, while others believe they should have it every year. It is also recommended that all women have a baseline screening mammogram at about age 35.

Colorectal Cancer

Colorectal cancer has only recently received more attention. This kind of cancer really deserves more focus on prevention, since it is one kind of cancer that truly may be decreased by preventive action. While the etiology of cancer of the colon and rectum is unclear, many things are known about ways of preventing colon cancer.

Assessment/Risk Factors for Colorectal Cancer

Risk factors for colon cancer include a family history, possibly a genetic risk factor, and a diet that is high in fat and low in fiber. Assessment of colon cancer includes yearly rectal examinations with a check for blood in the stools and sigmoidoscopy or colonoscopy beginning at age 50 (or earlier if a person has strong risk factors) at intervals dependent upon the specific risk factors of the individual.

Current Issues/Controversies

While colorectal cancer is receiving increasing attention recently, much more focus must be placed on this common form of cancer. Particularly because early and regular screening increases the likelihood of survival if cancer is detected, more public education must be directed toward a preventive approach to colorectal cancer.

Current Recommendations

Prevention includes several suggestions (*University of California at Berkeley Wellness Letter,* December 1998), as follows: (1) eating a diet that is low in fat and calories, high in fiber, high in β-carotene, calcium, folic acid, vitamins C and D; (2) decreasing alcohol intake; (3) avoiding smoking; (4) cooking without charbroiling or frying, trimming all visible fats from meats; (5) possibly taking low-dose aspirin; (6) exercising regularly; and (7) undergoing regular screening tests to detect precancerous polyps that can be removed before becoming malignant or, if malignant, before they spread.

Endometrial Cancer

Endometrial cancer, or uterine cancer, is another leading type of cancer in women.

Assessment/Risk Factors for Endometrial Cancer

The most direct way to detect endometrial cancer is with an endometrial biopsy or a dilation and curettage, as a pap smear often does not allow examination of endocervical cells. Those who have a major risk factor for endometrial cancer include women who have never had children; women who are obese, hypertensive, or diabetic; and women who are on estrogen replacement therapy that does not include progesterone to oppose the estrogen (Snyderman, 1996).

Signs/Symptoms of Endometrial Cancer

The major symptom of endometrial cancer is abnormal uterine bleeding. A particularly serious symptom is for a postmenopausal woman to experience abnormal bleeding, since endometrial cancer occurs most commonly in postmenopausal women.

Current Issues/Controversies and Recommendations

One important issue in relation to prevention of endometrial cancer is that many postmenopausal women believe that they do not need gynecological exams. Because of the importance of screening for endometrial cancer, which is associated with high survival rates if detected early, all women, regardless of being menopausal, must be encouraged to have annual gynecological exams.

Ovarian Cancer

Ovarian cancer is one of the more elusive cancers in that it often presents initially with no or few symptoms.

Assessment/Risk Factors for Ovarian Cancer

A family history of ovarian cancer puts a woman at higher risk than the general population for the development of this condition. Screening for ovarian cancer is problematic, as no cost-effective, accurate means for such screening exists today. Pelvic exams are very inaccurate, but combined with ultrasonography and the CA 125 laboratory test, the accuracy increases, but research has found that morbidity has not decreased significantly (Yon, 1995).

Signs/Symptoms of Ovarian Cancer

Very few symptoms accompany the early stages of ovarian cancer. With advanced cancer, a woman may experience ascites. Upon a pelvic examination, the practitioner may palpate an enlarged ovary, which could be an important sign of ovarian cancer.

Current Issues/Controversies and Recommendations

The biggest issue in relation to ovarian cancer is that more research is needed to understand the signs and symptoms better so that early detection will be possible with consequent greater survival rates. A recent issue is the implication that fertility drugs (clomiphene citrate, human menopausal gonadotropin) have been correlated with an increased incidence of ovarian cancer, but the research is inconclusive (Goldfien, 1998). Recommendations include that all women have annual pelvic examinations. Other screening examinations, such as blood tests, are still controversial regarding their accuracy.

Lymphoma

Lymphoma is a cancer of the lymphatic system. Non–Hodgkin's lymphoma is the more common type, and there are several forms of this kind of lymphoma.

Assessments/Risk Factors for Lymphoma

More needs to be learned about risk factors for development of lymphoma. Sometimes age is a risk factor, but this kind of cancer also occurs in young and middle-aged adults. No screening tests exist for lymphoma, although there are tests to confirm the diagnosis.

Signs/Symptoms of Lymphoma

The major symptoms of lymphoma include enlarged lymph nodes in the neck, underarm, or groin. These nodes are often painful and swollen and occur in conjunction with fever, fatigue, and weight loss. A physical examination will reveal palpable, enlarged lymph nodes.

Current Issues/Controversies and Recommendations

Because this kind of cancer is more elusive in that no specific screening tests are available, it is important to encourage women to seek consultation from health care providers if they notice any untoward symptoms that may be indicative of lymphoma. As with other cancers, early detection will increase one's chances of long-term survival.

Skin Cancer

Skin cancer is one of the most curable cancers if found early. Basal cell carcinoma is usually curable because it generally does not metastasize, although it can be disfiguring if not removed. Squamous cell carcinoma, while more serious than basal cell carcinoma, also has a very high cure rate. Melanoma is also curable if found early and removed, but this cancer, if not removed, aggresively metastasizes and can be fatal. Protection from the sun is essential.

Assessment/Risk Factors for Skin Cancer

One very important risk factor is a history of sunburns with peeling and continued sun exposure without protection of sunscreens. For melanoma, a family history contributes to risk. Also, the presence of many nevi and certain other skin lesions that may be considered precancerous (such as actinic keratosis) are considered to be risk factors.

Signs/Symptoms of Skin Cancer

The major sign/symptom of skin cancer is the presence of a skin lesion that has recently occurred or that has changed recently. For melanoma, the major signs include what is commonly referred to as "the ABCD" description: Assymetry, irregular Borders, multi-Colored, and Diameter greater than the size of a pencil eraser.

Current Recommendations

Protection from the sun is a major recommendation for all persons, but especially those who are fair skinned with light-colored eyes. Protection from the sun is achieved by staying out of the sun, or wearing wide-brimmed hats and other clothes to protect the skin, and/or wearing sunscreen with adequate sun protection factor (SPF). Routine skin examinations are also recommended, particularly for those at risk for skin cancer.

Current Controversies/Issues Related to Prevention of Skin Cancer

Questions may be raised as to what is an adequate amount of SPF to protect adequately against skin cancer. Alternative therapies for promotion of skin health include the use of vitamin E and lotions with other ingredients.

Cancer of the Urinary Bladder, the Pancreas, and the Cervix

Cancer of the urinary bladder, the pancreas, and the cervix comprise the eighth, ninth, and tenth most common forms of cancer in women.

Bladder Cancer

Bladder cancer usually is accompanied with symptoms of pain or burning with urination and blood present in the urine. Bladder cancer occurs more frequently in men than in women, but it is the eighth most common form of cancer in women. Bladder cancer is associated with smoking.

Pancreatic Cancer

Pancreatic cancer, which has been correlated with cigarette smoking, is a very elusive form of cancer, with few, if any, early signs and symptoms. Usually by the time the classic signs of sudden weight loss, abdominal pain, and loss of appetite occur, the cancer is well advanced. Unfortunately there are no screening tests for pancreatic cancer.

Cervical Cancer

Cervical cancer is highly curable because it grows slowly and is detectable through pap smears. Often very few symptoms accompany the development of cervical cancer, which is why it is so important to have regular screening examinations (pelvic exam and pap smear).

Examining the issue of women and cancer in general, without reference to specific kinds of cancers, raises some general issues for women and health care providers. Access to care, especially access to secondary prevention techniques (e.g., mammogram, colonoscopy, pap smear) cannot be assumed to be available equally to all women. The social context, therefore, presents an important and complex challenge in the provision of health-promoting care for women. Fears related to the meaning of the word *cancer* often preclude some women from even seeking care, due to the fear and anxiety of having to confront such a condition. Understanding women's psychological issues related to health promotion and prevention of cancer is essential in providing health care services that women will, in fact, use. A holistic approach to care considers these psychological issues as well as the development of scientific strategies for diagnosis and treatment. For example, understanding why women do not seek regular mammography elucidates important information as health care providers are challenged with encouraging optimal health promotion practices.

MUSCULOSKELETAL CONDITIONS

Some musculoskeletal conditions can be categorized under chronic conditions. Arthritis is one example and this condition is addressed under "Chronic Conditions."

NEUROLOGICAL CONDITIONS

Multiple sclerosis (MS) is a neurological disease that occurs twice as frequently in women as it does in men (Swain, 1996). The etiology of MS is unknown, but it appears that it occurs more commonly among those persons from Western European descent who live in temperate climate zones (Aminoff, 1997).

Signs/Symptoms of Multiple Sclerosis

Symptoms can include sensory abnormalities, blurred vision, sphincter disturbances, and weakness that may or may not be associated with spasticity (Aminoff, 1997). Because the disease has variable symptoms and is associated with many unknowns regarding long-term effects, Crigger (1996) has aptly addressed the issue of how to help women attain an adequate level of mastery despite the unknowns with which they are living.

INFECTIOUS CONDITIONS

Many sexually transmitted infections fall under the category of infectious conditions, but these infections are discussed in Chapter 3. Urinary tract infections are discussed in this chapter, however, as is human immunodeficiency virus (HIV), as these infections occur through multiple routes, including, but not limited to, sexual transmission.

Human Immunodeficiency Virus/Acquired Immune Deficiency Syndrome

Since the initial identification of the human immunodeficiency virus (HIV), the virus that causes acquired immune deficiency syndrome (AIDS), much progress has been made in understanding the etiology and progression of this virus. In the late 1970s and early 1980s this virus and disease were perceived as "gay men's afflictions." This notion developed because the first persons found to have the conditions were gay men who acquired the disease through homosexual relations. As a result of this perception, HIV and AIDS were not taken very seriously among the mainstream health professions and by society. Women, in fact, were not thought to be at risk for these conditions. With more research and consequent enlightenment and understanding about the AIDS disease, we learned that HIV is transmitted through blood and other body fluids, regardless of homosexuality or heterosexuality. Because gay men still were the predominant members of the population who were found initially to have contracted the disease, women were, for the most part, ignored as being at risk. Today, as we approach the new millennium, we understand that all of us are at risk for HIV/AIDS and women, in particular, have certain unique issues that must be addressed. These issues involve perinatal and breast-feeding transmission of the virus. Additionally, they involve issues of sexuality for women, as mentioned under "Prevention of Sexually Transmitted Diseases" in Chapter 3. Women must be vigilant in making sure that their male partners who may be at risk for HIV/AIDS consistently use condoms during all aspects of sexual relations. A recent article in the *New York Times* (December 4, 1998) reported that HIV in Subsaharan Africa is now believed to be present in one quarter of the population, with women being stigmatized and shamed by their male partners who, in fact, often are the ones who have transmitted the virus to the women.

Urinary Tract Infections

Urinary tract infections (UTIs) are very common in women, and older women are more susceptible than younger women to developing such infections (Robertson & Hebert, 1994). The offending bacteria usually originate in the vagina or rectum and can travel up the urethra to the bladder, the ureters, and the kidneys.

Assessment/Risk Factors

Sexual intercourse and the presence of vaginal infection as well as lowered estrogen levels may contribute to the development of a urinary tract infection. The woman may also experience suprapubic pain. Laboratory findings reveal an increased white blood cell count in the urine as well as the presence of bacteria, usually *Escherichia coli* (Robertson & Hebert, 1994).

Signs/Symptoms

The woman usually complains of dysuria, and urgency and frequency of urination.

Current Recommendations/Controversies

The usual traditional treatment for a UTI is with antibiotics. Herbal and homeopathic remedies have also been found to be useful in the management of UTIs.

AUTOIMMUNE CONDITIONS

Systemic lupus erythematosus (SLE) is an autoimmune disease of the connective tissue, in which the connective tissue is destroyed. Women are at a much higher risk than are men for this disease, with African American women at particular risk (Snyderman, 1996). SLE is a chronic condition that consists of several clinical symptoms, including a rash on the face that resembles a butterfly form over the bridge of the nose and across the cheeks; pain, swelling, and redness at various joints; skin sensitivity to sunlight; skin rashes; hair loss; anemia; fatigue; poor circulation to fingers and toes during cold or stress; bladder and kidney problems; nausea with or without vomiting; enlarged lymph nodes; and depression (Snyderman, 1996). While no cure exists for SLE, certain treatments can minimize discomforts associated with it. Such treatments include aspirin, avoidance of the birth control pill, avoidance of exposure to sun, exercise, following a low-fat diet, and getting enough rest.

REPRODUCTIVE FUNCTIONING

A separate chapter is devoted to reproductive and sexual health of women (see Chapter 3). It is helpful to note, however, that certain reproductive conditions may reflect other systemic conditions. Also, some sexually transmitted diseases may affect the body beyond only the sexual organs.

SUMMARY

For all of the women's physical health conditions described in this chapter, it is appropriate to summarize certain strategies for managing these conditions. While it is not always possible to prevent these various conditions, some may be preventable and most can be ameliorated to some extent by engaging in specific strategies. These strategies are categorized according to lifestyle or behavioral approaches, which include physical exercise and healthy nutrition, as well as cessation of smoking and stress-reduction techniques. For certain conditions, specific pharmacological or nonpharmacological (herbal, homeopathic, music, touch, acupuncture, biofeedback) treatments may be appropriate, as noted where applicable. Appropriate screening and early detection are also essential elements of health promotion and disease prevention. On a larger societal level, working to ameliorate oppressive conditions within the social context will improve the physical health and health care of women and of all individuals and communities. Understanding how social contextual issues influence one's health and health care is necessary in order to work toward developing useful strategies of addressing important health care issues. Understanding the myriad psychological issues associated with living with and managing specific physical health care conditions is also essential in working toward developing effective strategies of health care and a wellness approach to health care.

REFERENCES

Acheson, L.S., & Abelson, A.G. (1997). Osteoarthritis. In J.A. Rosenfeld (Ed.), *Women's health in primary care*. Baltimore: Williams & Wilkins.

American Cancer Society (1997). Cancer facts and figures.

American Dietetic Association and Canadian Dietetic Association (!995). Position statement: Women's health and nutrition. *Journal of the American Dietetic Association, 95*, 362–366.

Aminoff, M.J. (1997). Nervous system. In L.M. Tierney, S.J. McPhee, & M.A. Papadakis (Eds.), *Current medical diagnosis and treatment*. Stamford, CT: Appleton & Lange.

Arnstein, P.M., Buselli, E.F., & Rankin, S.H. (1996). Women and heart attacks: Prevention, diagnosis, and care. *Nurse Practitioner: American Journal of Primary Health Care, 21*(5), 57–58, 61–62.

Ashing-Giwa, K., & Ganz, P.A. (1997). Understanding the breast cancer experience of African-American women. *Journal of Psychosocial Oncology, 15*(2), 19–35.

Beckett, W.S. (1995). Lung cancer in women: Selected topics in epidemiology and prevention. *Journal of Women's Health, 4,* 637–643.

Beery, T.A. (1995). Gender bias in the diagnosis and treatment of coronary artery disease. *Heart and Lung, 24,* 427–435.

Brown, A.J. (1997). Diabetes: Prevention, treatment, and follow-up. In J.A. Rosenfeld (Ed.), *Women's health in primary care.* Baltimore: Williams & Wilkins.

Buchwald, D. (1995). Chronic fatigue syndrome. In D.P. Lemcke, J. Pattison, L.A. Marshall, & D.S. Cowley (Eds.), *Primary care of women.* Norwalk, CT: Appleton & Lange.

Crigger, N.J. (1996). Testing an uncertainty model for women with multiple sclerosis. *Advances in Nursing Science, 18*(34), 37–47.

Ferrary, E., & Parker-Falzoi, J. (1998). Common medical problems: Cardiovascular through hematologic disorders. In E.Q. Youngkin & M.S. Davis (Eds.), *Women's health: A primary care clinical guide.* Stamford, CT: Appleton & Lange.

Gibbons, E.F. (1995). Risk factors for coronary artery disease and their treatment. In D.P. Lemcke, J. Pattison, L.A. Marshall, & D.S. Cowley (Eds.), *Primary care of women.* Norwalk, CT: Appleton & Lange.

Goldfien, A. (1998). The gonadal hormones and inhibitors. In B.G. Katzung (Ed.), *Basic and clinical pharmacology* (7th ed.). Stamford, CT: Appleton & Lange.

Harvard Women's Health Watch, July 1998, page 1. Boston: Harvard Medical School.

Harvard Women's Health Watch, September 1998, page 2. Boston: Harvard Medical School.

Jensen, L., & King, K.M (1997). Women and heart disease: The issues. *Critical Care Nurse, 17*(2), 45–53.

Judelson, D.R., & Dell, D.L. (1998). The women's complete wellness book. New York: The Philip Lief Group, Inc., and The American Medical Women's Association.

LaCharity, L.A. (1997). The experiences of postmenopausal women with coronary artery disease. *Western Journal of Nursing Research, 19*(5), 583–607.

Moore, M.D. (1995). Commentary on smoking behaviors of women after diagnosis with lung cancer [original article in *Image: Journal of Nursing Scholarship, 27*(1), 35–41, by Sarna, L.]. *ONS Nursing Scan, 4*(4), 20–21.

Murdaugh. C. (1990). Coronary artery disease in women. *Journal of Cardiovascular Nursing, 4*(4), 35–50.

National Center for Health Statistics (1988). *Vital statistics of the United States, 1986* (Vol 2, Part A). Washington, D.C.: U.S. Government Printing Office.

New York Times (1998, Friday, December 4). Article on AIDS, 1.

Ornish, D. (1997). *Love and survivial: The scientific basis for the healing power of intimacy.* New York: HarperCollins Publishers.

Palmer, E.A. (1999). Family perspectives and experiences of having a school-age child with asthma. Unpublished doctoral dissertation, Duquesne University School of Nursing, Pittsburgh, PA.

Ringsberg, K.C., Segesten, K., & Akerlind, I. (1997). Walking around in circles: The life situation of patients with asthma-like symptoms but negative asthma tests. *Scandinavian Journal of Caring, 11*(2), 103–112.

Risser, N.L. (1996). Prevention of lung cancer: The key is to stop smoking. *Seminars in Oncology Nursing, 12,* 260–269.

Robertson, J.R., & Hebert, D.B. (1994). Gynecologic urology. In A.H. DeCherney & M.L. Pernoll (Eds.), *Current obstetric and gynecologic diagnosis and treatment* (8th ed.). Norwalk, CT: Appleton & Lange.

Smith, K.E., & Judd, H.L. (1994). Menopause and postmenopause. In A.H. DeCherney & M.L. Pernoll (Eds.), *Current obstetric and gynecologic diagnosis and treatment* (8th ed.). Norwalk, CT: Appleton & Lange.

Snyderman, N. L. (1996). *Dr. Nancy Snyderman's guide to good health for women over forty.* San Diego, CA: Harcourt Brace & Company.

Swain, S.E. (1996). Multiple sclerosis: Primary health care implications. *Nurse Practitioner, 21,* 40–54.

Thirlby, R.C. (1995). Evelution of a breast mass. In D.P. Lemcke, J. Pattison, L.A. Marshall, & D.S. Cowley (Eds.), *Primary care of women.* Norwalk, CT: Appleton & Lange.

United States Public Health Service Office on Women's Health (1998). Women's health issues: An overview. *Fact Sheet.*

University of California at Berkeley Wellness Letter (1998, September), *14*(12), 5.

University of California at Berkeley Wellness Letter (1998, December), *15*(3), 2–3.

Verdon, M.E. (1997). Respiratory diseases. In J.A. Rosenfeld (Ed.), *Women's health in primary care.* Baltimore: Williams & Wilkins.

Williams, F.H., & Kaul, M.P. (1995). Fibromyaligia and myofascial pain. In D.P. Lemcke, J. Pattison, L.A. Marshall, & D.S. Cowley (Eds.), *Primary care of women.* Norwalk, CT: Appleton & Lange.

Woods, N.F (1995). Women and their health. In C. Fogel & N.F. Woods (Eds.), *Women's health care: A comprehensive handbook.* Thousand Oaks, CA: Sage Publications.

Yon, J.L. (1995). Evaluation of pelvic masses and screening for ovarian cancer. In D.P. Lemcke, J. Pattison, L.A. Marshall, & D.S. Cowley (Eds.), *Primary care of women.* Norwalk, CT: Appleton & Lange.

Young, R.F., & Kahana, E. (1993). Gender, recovery from late life heart attack, and medical care. *Women and Health, 20*(1), 11–31.

CHAPTER 3

Sexual/Reproductive Health

Ellen Olshansky

Women's status as childbearer has been made into a major fact of her life.

—Rich, 1976, p. 11

While women's health is clearly more than women's reproductive health, which was the limited way in which women's health has been conceptualized in the past, sexual and reproductive functioning are important components of women's health. This book, therefore, devotes a chapter specifically to issues of the sexual and reproductive health of women. The chapter includes a discussion of issues related to sexuality, sexual identity, and sexual orientation; sexually transmitted disease prevention; conception and contraception issues and choices; infertility; and issues related to the menstrual cycle. Some of the sexual and reproductive health conditions noted in this chapter are described in more detail in some of the chapters in Part II, where specific treatments for these conditions are presented.

PROMOTION OF SEXUAL HEALTH

Promotion of sexual health in women requires that women and their health care providers understand and are sensitive to the variability in the definition of sexual health. A sexually healthy woman may be one who is involved in a monogamous heterosexual relationship or a monogamous lesbian relationship, or one who is not involved in a sexual relationship at all. In addition, a sexually healthy woman may be one who is involved in more than one sexual relationship and may be a woman who is heterosexual, lesbian, or bisexual. While we know that the risk of sexually transmitted diseases (STDs) increases with more sexual partners and the prevention of STDs is an important part of sexual health, sexual health also refers to the condition of a woman feeling fulfilled within her sexual relationships.

Women's sexuality has had and continues to evoke many and varied meanings. Often women's own sexuality was minimized, with women's sexual roles viewed as being to satisfy men's sexual desires. Words such as "frigid" or "asexual" were often used to describe women who were unable to or found it difficult to achieve orgasm through heterosexual intercourse. Masters and Johnson (1966) contributed important information about women's sexuality when they differentiated the vaginal orgasm from the clitoral orgasm, providing more understanding about women's sexuality and sexual pleasure. The illumination of the sexual response cycle (Masters & Johnson, 1966) provided further understanding of human sexuality and, specifically, particular issues relevant to women's sexuality. Since Masters and Johnson's classic work, others (Kaplan, 1979; Masters, Johnson, & Kolodny, 1988) have elucidated additional important information. The fact that women can have multiple orgasms and that women do not have an obligatory refractory period are two facts that differentiate their sexual response from that of men. Sexuality is part of a woman's overall health; therefore, it is important that health professionals understand unique aspects of women's sexuality.

Sexual orientation is part of overall sexual health. Homosexuality used to be considered pathological, according to professional groups in psychiatry, but recently the diagnosis of homosexuality was eliminated. The current belief is that homosexuality is simply one form of a person's sexuality. In fact, heterosexuality and homosexuality are believed to occur on a continuum, with bisexuality somewhere on the continuum. Many in the society, however, continue to believe that homosexuality is aberrant and, in fact, hate crimes have occurred and continue to occur based on this belief.

Women who are lesbians or who are bisexual face unique challenges. They are often ostracized by others, discriminated against in employment and social settings, and particularly within the health care system. According to a recent study reported by Hosaka in the *Pittsburgh Post-Gazette* (January 26, 1999), one of the biggest issues for lesbians is experiencing discrimination in the health care system and, therefore, feeling uncomfortable in accessing health care. Their physical health care needs are not necessarily different from those of heterosexual women, but the experience of seeking and receiving care is less adequate in meeting these needs. Since the focus for the past two decades has been predominantly on human immunodeficiency virus (HIV) and acquired immunodeficiency syndrome (AIDS) in relation to the gay community (even though the issues have been and are different for lesbians), and while deep concern continues in regard to HIV and AIDS, a desire to refocus attention on other aspects of health care has been voiced by health care providers and patients within both the gay and lesbian communities. Refocusing attention means developing a more comprehensive and empathic approach to the health and health care of lesbians, to include all aspects of their health concerns.

Another aspect of women's sexuality includes women who are not sexually active. They are sometimes referred to as being asexual, but that term is a misnomer, since sexuality is an inherent part of all persons regardless of the ways in which sexuality is expressed. Some women may choose a celibate life, while others desire a sexual partner but do not have one.

PREVENTION OF SEXUALLY TRANSMITTED DISEASES

A myriad of STDs exists, ranging from yeast infections to bacterial infections to viral infections that occur on a continuum from less serious to very severe. STDs pose a challenge to health because not only are they troublesome to a person who has contracted a particular disease, but they can be passed on to others, oftentimes unknowingly. This phenomenon becomes a public health hazard. It also becomes an important women's issue related to sexuality, as women must protect themselves from unwittingly contracting an STD from a partner as well as prevent transmitting a disease to a partner. Often, issues of sexual relations with men become complicated when men refuse to use condoms despite women's pleas to them to do so. Table 3–1 contains a summary of the common STDs, their symptoms, their complications, and their treatments. A separate section is devoted to HIV in Chapter 2, as this condition goes beyond only sexual transmission as the etiology and raises other issues that deserve attention.

Women's issues that are related to prevention and treatment of STDs include acceptance of women's sexuality by society and by health care professionals, understanding relational aspects of sexuality between women and men and between women and women, and understand-

Table 3–1 Summary of Sexually Transmitted Diseases

Type of STD	Treatment	Complications if Untreated
Gonorrhea	Antibiotics; sexual abstinence until treated	Cervicitis, salpingitis, urethritis
Chlamydia	Antibiotics; sexual abstinence until treated	Cervicitis, urethritis, bartholinitis
Pelvic inflammatory disease (PID)	Antibiotics; remove intrauterine device if present; bed rest; sexual abstinence until treated	Infertility
Mucopurulent cervicitis	Antibiotics; sexual abstinence until treated	Endometritis, salpingitis
Bacterial vaginosis	Metronidazole; antibiotics	PID postinstrumentation, postpartum, postsurgery
Trichomonal vaginitis	Metronidazole	Unknown
Candida vulvovaginitis	Antifungal agents	Not always transmitted sexually, but can be; complications unknown
Genital herpes	Antiviral therapy (palliative); sexual abstinence during presence of active lesions	Primary episodes may cause spontaneous abortion, neonatal herpes; premature birth; cesarean sections advised only if active lesions present in cervix or lower genital tract
Human papillomavirus	Palliative treatment with liquid nitrogen, trichloroacetic acid, podophyllin, laser therapy	Genital epithelial neoplasia; may cause anogenital or laryngeal papillomatosis in neonate
Syphilis	Antibiotics	Transmission to neonate; neurological disorders

Source: Reprinted with permission from E. Olshansky, The Reproductive Years, in *Women's Health: A Relational Perspective Across the Life Cycle,* J.A. Lewis and J. Bernstein, eds., p. 119, © 1996, Jones and Bartlett Publishers.

ing stigmas associated with STDs. Acceptance and understanding of these concepts are necessary in order for the health care providers optimally to meet the needs of women suffering from sexually transmitted diseases.

CONCEPTION AND CONTRACEPTION

The issue of birth control and family planning, while clearly involving both men and women, has traditionally been approached as a women's issue. While this approach makes sense in that it is predominantly women's bodies that are affected by the various contraceptive methods available, with some exceptions (e.g., condoms, vasectomy), and it is women who are the ones who become pregnant, it also raises troubling concerns. This approach has resulted in the prevailing medical and societal viewpoint that it is women who must be responsible for birth control and that birth control is only a "women's issue." Such an approach precludes men from having a voice in this issue and puts an undue burden on women. In terms of women's wellness, the various available birth control methods must be well understood in order for women to make intelligent decisions regarding which to use. Table 3–2 includes a summary of the currently available contraceptive methods, how they work, their side effects, their effectiveness, and warning signs associated with major concerns. Several important points deserve more detailed discussion, as follows.

Oral Contraception

Oral contraception, or "the pill," has become recognized as achieving a major social breakthrough for women in the 1960s. With the advent of this convenient and effective contraceptive method, women became much freer to engage in sexual relationships without undue fear of unwanted pregnancy, leading to what has been referred to as the "sexual revolution." In the early years of pill use, however, much higher doses of estrogen were used and, consequently, more frequent and more severe side effects occurred, with the most worrisome being cardiovascular effects. Unfortunately, women in Third World countries experienced even more of these side effects, as these women were often provided the pill in an effort for scientists to learn more about the effects of the pill before prescribing it for women in the United States or in Europe. From a holistic and global approach to women's wellness, it is essential that we be aware of this occurrence and that

Table 3–2 Summary of Contraceptive Methods

Type	Benefits	Side Effects	Contraindications
Spermicides	No systemic side effects; nonoxynol 9 may have some protection against STDs; can buy over the counter	Possible allergic reactions	Allergic reactions; unreliable in using (low user effectiveness)
Condoms	Possible prevention against STDs, particularly HIV; no systemic side effects; can buy over the counter	Possible allergic reaction to latex	Allergic reactions; unreliable in using (low user effectiveness)
Diaphragm and jelly/foam	No systemic side effects; nonoxynol 9 may have some protection against STDs	Possible bladder irritation and urinary tract infections (UTIs); possible allergic reaction to jelly/foam	Recurrent UTIs; allergic reaction to jelly/foam; unreliable in using (low user effectiveness)
Cervical cap	No systemic side effects; may be left in place for 48 hours without reapplying spermicide; may be able to fit a woman who cannot wear a diaphragm	Possible allergic reaction to jelly/foam	Cannot be worn during menses; may be difficult to insert; may be associated with cervical dysplasia; unreliable in using (low user effectiveness)
Contraceptive sponge	No systemic side effects; can buy over the counter	Possible bladder irritation; possible allergic reaction	Unreliable in using (low user effectiveness)
Oral contraceptives	Very reliable/effective; sex can be spontaneous; may be protective against endometriosis and ovarian cancer	Many potential systemic side effects	History of cardiovascular problems; hypertension; smoking
Intrauterine device	Very reliable/effective; sex can be spontaneous	Some IUDs associated with pelvic inflammatory disease (PID)	PID

continues

Table 3–2 continued

Type	Benefits	Side Effects	Contraindications
Norplant	Reliable; sex can be spontaneous; contraceptive effects last for several years	Various potential side effects to the hormone; changes in bleeding pattern; pain at insertion side	If desire pregnancy soon; long-acting
Depo-Provera	Reliable; sex can be spontaneous	Various potential side effects to the hormone; irregular bleeding; weight gain	If desire pregnancy soon; long-acting

Source: Reprinted with permission from E. Olshansky, The Reproductive Years, in *Women's Health: A Relational Perspective Across the Life Cycle,* J.A. Lewis and J. Bernstein, eds., p. 123, © 1996, Jones and Bartlett Publishers.

strong efforts be made to ensure that such occurrences do not happen again. Modern oral contraceptives consist of much lower estrogen doses and have many fewer untoward side effects, but caution and awareness still must prevail in terms of women's wellness issues and oral contraception.

Intrauterine Devices

The use of intrauterine devices (IUDs) has also led to major advances for women in providing effective contraception. The IUD, however, has been plagued with the recent memory of the effects of the Dalkon Shield (one particular brand of IUD) in causing pelvic inflammatory disease (PID) and resultant infertility in many women. For several years the IUD was taken off the market completely until a limited number of newer IUDs were recently reintroduced. These IUDs, which employ a small amount of progesterone or copper, are considered safe and highly effective (Grimes & Wallach, 1997), although, as with oral contraceptives, caution and awareness are always necessary in relation to use of an IUD.

The Diaphragm and Cervical Cap

The diaphragm combined with contraceptive cream or jelly has always been an effective method of birth control if used properly and consistently. The lower effectiveness rates of the diaphragm have been documented to be the result of improper and/or inconsistent use, rather than a lower theoretical effectiveness of the diaphragm. Before the advent of "the pill," the diaphragm was a very popular method of birth control. With the widespread popularity of the pill, the diaphragm became much less popular among women, but has continued to be a reliable and available method for women. While the diaphragm is a barrier method of contraception, it is not considered to be a "barrier" to the transmission of HIV in the same way that the condom is considered to be. The diaphragm does not allow a tight enough fit over the cervix and, even though the contraceptive jelly or cream decreases chances of transmission, it is not considered as effective as the condom in conjunction with contraceptive foam in decreasing such transmission.

The cervical cap is another form of barrier contraception for women. The cervical cap is much smaller than the diaphragm and fits more tightly directly over the cervix. The advantage of the cervical cap is that it can be left in place longer, allowing for multiple instances of sexual intercourse more spontaneously. The fact that the cervical cap covers the cervix, however, leads health care providers to be wary of advising women to leave it in for long periods of time because of concern about developing toxic shock syndrome.

The Condom

The condom, while traditionally a male method of birth control, has gained great popularity recently because of its association with decreasing the risk of transmission of STDs, particularly HIV. The condom is best used in conjunction with contraceptive foam. Condom use has encouraged men to take an active responsibility in regard to contraception and prevention of STDs. Not all condoms, however, are male methods of birth control. A very recent addition to the repertoire of contraceptive methods is the female condom, which is a barrier method that covers the cervix, the walls of the vagina, and the labia, also serving as a barrier to the transmission of STDs, particularly HIV/AIDS.

Injectable and Implantable Forms of Contraception

Two other contraceptive methods, categorized under injectable forms, deserve mention. Depo-Provera consists of an injection of progesterone, providing highly effective contraception for a 3-month period. Norplant consists of inserting Silastic capsules that contain progesterone, just under the surface of the skin in the upper arm. This method provides highly effective contraception for 5 years.

The above points have been in regard to contraception. The issue of conception also deserves some mention. For many women, conception is voluntary, desired, and planned. For others, however, conception is neither desired nor planned. There has been an epidemic of teenage pregnancies; while some of these pregnancies were planned, the majority were not. Even among those that were desired, the teenagers desiring them did so in the hopes of finding a way out of loneliness, poverty, or in the hopes of finding a marriage partner. When these outcomes did not occur, the teenagers were confronted with even more complex problems and challenges. Many of these young women have difficulty completing their education, finding fulfilling careers, and developing a strong sense of themselves because of the challenges they face in raising children. This is a women's issue in that most of the time the fathers are not involved and are much less affected by the situation. Therefore, assisting women with choices regarding abortion or relinquishing a child for adoption, are part of providing women's health care.

INFERTILITY

The other end of the continuum from the above discussion is that of involuntary childlessness, or infertility. Infertility is estimated to occur in one out of six U.S. couples (Martin, 1994). The causes of infertility are evenly distributed among men and women (see box "Causes of Infertility"), but infertility is commonly perceived as a women's issue. While recently more attention has been directed to men and reproduction, the predominant social view in the United States is that parenting/mothering is mostly a woman's role. Little girls often grow up symbolically rehearsing their future as mothers (Olshansky, 1987), and women who find themselves to be infertile often take on a central identity of themselves as infertile (Olshansky, 1987, 1996). This iden-

---

Causes of Infertility

Female factors—45%
    Ovulatory problems   —18%
    Tubal problems   —14%
    Endometriosis   — 7%
    Cervical mucus problems   — 6%

Male factors—23%
    Sperm problems   —21%
    Other male problems   — 2%

Interactive and unexplained factors—32%
    Including coital problems
    Antisperm antibodies

Source: Adapted with permission from L. Speroff, R.H. Glass, and N.G. Kase, *Clinical Gynecologic Endocrinology and Infertility,* 4th Ed., p. 518, © 1989, Williams and Wilkins.

---

tity affects their sense of self as other, more positive aspects of their identities are pushed to the periphery.

Infertility treatment has raised some very complex issues for women's wellness. From a medical perspective, concern exists about potential side effects of the various drugs used in treatments. Clomiphene citrate has been implicated in possibly being correlated with the development of ovarian cancer in women who use this drug for extended time periods, although the findings are inconclusive (Goldfien, 1998). From a social-psychological perspective, infertility treatment has raised issues about what constitutes a family, the importance of being a biological parent versus an adoptive parent, and issues related to disclosure of birth parents. In addition, psychological stresses of infertility, while often relieved if treatment is successful, may be exacerbated as individuals and couples find it more and more difficult to stop treatment and resolve their infertility because newer treatments continue to be provided and available. Despite the increased availability of treatments, however, many of the expensive and highly technological treatments are available only to those who can afford the high costs. Infertility treatments, particularly the highly technological treatments such as in vitro fertilization (IVF) are rarely covered by insurance companies. This inequitable availability creates women's issues that are related to socioeconomic status as well as prevailing social norms about who are considered to be "appropriate" parents. Sometimes treatment is withheld from single women or from lesbians as health care providers play the role of "gatekeeper" in deciding who is fit to be a parent.

MENSTRUAL CYCLE ISSUES

Many women's physical conditions are correlated with the menstrual cycle, as this monthly cycle involves hormonal changes that lead to physiological changes. While these changes are considered normal, many women suffer untoward consequences that deserve attention from the medical community.

Menarche

Menarche is one phase in a woman's life cycle that deserves more understanding among health care providers. While menarche is clearly a normal part of a woman's life, it is also a time of complex psychosocial feelings and experiences as well as dramatic physical changes in a woman's body.

Premenstrual Syndrome

Premenstrual syndrome also deserves more understanding among health care providers. Many women complain of certain symptoms that occur shortly before their menses. Some of these symptoms are simply annoying, while others are more distressing. For years, women's concerns around the menstrual cycle were dismissed by the medical community, but recently the term *premenstrual syndrome* has been developed to describe these cyclical symptoms that women experience. The acknowledgment of this syndrome has allowed systematic, scientific research that has resulted in a better understanding of the syndrome and of ways to alleviate the distressing symptoms associated with it. Recent research has revealed a pattern called "premenstrual magnification syndrome" (Mitchell, Woods, & Lentz, 1994), which reflects the complexity of symptoms during this premenstrual period that were previously dismissed as being "all in a woman's head." One caveat of this research, however, is that health care professionals must be careful not to label all women as unable to perform certain duties or responsibilities because of their monthly menstrual cycle. It is important that the symptoms not be exaggerated.

The menstrual cycle can often be irregular, reflected in several variations. These variations are menorrhagia, meaning heavy or prolonged flow; hypermenorrhea, meaning very light flow that sometimes consists simply of "spotting"; metrorrhagia, or bleeding between menses; polymenorrhea, or too frequently occurring menses; menometrorrhagia, or irregular intervals of bleeding; oligomenorrhea, meaning menses that occurs at more than 35-day intervals; and contact bleeding, or postcoital bleeding (Gerbie, 1994).

Menopause

Issues around menopause have also recently received increasing attention from the health care community and continue to need more investigation and understanding. Menopause, as menarche, is a normal stage in a woman's life. Menopause is the point at which a woman has ceased menstruating for at least 1 year. The perimenopausal period, however, includes the transition from premenopause to menopause, usually a span of a few years when menopausal symptoms begin even though a woman has not yet reached a full year of no menses. Accompanying this normal stage, however, are certain changes in a woman's body and psyche that require attention. Physical changes occurring as a result of decreasing estrogen production include, among others, osteoporosis, decreased vaginal lubrication, thinning of the labia and vaginal tissue, and hot flashes. The decreased estrogen production places women at higher risk for cardiovascular disease due to hyperlipidemia. Decreased vaginal lubrication, thinning of the labia and vaginal tissues, and hot flashes are common and very annoying and uncomfortable symptoms that many perimenopausal women experience. Women suffer these symptoms to varying degrees and not all women experience them in the same way. The box "Common Menopausal and Perimenopausal Symptoms" includes a summary of common symptoms of perimenopause and menopause.

Osteoporosis is a condition that deserves more attention. With age and decreasing estrogen production, resulting in decreasing calcium production as well, the bones become more brittle and more prone to fractures. Brittle bones pose a serious threat to women's health, particularly in older women, who might fall and suffer severe fractures, such as of the pelvic bones.

> **Common Menopausal and Perimenopausal Symptoms**
>
> Hot flashes
> Sleep disturbances
> Genitourinary problems, including some sexual difficulties
> Skin changes
> Loss of muscle strength
> Bone loss
> Decreased memory
> Depression

The risk of cardiovascular disease that sharply increases at menopause also raises a serious health issue for women. Prior to menopause, heart disease risks for women have received little if any attention, but after menopause this risk is equal to or greater than that of men.

SUMMARY

This chapter has presented an overview of the most common women's reproductive health conditions. Again, in keeping with a holistic approach, these conditions must be understood and assessed within each woman's physical and psycho-social-cultural-spiritual context.

REFERENCES

Gerbie, M.V. (1994). Complications of menstruation: Abnormal uterine bleeding. In A.H. DeCherney & M.L. Pernoll (Eds.), *Current obstetric and gynecologic diagnosis and treatment* (8th ed.). Norwalk, CT: Appleton & Lange.

Goldfien, A. (1998). The gonadal hormones and inhibitors. In B.G. Katzung (Ed.), *Basic and clinical pharmacology* (7th ed.). Stamford, CT: Appleton & Lange.

Grimes, D.A., & Wallach, M. (1997). Modern contraception: Updates from the Contraception Report. Totowa, NJ: Emron.

Hosaka, T. (1999, January 26). Affirmation: Advocates praise study that finds special health challenges faced by lesbians. Pittsburgh, PA: *Pittsburgh Post-Gazette*.

Hull, M.G.R., Glazener, C.M.A., Kelly, N.J., Conway, D.I., Foster, P.A., Hinton, R.A., Coulson, C., Lambert, P.A., Watt, E.M., & Desai, K.M. (1985). Population study of causes, treatment, and outcome of infertility. *British Medical Journal, 291*, 1693.

Kaplan, H.S. (1979). *Disorders of sexual desire*. New York: Simon & Schuster.

Martin, M. (1994). Infertility. In A.H. DeCherney & M.L. Pernoll (Eds.), *Current obstetric and gynecologic diagnosis and treatment* (8th ed.). Norwalk, CT: Appleton & Lange.

Masters, W., & Johnson, V. (1966). *Human sexual response.* Boston: Little, Brown and Company.

Masters, W., Johnson, V., & Kolodny, R. (1988). *Human sexuality* (3rd ed). Boston: Little, Brown and Company.

Mitchell, E. S., Woods, N. F., & Lentz, M. J. (1994). Differentiation of women with three perimenstrual symptom patterns. *Nursing Research, 43,* 25–30.

Olshansky, E. (1996). Theoretical issues in building a grounded theory: Application of an example of a program of research on infertility. *Qualitative Health Research, 6,* 394–405.

Olshansky, E. (1987). Identity of self as infertile: An example of theory-generating research. *Advances in Nursing Science, 9*(2), 54–63.

Rich, A. (1976). *Of woman born.* New York: W.W. Norton & Company.

Speroff, L., Glass, R.H., & Kase, N.G. (1989). *Clinical gynecologic endocrinology and infertility* (4th ed.). Baltimore: Williams & Wilkins.

CHAPTER 4

Psycho-Social-Cultural-Spiritual Health

Ellen Olshansky

> *The challenge before us is to create effective health policy and health delivery that accommodate the racial, economic, cultural, and ethical issues affecting health care delivery to distinct groups and subgroups of women of color.*

> —Adams & Williams, 1995, p. 1–2

When the notion of women's health is discussed, the aspect of physical health is usually the first thing that comes to mind. The previous two chapters provide an overview of women's physical health, emphasizing that physical health, including women's reproductive health issues, while essential to women's well-being, is not all of women's health. And, as with physical health, psychosocial health does not exist separately from the total health and well-being of women. In the interest of addressing the complex issues related to psychosocial well-being, however, a separate discussion is warranted.

While it is important to allot a separate section related to psychosocial well-being, it is somewhat paradoxical that this chapter does not separate psychological health from social, cultural, and spiritual health. While each of these aspects of women's health has been traditionally conceptualized as separate entities, it is extremely difficult, if not impossible, to view these as separate aspects. In the spirit of holism, women's psychological health occurs within a relational and contextual context that includes social, cultural, and spiritual aspects. All of these aspects together, occurring in a simultaneous and interrelated manner, are integral to women's well-being. This chapter reviews issues related to women's psychosocial health, with an emphasis on relational, cultural, and spiritual aspects of women's psychological health. The emphasis on relational concepts reflects the newer work on women's psychological development, particularly the work of J.B. Miller (1986) and her colleagues at the Jean Baker Miller Training Institute at the Wellesley Centers for Women (Jordan, Kaplan, Miller, Stiver, & Surrey, 1991; Jordan, 1997; Miller & Stiver, 1997) and Gilligan (1982) and her colleagues (Gilligan, Rogers, & Tolman, 1991). Lewis and Bernstein (1996) applied a relational theory model, based on this work, to understanding women's lives, with emphasis on all stages of the life cycle. Ruzek (1997), in a recent work with colleagues Olesen and Clarke, also emphasized the importance of social and cultural factors as contributing to women's well-being.

In the past, healthy psychological development was measured against the norms that were determined based on male models. Classically, the attainment of autonomy and individuation defined healthy psychological growth, with relational (classically attributed to females) aspects of nurturance, dependency, and caring associated with a less actualized individual. The recent work of the Stone Center at Wellesley College and the work of scholars at Harvard University represent newer models of psychological development that are based on women's experiences and that incorporate relational aspects of psychological growth. This work has contributed to a more complex and insightful understanding of adult development, both male and female. One caveat, however, that is important to consider when understanding and analyzing these newer approaches is the potential for "essentializing" women, that is, categorizing or stereotyping women according to "women's characteristics" of relational behavior. Not all women behave in the same manner and to categorize women as a uniform group negates the important differences among women based on such variables as race, class, and sexual orientation. In addition, some men demonstrate "relational" characteristics. Thus, while these newer models of women's psychological development are presented with the goal toward understanding women's (and men's) psychology in a more complex and compassionate manner, this important caveat must be incorporated into such understanding. A difficult challenge to health care providers for women is to be able to view women's health as unique and different from men's health while, at the same time, to appreciate and understand the differences among women. The women's health movement of the 1960s and 1970s was predominantly based on experiences of white, middle-class, heterosexual women. Only recently has attention been paid to the interests and concerns of women of color, of poor women, and of lesbians. The intent of this chapter is to focus on the important differences among women based on sociocultural variations in order to understand better the health concerns and needs of all women. The issue of differences in sexual orientation is addressed in Chapter 3.

According to these newer models of psychological development, interpersonal relationships are considered essential for healthy psychological growth. Not all relationships, however, are healthy. Aspects of healthy relationships include a combination of mutuality, empathy, and reciprocity that leads to connections that are growth fostering for both persons engaged in the relationship. The concept of relationships as being key to health is supported by others, most recently by Ornish (1998) in his work on intimacy and health and by Borysenko (1996), in her work on women's development. In emphasizing health promotion and the attainment of high-level wellness, encouraging relationships is essential. This approach differs from the classic psychoanalytic belief that autonomy and individuation were the key components of a psychologically healthy person. These newer models do not reject the notion of individuation, but they moderate such separateness with connectedness.

Another key aspect of these newer models of women's psychological development includes the strong emphasis on social and cultural context. Mirkin (1994) reconceptualized an approach to understanding women's psychology from a feminist perspective by emphasizing context as a central concept to which attention must be paid in order to assist women in achieving their highest potential for psychological health. For example, eating disorders and sexual problems are found to have roots not only in women's intrapsychic selves, but in their social and cultural contexts, as they are influenced by and influence women's intrapsychic selves. Women who live in poverty or within a context in which racism affects their daily lives experience these contexts as influencing their health. This notion is similar to the central tenets of symbolic interaction theory (Blumer, 1969), which states that persons construct meaning based on the interpretation of interactions they have with one another and with themselves within a social context.

Key concepts to understanding this chapter include connectedness, mutuality, authenticity, reciprocity, empathy, social support, and context. These concepts are discussed briefly here, but are addressed in greater detail in Chapter 5 of this book. **Connectedness** refers to a process of a person's feeling a bond or attachment to another person. **Authenticity** is a condition in which a person is able to be self-reflective, to know herself, and to represent herself to others in a way that reflects her true self without feeling a need to "cover up" aspects of her self. **Reciprocity** refers to one aspect of connectedness, in which the feeling of attachment is reciprocated (is experienced by both members of the relationship). **Mutuality** is very similar to the concept of reciprocity, in which there is a simultaneous feeling of caring and concern for the other person in the relationship. **Empathy** reflects an ability to take on the perspective of the other person within the relationship and to have a sense of what the other person is feeling. **Social support** refers to those persons significant to a woman who are supportive of and helpful to her, particularly in times of need. **Context** reflects the social and cultural aspects of one's life that influence how a person experiences feelings and events and makes meaning of such feelings and events.

Many of these concepts are key in the formulation of "relational theory," developed by the founding members of the Stone Center as they have worked to explain how women develop healthy psychological selves. Each of the topics presented in this chapter is discussed in relation to these newer models of women's psychosocial health.

DEVELOPING A SENSE OF SELF AND SELF-ESTEEM

Relational theory emphasizes that psychological growth occurs within the context of relationships, and psychological growth is reflected in the development of a sense of self and self-esteem. By being in relationships with others, one develops a stronger sense of self. That is, through a mutually empathic relationship with another person, each person is confirmed/validated for her thoughts and feelings. A relationship that is not mutual and that is not empathic, however, may have a very different effect by creating the sense within a person of being dismissed for her feelings and thoughts. The study by Jack (1991) of women and depression supports this notion of the influence of relationships on one's sense of self. She demonstrated, in her qualitative study, that women who were in unhealthy relationships with men (in which each woman's own needs were not met despite her striving constantly to meet her partner's needs) experienced depression as a consequence.

MANAGING MULTIPLE ROLES

The ability to manage multiple roles is directly linked to relational theory in that all persons live and function within a context of other people. Therefore, multiple roles are created vis-à-vis these other persons. A woman may take on the role of mother, wife, partner, friend. Each of these roles is specifically defined in relation to significant other persons. The ability to manage these multiple roles does not occur in a vacuum, meaning that this ability does not occur without interaction from others within the woman's social context. The study by Hochschild (1989) of women who work outside the home indicates that most of these women come home from work and then engage in a "second shift" of work, consisting of routine housekeeping, roles normally designated to women within this sociocultural context. Hochschild's study is an example of why it is essential to include a description of social context in order to understand women's experiences of managing multiple roles.

STRESS MANAGEMENT

Managing stress seems to be a constant problem faced by women. Domar and Dreher (1996) described stress as being a primary concern of women, particularly as a consequence of the challenge of managing multiple roles. Stress can result from role overload; living in a fast-paced society with multiple and varied responsibilities; and, for some, awareness of the "haves" while one is a "have-not."

Stress also often occurs as a consequence of fear related to physical concerns. Domar and Dreher (1996) described several situations in which women were concerned about diagnoses, such as possible breast cancer or cervical cancer and, in response to their fears, experienced a stress response described as the "flight or fight syndrome" (p. 9). This common syndrome consists of physical symptoms that occur in response to psychological fears.

One concept that is overarching here is that stress occurs within a societal context and that it is often one's experience in relation to this societal context that influences one's stress level. In other words, what might be considered stressful for one woman may be considered "challenging" to another, wherein she welcomes this new venture. Also, role overload for some women may be managed by hiring someone to take care of household tasks, a luxury that is not afforded to women of a lower socioeconomic class, emphasizing the importance of understanding the social context as it relates to management of stress.

PREVENTION OF DEPRESSION, ANXIETY, AND OTHER MOOD DISORDERS

Multiple theories exist to explain the origins of depression and other mood disorders. There are psychodynamic theories of depression, cognitive theories, behavioral theories, and interpersonal theories. Relational theory provides a plausible explanation based on the idea that women may become depressed as a result of suppressing their authentic selves. This suppression of their authentic selves can occur in response to efforts to maintain relationships by neglecting their own needs and sense of self (Jack, 1991). This suppression of their authentic selves can also occur in response to suppressing their own sadness due to lack of validation of these feelings (Miller & Stiver, 1997). Often women's psychological responses to stresses or their emotional expressions are dismissed by others or, at least, minimized. As a result, women lack validation for their feelings, and consequently become critical of themselves for having the feelings rather than confronting their authentic thoughts and feelings and seeking appropriate care for distressing thoughts and feelings.

PREVENTION OF EATING DISORDERS

The etiology of eating disorders is complex and not completely understood, but taking a relational approach provides a very plausible and useful way of conceptualizing this devastating women's health problem. Women, and young adolescent girls in particular, define themselves largely in terms of their body image. Their definition of body image is based largely upon societal "norms," or, more accurately, their perception of societal norms. In a world where thinness is portrayed as a goal to the extent that it becomes more important than body functioning, young women become caught up in a drive to attain such thinness at all cost, including, at the extreme, their lives. The fact that eating disorders do not seem to exist in developing countries leads many scholars to ask about what, specifically, exists within a more affluent culture that lends itself to eating disorders. Gender issues are apparent, too, in that the large majority of persons who suffer from eating disorders are women. One argument can be made that in this male-dominated society, physiological "norms" are established based on the patriarchal culture. At puberty, as Surrey (1984) described in a working paper from the Stone Center, girls develop proportionately more fat than do boys, who develop more muscle. Fat comes to be looked upon as something to reduce, often to an extreme extent, based on lack of knowledge of female physiology. Females need a certain amount of fat to maintain normal menstrual cycles and fertility, but the focus instead is on the notion that fat is a negative, something to be rid of.

To prevent eating disorders in women, it is critical to comprehend women's own perceptions of their bodies, specifically their body image, with the goal of understanding the etiology of eating disorders.

PREVENTION OF SUBSTANCE ABUSE (ALCOHOL, DRUGS, TOBACCO)

Substance abuse is another very serious problem for women. This issue is quite complex, particularly when it is not limited to women only, but to women and their children, specifically the issue of pregnant women using crack/cocaine. Taking an empathic approach to women, Kearney (1998) has studied the experience of mothers addicted to crack/cocaine, finding that despite their addiction, they do have maternal feelings toward their children. Understanding women's addictive behaviors is best accomplished by making an effort to understand these women's social contexts and their own perceptions of their lives and their situations. Rather than blaming women for their destructive behaviors, it may be much more effective to demonstrate an empathic approach to their situation and to try to work *with* the women as allies rather than as adversaries.

PREVENTION OF ABUSE AND VIOLENCE WITHIN RELATIONSHIPS

The issue of violence against women has only recently been taken seriously. Much more needs to be studied and understood about this devastating phenomenon. One way of understanding the occurrence of violence against women is from a relational perspective. A relational perspective includes a focus on the social context within which women form and maintain relationships. In our current patriarchal social context, men are certainly more dominant and stronger than women. Swift (1987) noted that institutional authorities, namely "police, prosecutors and judges, the clergy, and physicians . . . have a cumulative record of disbelieving the women and exercising their authority to maintain the status quo—that is, to return the woman to the battering situation" (p. 3).

One question that is often asked is why women stay in battering relationships. Taking a relational approach to answering this question, more light can be shed to assist in understanding why, in fact, women do stay in these destructive relationships. As Landenburger (1989) found in her research, women are often trapped in these relationships as they experience a shrinking self, a self that is defined by being in a relationship. For these women, by even contemplating leaving this significant relationship they risk losing their selves even more.

To be able to prevent violence against and abuse of women, it is critical that we understand women's experiences of this phenomenon. Interventions can then be developed that are sensitive and empathic toward women, creating a better chance of achieving an effective outcome.

KEY ISSUES RELATED TO SOCIOCULTURAL ASPECTS OF WOMEN'S HEALTH

To appreciate women's lives and women's health from a holistic, comprehensive perspective, understanding the social-cultural aspects is integral to such an appreciation. This understanding is particularly key in terms of a relational approach to women's psychological development where, as emphasized previously, the social and cultural contexts are so important. Several aspects of the social-cultural context are discussed in this section, as they are relevant to an understanding of women's psychological health.

Social Attitudes toward Women

Views toward women have changed significantly, as evidenced by more women in elected office, more women in professions previously dominated by males, and more women taking leadership roles within society. These examples, however, are overt. On a covert level, it is difficult to assess the degree to which views of women by society have changed. Societal views incorporate views held by men of women, but also views held by women of themselves. An important question to ask is whether, in fact, women's views of themselves have changed and whether individual men do, in fact, perceive women as their equals. While policies toward women may have changed, attitudes may lag behind. One important example of how social attitudes toward women may influence women's psychosocial health is in the area of reproduction. Women who choose to be childfree are often ostracized by others who believe that these women have foresaken an important responsibility, that of reproduction. Other women who desperately want to conceive and bear a child are unable to do so because of infertility; these women often feel "incomplete" as women in not being able to fulfill what they and others perceive to be their expected role.

Women in Communities

Following relational theory, it makes sense that women do live and thrive within communities rather than in isolation. Some women, however, have stronger community ties than others, while some women may suffer a sense of isolation in their day-to-day lives. Certain cultural groups emphasize community very strongly. Women who are less connected to others may endure a more isolated existence, perhaps developing a greater dependence on their spouse or partner, if they have one. With the evidence for the importance of healthy interpersonal relationships in achieving a high level of wellness, it is clearly important that health care providers assess and understand the degree to which women are engaged in such healthy relationships or, conversely, the degree to which they lack such relationships or are perhaps involved in unhealthy, destructive relationships.

Women of Various Cultural/Ethnic Backgrounds

While we are currently paying more attention to diversity within women's groups, the overwhelming concerns of women have been addressed based on white, middle- to upper-class, heterosexual women. Recent scholars such as hooks (1984), Lorde (1994), Adams and Williams (1995), Saran (1993), Avery (1994), and others have raised important and complex issues pertaining to women of color. They have challenged the previous lack of sensitivity to cultural differences. One very important point is our traditional notion of "other" backgrounds. The connotation underlying such language is that "other" is not normal, but instead is marginalized because of being different. A huge and important challenge for us to confront is to work toward reconceptualizing how we view diversity with a goal toward including difference within the margins rather than outside the margins, making diversity the norm rather than the exception (or the "other").

Women of Various Economic Backgrounds

Economic status is a very important variable in influencing one's level of wellness. This is particularly true in our current climate of increased health care costs. With the wide gap between the rich and the poor of this nation, much inequality exists in access to health care and other services. In the 1970s and 1980s the term *feminization of poverty* was often used to refer to the fact that women, overwhelmingly, suffered from poverty within our society. Currently, women have made some gains in the economic system, but they continue to earn significantly less money than their male counterparts.

Incarcerated Women

The health care needs of women in prisons have been sorely neglected. Recently, however, Coll and Duff (1995) developed a Women in Prison Project, as part of the services offered through the Stone Center for Developmental Services and Studies at Wellesley College in Massachusetts. Their 15-month project provided needed insight into incarcerated women's health care needs. Their findings consisted of a summary of the women's health care needs as well as suggestions for future interventions with these women. The women's needs were categorized according to those needs identified by the staff at the Department of Corrections and those needs identified by the women themselves. The staff noted two major categories of needs, consisting of economic self-sufficiency, referring to educational and job skills, and psychosocial needs, consisting of treating of substance abuse and promoting emotional well-being. The women noted that they were concerned with obtaining further education, and particularly the need to address their previous traumatic situations, involving such occurrences as losing their parents during the women's own childhood and experiencing verbal, sexual, and physical abuse

Issues of Access to Health Care

As described in several of the above sections, unequal access to health care presents a major barrier to women's health and wellness. When health promotion is emphasized with a focus on prevention and early detection of diseases, it is imperative that equal and strong access to health services exists for all persons. Unfortunately, equal access does not exist.

Discrimination in Health Care

Discrimination in health care is part of unequal access to care, but discrimination consists of other aspects. A woman may have good access to health care services, but the health care providers within those services may discriminate against her. For example, a lesbian may receive less-than-adequate care because of negative feelings toward her by a health care provider. A woman of color may also receive less-than-adequate care. Sometimes this less-than-adequate care results from lack of understanding of the specific health care needs of particular groups, but often this lack of understanding is a direct consequence of not directing attention to this much-needed area. As a result of experiencing discrimination within the health care system, those persons discriminated against will tend to seek care less often and less regularly.

Stereotyping and Its Influence on Health Care

While emphasizing cultural differences and the importance of embracing diversity within groups of women, it is simultaneously extremely important that we are careful not to stereotype individuals based on their ethnicity or cultural group. In order to be culturally competent, we must be aware not only of cultural differences but also of individual differences within cultural groups. It is important that we talk with, listen to, and assess individuals as individuals, while being sensitive to their sociocultural group affiliation without making assumptions for which no evidence exists (Lipson, 1996).

KEY ISSUES RELATED TO SPIRITUAL ASPECTS OF WOMEN'S HEALTH

Women's spiritual health is an important aspect of their overall health, contributing to a holistic understanding of wellness. M. A. Miller (1995) described spirituality as a belief in persons regarding something greater than oneself. She also stated that spirituality can be present in a person without that person's identifying with a religious group, but is a quality that seeks to find meaning in life and in the world. As such, the spiritual dimension in one's life is an important part of one's overall health; hence, a holistic approach to health includes recognition and understanding of that dimension. Miller (1995) described how women's experiences of childbearing are often influenced by their spiritual beliefs. She also mentioned the concept of "spiritual feminist healing" (p. 261), a philosophy in which women are viewed as possessing natural healing knowledge.

The above issues have relevance to women as a group, but also to specific groups of women based on social status and/or culture. Attention to cross-cultural aspects of women's psychological health and well-being provides a more complex understanding of women's psychosocial health. For example, violence against women is a worldwide phenomenon, but it may take various forms in different cultural groups. Clearly much more research is needed on cultural issues related to women's psychosocial health, particularly as we emphasize the development of cultural competence as a central part of health care.

To summarize the emphasis in this chapter, the most important concept is that it is essential that we understand women's own perceptions of their experiences of these psychosocial issues and how these issues affect their own wellness. Only by understanding women's experiences can we provide empathic and effective care in an effort to improve the quality of their psychosocial-cultural-spiritual wellness.

REFERENCES

Adams, D.L., & Williams, B.S. (1995). Introduction. In D.L. Adams (Ed.), *Health issues for women of color: A cultural diversity perspective*. Thousand Oaks, CA: Sage Publications.

Avery, B.Y. (1994). Breathing life into ourselves: The evolution of the national black women's health project. In E.C. White (Ed.), *The black women's health book*. Seattle, WA: Seal Press.

Blumer, H. (1969). *Symbolic interactionism: Theory and method*. Chicago: University of Chicago Press.

Borysenko, J. (1996). *A woman's book of life: The biology, psychology, and spirituality of the feminine life cycle*. New York: Riverhead Books.

Coll, C.G., & Duff, K.M. (1995). Reframing the needs of women in prison: A relational and diversity perspective. Final Report to the Stone Center, March 1995.

Domar, A.D., & Dreher, H. (1996). *Healing mind, healthy woman*. New York: Dell Publishing.

Gilligan, C. (1982). *In a different voice: Psychological theory and women's development*. Cambridge, MA: Harvard University Press.

Gilligan, C., Rogers, A.G., & Tolman, D.L. (1991). *Women, girls and psychotherapy: Reframing resistance*. New York: Harrington Park Press (Haworth Press, Inc.).

Hochschild, A. (1989). *The second shift: Working parents and the revolution at home*. New York: Penguin Books.

hooks, B. (1984). *Feminist theory: From margin to center*. Boston: South End Press.

Jack, D. C. (1991). *Silencing the self: Women and depression*. Cambridge, MA: Harvard University Press.

Jordan, J.V. (1997). *Women's growth in diversity: More writings from the Stone Center*. New York: Guilford Press.

Jordan, J.V., Kaplan, A.G., Miller, J.B., Stiver, I.P., & Surrey, J.L. (1991). *Women's growth in connection: Writings from the Stone Center.* New York: Guilford Press.

Kearney, M.H. (1998). Truthful self-nurturing: A grounded formal theory of women's addiction recovery. *Qualitative Health Research, 8,* 495–512.

Landenburger, K. (1989). A process of entrapment in and recovery from an abusive relationship. *Issues in Mental Health Nursing, 3,* 209–227.

Lewis, J.A., & Bernstein, J. (1996). *Women's health: A relational perspective across the life cycle.* Sudbury, MA: Jones and Bartlett Publishers.

Lorde, A. (1994). Living with cancer. In E.C. White (Ed.), *The black women's health book.* Seattle, WA: Seal Press.

Lipson, J. (1996). Culturally competent nursing care. In J.G. Lipson, S.L. Dibble, & P.A. Minarik (Eds.), *Culture and nursing care: A pocket guide.* San Francisco: University of California San Francisco Nursing Press.

Miller, J.B. (1986). *Toward a new psychology of women.* Boston, MA: Beacon Press.

Miller, J.B., & Stiver, I.P. (1997). *The healing connection: How women form relationships in therapy and in life.* Boston, MA: Beacon Press.

Miller, M. A. (1995). Culture, spirituality, and women's health. *Journal of Obstetric, Gynecologic, and Neonatal Nursing, 24,* 257–263.

Mirkin, M.P. (1994) *Women in context: Toward a feminist reconstruction of psychotherapy.* New York: Guilford Press.

Ornish, D. (1998). *Love and survival: The scientific basis for the healing power of intimacy.* New York: HarperCollins Publishers.

Ruzek, S.B. (1997). Women, personal health behavior, and health promotion. In S.B. Ruzek, V.L. Olesen, & A.E. Clarke (Eds.), *Women's health: complexities and differences.* Columbus: Ohio State University Press.

Saran, A.R. (1993). My guardian spirits. In B. Bair & S.E. Cayleff (Eds.), *Wings of gauze: Women of color and the experience of health and illness.* Detroit: Wayne State University Press.

Surrey, J.L. (1984). Eating patterns as a reflection of women's development (work in progress). Wellesley, MA: The Stone Center, Wellesley College.

Swift, C.F. (1987). Women and violence: Breaking the connection (work in progress). Wellesley, MA: The Stone Center, Wellesley College.

CHAPTER 5

Goals for Women's Wellness

Ellen Olshansky

As far as your health goes, there's no time like the present to begin!

—Alles, 1996, p. xi

In keeping with the holistic, integrated perspective of this book, this chapter includes various goals for women's wellness that, together, comprise a comprehensive and integrated whole, reflecting a holistic view of wellness. It is important to consider that health for one woman may be somewhat different as compared with another woman, as viewed by the individual women themselves. Their meaning of health is highly influenced by their own physical limitations, social context, cultural, psychological, and spiritual issues.

DEVELOPING AND MAINTAINING BALANCE, PERSPECTIVE, AND PRIORITIES

When I am in balance, I see the best in every situation and feel grateful. My heart is at peace. When I am in balance I see the best in others, and the magic of self-in-relation becomes a reality as each of us comes more fully into being.

—Borysenko, 1996, p.138

One very important goal in the attainment of maximum wellness is to achieve a sense of balance and perspective, while maintaining one's priorities in life. This goal refers to the ability to see beyond one issue even if that issue is, at the time, all-encompassing. This goal is reflective of the larger, more esoteric goal of finding meaning and satisfaction in one's life and managing stressful life situations.

Balance refers to equilibrium, stability, and harmony. It is a state or condition of being able to juggle various aspects of one's life and one's self. **Perspective** refers to the notion that all objects and events occur in relation to other objects and events. It is the ability to take on a comprehensive and expansive view of these objects and/or events within the context of their relationships to one another. **Priorities** refer to the notion that decisions often must be made regarding the importance of some things in relation to others. Priorities are determined relative to others. The ability to set priorities reasonably influences the degree of balance and perspective that one attains. By combining each of these concepts, we can see the importance of things or events as they are related to other things or events, with the goal being to achieve a state of harmony or equilibrium among the various things or events. From a wellness and health-promotion perspective, a woman's ability to develop and maintain such harmony and equilibrium will contribute to a greater sense of well-being.

One of the hallmarks for contemporary women is being bombarded with multiple and simultaneously competing responsibilities. The ability to juggle and balance these responsibilities in a manner that reflects a woman's priorities can be a difficult, if not overwhelming, task. This goal is related to the ability to develop and maintain balance and perspective in that priorities are determined based upon how all responsibilities are related to one another. Only by having a perspective on what, in fact, these competing responsibilities are can a woman then decide which responsibilities are of utmost importance at a particular place and time. Balance and perspective are important as women take on simultaneous, multiple, and varied roles and tasks. Being able to keep each of the various roles in perspective relative to the other roles and to balance all of the responsibilities will contribute to a greater sense of well-being. The aspects of life that an individual woman must balance may be very different for a particular woman as compared with another woman. For example, a woman living in poverty is challenged to balance aspects related to survival of self and family while an upper-class woman has different kinds of challenges. How one balances this myriad of roles is key in understanding the degree to which they enjoy a sense of well-being.

Balance and perspective refer to other aspects of women's lives besides the issue of taking on and maintaining multiple roles. These concepts are also related to one's ability to distribute mental and physical energy among varied aspects of one's life in a way that allows for maximum productivity and enjoyment or satisfaction of these varied aspects.

Clearly, in relation to health, the ability to maintain balance, perspective, and priorities is essential. For example, in order to set aside time for daily exercise in the pursuit of high-level wellness, such exercise must become a priority and a balance of other priorities must be achieved in order to allow the needed time to engage in this activity. Another example involves allowing time for relaxation and stress management. Being able to organize one's time and set priorities to meet responsibilities will then enable one to have time for relaxation and attention to dealing with managing stressful issues in one's life. A woman's particular life situation and social context will strongly influence the ability to achieve such balance, as many women, on a daily basis, face overwhelming constraints and serious challenges to developing balance.

One important goal, then, for achieving a high level of wellness is to attain the ability to develop and maintain balance, perspective, and priorities in one's life. Health-promotion efforts should address this goal by assisting women in developing strategies to do so. Such strategies will only be effective, however, if the individual context of a woman's life is accounted for and integrated into these strategies. It will not be helpful, for example, to encourage a woman to join a health club to get needed exercise when she is struggling to earn enough money to put food on the table for her family. From a holistic perspective, therefore, a health care provider must be aware of and sensitive to the social context within which women seek health.

Borysenko (1996) described two types of balance, which she termed *inner balance* and *outer balance.* Inner balance is a state within the mind wherein one experiences "mindfulness," or a sense of natural creativity and synchronization with a larger whole (Borysenko, 1996). Inner balance and mindfulness refer to meaning-making within oneself. Outer balance refers to a woman's ability to organize her priorities so that she can feel more positive about the balance she has created. For example, being able to juggle multiple roles and responsibilities and feel good about those roles rather than overwhelmed reflects an outer balance. Achieving this balance is more complicated than simply arranging priorities; it also means developing a sense or a feeling that these priorities are "right" regardless of what others may expect. A societal example that applies very well to women is the common notion that women must be at home to raise children, and if a woman works outside the home she is taking away time that should be devoted to the children. Some women, however, may have established relationships with partners wherein each partner shares equally in the raising of children and can devote equal time to career endeavors as well. If a woman has achieved an outer balance, she has been able to develop an attitude toward her own constructed priorities that reflects a positive feeling about how those priorities are balanced in her life. This mental attitude, then, leads to a sense of inner balance as well.

The above discussion indicates that the concept of balance is closely interrelated with the concept of developing priorities. The degree to which priorities are organized is a reflection of the degree to which balance is achieved. The concept of perspective transcends both balance and priorities, as perspective is really a state that is achieved through developing healthy priorities and balance. In terms of optimal wellness for women, the goal of developing such priorities and balance underlies the larger goal of achieving a healthy perspective in one's life: a perspective in which a woman sees herself as having achieved an order and a place for each priority, but which also allows room for change in priorities as needs change. Thus, this perspective is dynamic, allowing the woman to change and grow in relation to changes within herself and her family and environment.

As part of developing and maintaining balance, perspective, and priorities, women need to develop strategies to make time for themselves. In this instance, effort must be paid to developing a balance between having time for personal relationships with friends and family and having time for oneself. Sometimes just sitting and reading a newspaper or a book or taking a walk alone can be very important in helping a woman have time for self-reflection. Setting aside time for exercise (as emphasized under "Developing and Maintaining a Physically Healthy Body") by making exercise a priority in one's busy life is another way of attaining balance. Balance, therefore, can also be conceptualized as organizing one's time for both relational and individual activities: setting aside time for friends and family as well as setting aside time for oneself. When a woman is able to prioritize important aspects of her life and keep things in a reasonable perspective, the likelihood of living a balanced life is greatly enhanced and, consequently, a greater sense of well-being is also enhanced.

In order to achieve balance and perspective and maintain priorities, a woman must be able to manage stress effectively. Conversely, the ability to achieve balance, perspective, and priorities is essential in and of itself in contributing to the ability to manage stress. Therefore, the strategies for achieving these three goals will also contribute to managing stress. Individual women will develop their own strategies for managing stress, which may include one or some of the strategies described in Part III of this book.

Stress is a fact of everyday life for all persons. The form and degree of stress, however, differ. The goal is not to eliminate stress completely, as that is not realistic nor is it even desirable. A certain amount of stress serves as a stimulus for action. The important aspect of how women deal with stress in their lives is how they can manage it and can thrive despite its presence. How stress is identified and defined by women varies greatly among individual women. As emphasized throughout this chapter, individual women live in differing contexts and experience differing life circumstances, posing particular challenges for particular women. Thus stress is identified and defined differently and, therefore, managed differently for individual women. Strategies for managing stress must be developed that are effective for a particular woman.

DEVELOPING AND MAINTAINING HEALTHY RELATIONSHIPS WITH OTHERS

In short, the goal is not for the individual to grow out of relationships, but to grow into them. As the relationships grow, so grows the individual.

—Miller & Stiver, 1997, p. 22

Another major goal for women as they seek to attain a high level of wellness is to develop and maintain healthy relationships with others. For this reason, a chapter devoted to how women develop such relationships is warranted. Current research reveals that healthy relationships are critical factors that contribute to a woman's psychological health (Ornish, 1997). Northrup (1998) noted that healthy relationships are important for the development of self-esteem in women. While a separate section is devoted to self-esteem, the concept of relationships also deserves focused attention, as relationships influence a woman's sense of well-being. A very important point here is that these relationships must be healthy. An unhealthy relationship can, in fact, be detrimental to a woman's well-being, as described by Johnson (1991). For example, an abusive relationship with a spouse or partner is destructive. Even more subtle examples, however, are important. A woman whose spouse dismisses her concerns or is uninterested in her daily activities and in her thoughts and ideas will experience a detrimental effect on her own sense of well-being. This chapter addresses the key elements of a healthy relationship and discusses why it is so important to develop and maintain such relationships.

A healthy relationship is one that is connected, empathic, and mutual. These concepts are derived from the work of Miller (1986) and colleagues at the Stone Center at Wellesley College (Jordan, Kaplan, Miller, Stiver, & Surrey, 1991; Jordan, 1997; Miller & Stiver, 1997), and build on the description presented in Chapter 4. A more detailed description and analysis of these concepts are included in the next section.

Description of Healthy Relationships

The entire concept of relationships has always been integral to understanding one' psychological health and, in turn, one's physical health, since we know that psychological and physical health are interrelated. Most psychological developmental models, however, have been constructed based on the study of males and have, consequently, emphasized the importance of individuation, separation, and autonomy to a much larger degree than the importance of relationships. In fact, healthy adults have usually been defined as those persons who have successfully "separated" from their families of origin, in particular their mothers, and have developed "autonomous" selves. The importance of relationships has been minimized in these predominating theories. Relationships, in fact, have been de-emphasized as often reflecting an unhealthy "dependency" on the part of the person involved in and valuing such relationships. Recently, however, theories of psychological development have focused particular attention toward women and have emphasized the importance of relationships as central in attaining a healthy psychological self. The work of the scholars at the Stone Center at Wellesley College (Jordan, 1997; Jordan et al, 1991; Miller, 1986; Miller & Stiver, 1997) and at Harvard (Gilligan, 1982), as well as the work of Jack (1991) and the earlier work of Chodorow (1978) reflect this shift in emphasis toward healthy relationships as key in developing healthy psychological selves. While this recent work has focused on women, the belief is that these theories are relevant to men's psychological development as well.

Elements of Healthy Interpersonal Relationships

This section describes the key elements of healthy interpersonal relationships, followed by a discussion of how such healthy relationships are central to healthy psychological development. Five main concepts, building on Chapter 4, are described: connected, empathic, mutuality, authenticity, and reciprocity. One outstanding feature of all of these concepts is how highly interrelated they are with one another. The presence of one concept automatically means that the others must be present. In other words, a connected relationship cannot exist without the presence of empathy, mutuality, authenticity, and reciprocity. The same is true for each of these concepts.

Connected refers to the notion that individual persons do not live and function in isolation from others. Furthermore, healthy relationships involve a sense of being a part of another person, whether that be sharing certain ideas and values or sharing certain feelings. There is a certain subjectiveness in the definition of connected, which makes it difficult to define clearly, but this subjective sense of being connected to someone else is a very important part of being in a healthy relationship with another person. It is, in fact, the perception that one has of being and feeling connected to another person that is of such importance. Belenky and colleagues (1986) emphasize connectedness in relation to ways of knowing, with direct reference to women and how women come to know and make meaning of phenomena in their lives. Knowing, making meaning, and developing healthy psychological selves develop within the context of connected relationships with others.

Empathy is related to connectedness in that it refers to a sense of sharing subjective feelings with another person. While one person can never exactly feel and know how another person is experiencing something, a person can have a sense of sharing some of the experience and can express this sense through an empathic approach of communicating and relating to another person.

Mutuality is a dynamic condition in which two or more persons simultaneously experience situations together. One person does not experience something in complete isolation of another person, even though no two persons experience something in exactly the same manner.

Authenticity is a condition in which a woman is able to know herself through self-reflection and, in turn, can present herself to others in a manner that truly represents her genuine thoughts and feelings. In addition, a degree of comfort exists in being genuine with others, which is related to having a strong sense of oneself.

Reciprocity is very similar to mutuality in that there is a sense of experiencing something together. Reciprocity, however, emphasizes and highlights the "back-and-forth" nature of a relationship, or the "give-and-take" that occurs in relationships.

One challenge in the above descriptions of healthy relationships is to maintain the importance of a certain degree of individuality and autonomy for all persons. It is important to note that even though relationships are highly emphasized in these newer models of women's psychological development, this does not mean that individuation and autonomy are not important at all. To the contrary, an individual's sense of self and ability to think for oneself is essential to one's healthy psychological development. One's autonomy and sense of self, however, are not independent of one's healthy relationships with others. Underlying relational theory is the notion that through the development of healthy relationships one can develop a healthy psychological independent, while simultaneously interdependent, self. In some ways the major goal emphasized in this chapter is similar to the goal emphasized under "Developing and Maintaining Balance, Perspective, and Priorities," in that a healthy woman is one who has attained a balance between independence and interdependence.

The scholars at the Stone Center have effectively argued that relationships are central factors in women's healthy psychological development and, thus, in women's well-being. These findings are supported by others, who have also demonstrated that healthy relationships may affect one's physical well-being. The development and maintenance of healthy relationships is, therefore, a key goal for achieving wellness.

DEVELOPING AND MAINTAINING A SENSE OF SELF

Rediscovering the girl within appears to be the key to women's identity.

—Hancock, 1989, p. 25

The concept of self-esteem evokes many different meanings. What do we know about self-esteem? How much of this knowledge is based on studies of women? What factors contribute to or detract from a woman's self-esteem? Are we using self-esteem interchangeably with sense of self? This section addresses the concepts of self-esteem and sense of self in an effort to delineate for women the importance of the goal of developing and maintaining a strong sense of themselves.

Research shows that one's sense of self very much influences other aspects of one's self and one's health. The extent to which an individual thinks well of herself and has confidence in herself may have an influence on her abilities to perform everyday functions. While the newer models of women's psychological development emphasize women within the context of relationships with others, the concept of self remains central. The notion in these newer models is that women develop a strong sense of themselves within the context of healthy interpersonal relationships. Previous chapters in this book have described healthy relationships and have outlined the importance of such relationships. This current chapter focuses on the development of one's self, with attention to the goal for women of developing a strong sense of self or a healthy self-esteem.

Self-esteem has, in many ways, become a word of the "pop culture," as many self-help books and activities are geared toward increasing one's self-esteem. As a result, the term *self-esteem* has many different connotations and sometimes self-centeredness is one of these connotations, with a very negative association attached to the idea put forth by the "me generation." The intent of this chapter, however, is to present the concept of self or self-esteem as a fundamental basis upon which people develop a sense of well-being and health. Underlying this intent is the notion that women who have a healthy sense of self will be healthier in a holistic way and will be able to better contribute to society as well as reap the benefits of good health.

Sanford and Donovan (1984) interviewed women and discovered six common problems associated with self-esteem. These problems included: (1) women lacking knowledge of themselves and how they, in fact, identify themselves; (2) women minimizing who they are and their importance; (3) women perceiving themselves to be failures in most areas; (4) women minimizing the importance of things that they are good at; (5) women experiencing "self-concept dislocation" (Sanford & Donovan, 1984, p. 17) where they have gone through an event that has contributed to a new and lowered self-esteem; and (6) women readjusting their own image of who they would like to be.

From a societal perspective, we can understand where women have often pushed aside their selves in an effort to maintain their traditional roles as wives and mothers. The work of Jack (1991), *Silencing the Self,* is very useful for understanding some important issues for women. Jack (1991) aptly addressed women's sense of themselves in her study of depressed women in unhealthy relationships with men. She found that all the women in her study suppressed their own needs and desires as they worked hard to meet the needs of their spouses in order ultimately to maintain their relationships with their spouses, even though those relationships were not healthy and were, in fact, detrimental to their psychological health. In these cases the lack of a strong sense of self precluded them from leaving these unhealthy relationships, thus fostering more negative effects on their self-esteem. Ironically, however, we also know that it is the presence of a healthy interpersonal relationship that contributes to the development of one's sense of self and self-esteem. Thus, the cause-and-effect relationship here is not linear, but very circular (something inherent in taking a holistic approach to health and health care). What this means for our understanding of women's self-esteem is that we cannot even begin to understand it and even less to assist women in attaining a healthy self-esteem without understanding the social-cultural context of each individual woman.

The study by Hancock (1989) of 20 women's experiences as they grew from adolescence to adulthood revealed the important finding that these women developed a sense of self, which, during adolescence, became submerged or pushed aside. Consequently, as these women became adults, they struggled with reclaiming their sense of self. This finding is similar to Jack's work of depressed women who submerged their sense of self in order to maintain a relationship with a man, later struggling to reclaim their own sense of self and, in turn, overcome their depression.

Both Hancock (1989) and Jack (1991) have emphasized the need for women to reclaim their authentic selves that have likely been suppressed or submerged, particularly during adolescence and during efforts to maintain unhealthy and possibly destructive relationships. The ability to become self-reflective and to work through difficult issues during a woman's past will contribute greatly to her eventual ability to develop authenticity in relation to others and to feel confident in relation to oneself.

The goal of developing a strong sense of oneself, then, consists of several factors: **self-esteem**, **self-reflection**, and engaging in **healthy interpersonal relationships**.

DEVELOPING AND MAINTAINING A PHYSICALLY HEALTHY BODY

Living in strength gives us no need to wear armor, but the courage to reveal ourselves as we are.

—Andes, 1995, p. 20

Physical health, while not separate from psychological, emotional, and spiritual health, is an integral part of overall health for women and, thus, a separate section is devoted to the goal of developing and maintaining a healthy body. The goals of physical health include **strength, endurance, functionality**, and **prevention of acute and chronic illnesses**. In examining these goals, it is very important to consider each individual person's own views of her own health, with an emphasis on her own strengths rather than weaknesses or lacks (Pender, 1996). Achieving these goals in conjunction with the other goals outlined in this section of the book contribute to an overall sense of well-being for women. Each of these goals related to physical health is described in this section.

Strength refers to the condition of the muscles in the body. The muscles, according to Andes (1995) are "active" tissues because they increase metabolism, assisting one to burn up greater numbers of calories to maintain a healthy weight.

Endurance is related to strength in that it refers to the length of time a woman can exert extra effort. Clearly, greater strength will lead to greater endurance capability.

Functionality refers to the degree to which a woman can carry out tasks needed to live a high-quality life.

Prevention of acute and chronic illnesses refers to the ability to resist illnesses. It also, however, refers to the ability to detect illnesses or disorders early enough that they can be treated. Cancer is an excellent example of the importance of early detection, which is a central tenet of health promotion. A holistic approach to health promotion includes making use of our greatly expanding ability within health care to detect and treat cancers at an early and potentially curable stage, as well as to engage in measures, to the extent possible, to prevent these cancers from occurring in the first place.

Taken together, the attainment of all four goals for women's wellness will contribute to an overall sense of well-being. Part II of this book describes various modalities for achieving a higher level of wellness.

REFERENCES

Alles, W.F. (1996). Foreword to Stanford Center for Research in Disease Prevention in Partnership with the Stanford Alumni Association (Eds.), *Fresh start: Real health, real results for real people.* San Francisco: KQED Books.

Andes, K. (1995). *A woman's book of strength: An empowering guide to total mind/body fitness.* New York: Berkley Publishing Company.

Belenky, M., Clinchy, B., Goldberger, N., & Tarule, J. (1986). *Women's ways of knowing: The development of self, voice, and mind.* New York: Basic Books.

Borysenko, J. (1996). *A woman's book of life: The biology, psychology, and spirituality of the feminine life cyle.* New York: Riverhead Books.

Chodorow, N. (1978). *The reproduction of mothering.* Berkeley: University of California Press.

Gilligan, C. (1982) *In a different voice: Psychological theory and women's development.* Cambridge: Harvard University Press.

Hancock, E. (1989). *The girl within.* New York: Fawcett Columbine.

Jack, D. (1991). *Silencing the self.* Cambridge: Harvard University Press.

Johnson, K. (1991). *Trusting ourselves: The complete guide to emotional well-being for women.* New York: The Atlantic Monthly Press.

Jordan, J.V. (1997). *Women's growth in diversity.* New York: Guilford Press.

Jordan, J.V., Kaplan, A.G., Miller, J.B., Stiver, I.P., & Surrey, J.L. (1991). *Women's growth in connection.* New York: Guilford Press.

Miller, J.B. (1986). *Toward a new psychology of women.* Boston: Beacon Press.

Miller, J.B., & Stiver, I.P. (1997). *The healing connection: How women form relationships in therapy and in life.* Boston: Beacon Press.

Northrup, C. (1998). *Women's bodies, women's wisdom: Creating physical and emotional health and healing.* New York: Bantam Books.

Ornish, D. (1997). *Love and survival: The scientific basis for the healing power of intimacy.* New York: HarperCollins Publishers.

Pender, N. J. (1996). *Health promotion in nursing practice* (3rd ed.). Stamford, CT: Appleton & Lange.

Sanford, L.T., & Donovan, M.E. (1984). *Women and self-esteem.* New York: Penguin Books.

PART II

Integrated Strategies To Meet the Goals

Ellen Olshansky

Part II presents an array of strategies used in promoting and maintaining women's health and wellness. In keeping with the focus of the entire book, Part II includes an integrated approach to women's health by including both traditional and complementary health care strategies. The intent is to provide the reader with several suggested approaches, in the hopes that an individualized plan of care can be devised for each individual woman, based on her own needs and goals.

Chapter 6 presents a conceptual introduction to these overall approaches, followed by Chapters 7 through 18, which include specific approaches and strategies. As stated earlier in this book, the goal is not to prescribe a plan of care, but rather to provide options, based on the strategies presented, for various plans of care.

A comment on pain management is important here. Because pain is a common symptom of many illnesses and conditions, it has not been delineated as a separate category. It is helpful to note, however, that a variety of approaches to pain exist and that all the therapies included in Part II address pain management in some way. These approaches are mentioned where appropriate.

Historical Background to Integrated Strategies for Women's Wellness

Natalie Pavlovich and Christine Meyer

> *The ultimate goal of the investigations of alternative medical practices is to integrate validated alternative medical practices with current conventional medical practices.*

—Dossey & Guzzetta, 1995, p. 11

Alternative medicine was initially defined by Eisenberg et al. (1993) as "medical interventions not taught widely at United States medical schools or generally available at U.S. hospitals" (p. 246). In Europe these kinds of therapy are called *complementary,* but in the United States, depending upon one's views, they may be termed *Eastern, unconventional,* or *quackery* (Brown, Cassileth, Lewis, & Renner, 1994; Hufford, 1995; Mayo Clinic, 1993). Other common expressions are *folklore, natural,* and sometimes *traditional* (Swackhamer, 1995). In the literature, however, the connotative meaning of the term *traditional* seems to depend mostly upon the author's orientation. That is, *traditional* can refer either to the art of healing that was customarily practiced and passed down for thousands of years or to Western medicine that is rooted in the scientific method. Nevertheless, since the early 1990s, the terminology has gradually evolved from *alternative,* a label that implies an incompatible or *either/or* stance; to *complementary,* an expression that suggests a cooperative, but a subordinate relationship; to *integrative,* a term that denotes a balanced and interdisciplinary blending of the best from both perspectives for the highest good of the patient (Dossey, 1995). Thus, *integrative* or *integrated* is the term used in this book to reflect an overall comprehensive approach to health and health care. All of the chapters in Part II of the book, together, comprise an integrative approach to the health and health care of women, as both conventional approaches (e.g., pharmacological therapy) and complementary approaches (e.g., herbal and homeopathic remedies) are included in an effort to develop a comprehensive, integrated overall approach.

BACKGROUND

As we approach the twenty-first century, an integrative approach to health and health care will increase. For centuries, each civilization practiced its folk medicine, which later became known as home remedies. These home remedies used natural substances, specifically plants, which were easily obtainable from one's environment. These remedies were prepared in a variety of ways, such as compresses, teas, creams, poultices, or ointments from the various parts of the plant (i.e., seeds, roots, stems, bark, leaves, flowers, or fruits).

For the purposes of introducing the particular chapters of the book that focus on less conventional approaches, the term *complementary* will be used. The majority of this introductory chapter focuses on the history and philosophy of these complementary approaches, since much less has been written about them in the United States.

In world civilization, natural substances, such as herbal remedies, became very popular in most European and Eastern countries (India and China) before becoming accepted in the United States. Recently this movement toward natural therapies has emerged in the United States. The general public is seeking an increasing amount of care from complementary practitioners (Dickstein, 1999; Spencer & Jacobs, 1999). A survey showed that greater than a third of United States citizens have used complementary health approaches (Eliopoulos, 1999). The number of Americans using different types of complementary modalities and the frequency of use have increased dramatically in the past ten years. A national survey conducted by Eisenberg and colleagues (1998) of 2,055 adults revealed that the rate of use of those who have used at least 1 of 16 complementary modalities grew from 33.8% in 1990 to 42.1% in 1997 ($P \leq 0.001$). Other surveys and studies support these findings. For instance, the landmark report on public perceptions of alternative care (Landmark Healthcare and Interactive Solutions, 1998), for which 11,500 Americans were interviewed in 1997, obtained similar results; that is, 42% have used some type of complementary intervention in the past year. Further support is provided by another random survey of 1,000 Americans by the Stanford Center for Research in Disease Prevention (SCRDP, 1998). This survey indicated that 69% had used some type of complementary intervention. In a study by Burg, Hatch, and Neims (1998), 62% of 1,012 Florida residents reported that they had used 1 or more of 11 complementary modalities. This study also revealed that the respondents who tended to use more of these therapies were women, unmarried persons, those with a regular health care provider, and those who rated their health as poor (Burg, Hatch, & Neims, 1998).

This trend among consumers has contributed to public pressure that has influenced health care professionals to incorporate complementary remedies into their practices. Boucher and Lenz (1998) studied 109 physicians and found that 65.1% believed that many of the complementary therapies can be useful for specific diseases and that 64% would recommend or refer a patient to an integrative practitioner. Astin, Marie, Pelletier, Hansen, and Haskell (1998) examined surveys of orthodox doctors concerning their beliefs, patterns of referral, and professional use of five of the most prevalent complementary therapies between 1982 and 1995. Of the five therapies, physicians referred patients for acupuncture the most (43%) and considered acupuncture to be most efficacious (51%) (Astin et al., 1998). Most of the studies indicated that the patient's request for education and referral to complementary practitioners is the primary motivation for physicians' interest in these modalities (Boucher & Lenz, 1998). Today consumers are questioning their health care providers about other ways to treat their symptoms or conditions, and many providers are giving the consumer a wider range of choices regarding treatment. These choices include herbal remedies, homeopathic remedies, or traditional Chinese medicine (TCM) that predominately uses herbs. This openness to alternative approaches to health care has been substantiated by the recent publication in the *Journal of the American Medical Association* (Garn, 1998), reporting survey results that ranked alternative/complementary medicine among the top three subjects that the journal planned to address in future issues. Garn further stated that the survey findings indicated that physicians were communicating to their patients their own interest in complementary therapies.

In the 1970s, registered nurses recognized the value of complementary therapies in the healing process. Nurses always have focused on the patient as the center of their work. Through this focus, they saw the suffering, hopelessness, and helplessness of many patients as they underwent processes of illness and terminal conditions. Consistent with their holistic perspective in helping patients, these nurses began expanding their skills in healing therapies to include touch, body work, herbology, and homeopathy. Nurses recognized that these modalities not only helped a patient's physical needs, but also were beneficial to a patient's mind and spirit. These nurses, interested in holistic approaches, decided to form a professional organization that supported their common interests. In 1973, The American Holistic Nurses Association (AHNA) was established. The term *holistic* referred to wellness, and to harmony among body, mind, and spirit within a context of an ever-changing environment (Fasano-Ramos, 1999). AHNA was the first professional nursing organization to initiate certificate programs in holistic nursing, healing touch, interactive imagery, and aromatherapy. They offered seminars, workshops, and conferences throughout the nation so that professional registered nurses not only would be better informed, but also knowledgeable and skilled in the particular modality. Academic nursing programs are now offering courses in topics related to natural health in the professional curricula, in both undergraduate and graduate programs. Finally, nurses have been sharing their knowledge and experiences in complementary therapies through their professional publications via books, journals, and newspaper columns (Rew, 1999).

Pharmacists, too, have begun expanding their practices, and their pharmaceutical sites now include natural wellness sections that promote natural health products, including herbal remedies, homeopathic remedies, and nutritional supplements. Along with this rapid growth in consumer interest, pharmacists are seeking additional knowledge by attending seminars, courses, or workshops in order to expand their educational base in integrated approaches to health and to learn more about the natural substances. This continuing education has allowed pharmacists to conduct client assessment and counseling services for a fee (Patel, 1999). Meanwhile, courses offered within pharmacy curricula are beginning to incorporate information about herbal remedies.

Concurrently, some insurance companies have begun to provide coverage for selected complementary modalities. These insurance companies include coverage for acupuncture, massage, and chiropractic treatments. Initially, health care insurance plans did not provide for chiropractic coverage. Today the insurance companies cannot discriminate against doctors. That is, a chiropractor who is viewed as "doctor" of chiropractic and who is licensed, like a medical doctor, is eligible for coverage. Therefore, most major health care plans include chiropractic services. In 2000 Medicare will cover chiropractic spinal adjustment and spinal manipulation within the need for X-rays.

In the 1990s, the federal government responded to the public's demand for complementary approaches to health. The first evidence of this response was in 1991, when the American government appropriated funds to establish the Office of Alternative Medicine (OAM) at the National Institutes of Health (NIH). The creation of this significant federal agency became a reality in 1993 (Spencer & Jacobs, 1999). In 1998 the American Congress allocated an increase of $8 million in the OAM budget. These funds offered grant awards for research studies focusing on complementary modalities for improvement of health (Prevention, 1998).

The passage of the 1999 Omnibus appropriations bill, signed by President Clinton on October 21, 1998, established the National Center for Complementary and Alternative Medicine (NCCAM), which replaced the former Office of Alternative Medicine. This expansive structural change encompassed a broader perspective than the former OAM. The purpose of NCCAM is to conduct and support basic and applied research and training to disseminate information to practitioners and the general public. The government is also examining and analyzing the effects of complementary remedies on cost of current prescription drug bills (Shealy, 1996).

Increasing numbers of studies are being conducted on professional health care providers' personal use of complementary therapies. A recent study by Burg, Kosch, and Neims (1998) of 764 faculty members employed in six schools of health sciences at the University of Iowa revealed that more than half had used one or more such therapies. Faculty in the school of allied health reported the highest use, followed by the schools of nursing, dentistry, pharmacy, veterinary medicine, and medicine. The results also indicated that female physicians were more likely than male physicians to use such therapies ($P \leq 0.001$) (Burg et al., 1998).

THE PHILOSOPHICAL AND PRACTICAL BASES FOR THE CURRENT TREND TOWARD INTEGRATING HEALTH CARE APPROACHES

In 1998, Austin reported that most individuals used complementary remedies because these remedies were consistent with their own beliefs, their values, and their philosophical perspectives regarding health. This rapidly growing shift in health care approaches can be understood from a philosophical perspective as well as a practical perspective.

From a philosophical perspective, the traditional Western approach to health is characterized by its focus on the "part" of the individual rather than the "whole" individual. That is, traditional health care providers emphasize portions of the individual's body, sections of the individual's human experiences, or particular aspects of a person's life. Contrary to such a focus, holistic or integrative practitioners emphasize that the whole is greater than the sum of its parts. In other words, the whole cannot be reduced to parts without losing a significant portion in the process, especially in alleviating symptoms and ailments. In totality, healing occurs in the entire or "whole" self. This perspective is viewed as synthetic or holistic (Moskowitz, 1980). Holism became a popular term for describing this comprehensive approach to health care. In this view, the entire person—the physical, mental, emotional, cultural, and spiritual aspects—is considered in the application of healing modalities. For instance, we know that many ailments begin with the emotions and the mind. Today, stress is the cause for several symptoms, such as tiredness, lack of energy, depression, headaches, constipation, irritability, and anxiety (Kassin, 1998; Lahey, 1998). Integrative health practitioners constantly strive to maintain foremost in their approaches that the mind and body are interconnected (Hammond, 1995). Murray and Pizzorno (1998) pointed out the importance of recognizing the interconnections among body, mind, emotions, social factors, and environment as these aspects, all together, contribute to one's state of health.

Another important aspect of this philosophical perspective is the focus on information. Integrative practitioners emphasize subjective information, such as how the patient is responding to particular symptoms or ailments. This subjective information, along with objective information such as laboratory test results, provides the practitioner with a total profile of the patient.

In looking closer at the patient-provider relationship, in the traditional approach this relationship is often one-sided. That is, the provider listens initially to the patient as she describes her health problem, then makes a diagnosis or assessment, and quickly determines the medical plan (usually consisting of drugs, necessary tests, and specific treatments). While many traditional practitioners emphasize a more reciprocal relationship with the patient, integrative practitioners consider the interpersonal relationship to be a key part of the healing.

Both the consumer and the practitioner participate in the relationship equally, as the integrative practitioner views caring and empathy to be central to the healing process (Murray & Pizzorno, 1998).

From a practical perspective, the traditional health practitioner relies heavily on prescribed medications or allopathic drugs. It was reported that in 1996, 2.2 million Americans developed adverse reactions to Food and Drug Administration (FDA)-approved drugs (Gormley, 1998). Furthermore, in that same year, 108,000 Americans died in hospitals from FDA-approved drugs (Gormley, 1998). While adverse effects are also possible with herbal or homeopathic remedies, it cannot be assumed that all FDA-approved drugs are completely safe.

SUMMARY

More and more women today are taking control of their own health needs as well as the health needs of their families (Loecher, 1997). Women are becoming more informed, more discerning, and more selective as to how they care for their health. Consumers seek out information about their health through self-help literature, workshops, seminars, word of mouth, and the Internet. Meanwhile, publications on natural approaches are featured in major newspapers, journals, and broadcast media. Consumers will continue to seek out timely and accurate health information as we enter the next millennium. The various complementary modalities are making inroads among both consumers and professionals. The general public has become the driving force behind recent trends to consider the complementary health arena, in an effort to develop a truly integrative health care system. The American Congress has been instrumental in allocating funds for the establishment of the Office of Alternative Medicine, known today as the National Center for Complementary and Alternative Medicine. This trend toward integrated health has led professional schools at universities and colleges to introduce courses on complementary modalities into their health-related professional curricula. Health care professionals are seeking knowledge and training in these modalities. At the same time, many professional organizations are sponsoring conferences, workshops, and seminars to further educate professionals who have been practicing in the discipline for many years. Together, these health care professionals are becoming open, alert, and sensitive to the consumers' needs for a combination of alternative and conventional therapies, namely for an integrated approach to health and health care. The intent of the next chapters is to present an array of health care approaches and modalities in an effort to assist nurses and other health care providers in developing integrative strategies for health and health care of women.

REFERENCES

Astin, J.A., Marie, A., Pelletier, K.R., Hansen, E., & Haskell, W.L. (1998). A review of the incorporation of complementary and alternative medicine by mainstream physicians. *Archives of Internal Medicine, 158,* 2303–2310.

Austin, J. (1998). Why patients use alternative medicine: Results of a national study. *Journal of the American Medical Association, 279,* 1548.

Boucher, T.A., & Lenz, S.K. (1998). An organizational survey of physicians' attitudes about and practice of complementary and alternative medicine. *Alternative Therapies in Health and Medicine, 4*(6), 59–65.

Brown, H., Cassileth, B.R., Lewis, J.P., & Renner, J.H. (1994, June 15). Alternative medicine—or quackery. *Patient Care,* 80–98.

Burg, M.A., Hatch, R.L., & Neims, A.H. (1998). Lifetime use of alternative therapy: A study of Florida residents. Personal use of alternative medicine therapies by health science center faculty. *Southern Medical Journal, 91,* 1126–1131.

Burg, M.A., Kosch, S.G., & Neims, A.H. (1998). Personal use of alternative medicine therapies by health science center faculty [letter to the editor]. *Journal of the American Medicial Association, 280,* 1563.

Dickstein, L. (1999). A guide to natural health. *Psychology Today, 32*(2), 37–52.

Dossey, B.M., & Guzzetta, C.E. (1995). Holistic nursing practice. In B.M. Dossey, L. Deegan, C.E. Guzzetta, & L.G. Kolkmeier (Eds.), *Holistic nursing: A handbook for practice* (2nd ed.). Gaithersburg, MD: Aspen Publishers, Inc.

Dossey, L. (1995). A journal and a journey. *Alternative Therapies in Health and Medicine, 1*(1), 6–9.

Eisenberg, D.M., Davis, R.B., Ettner, S.L., Appel, S., Wilkey, S., Rompay, M.V., & Kessler, R.C. (1998). Trends in alternative medicine use in the United States, 1990–1997. *Journal of the American Medical Association, 280,* 1569–1575.

Eisenberg, D.M., Kessler, R.C., Foster, C., Norlock, F.E., Calkins, D., & Delbanco, T.L. (1993). Unconventional medicines in the United States. *New England Journal of Medicine, 328,* 246–252.

Eliopoulos, C. (1999). *Integrating conventional and alternative therapies: Holistic care of chronic conditions.* St. Louis: Mosby.

Fasano-Ramos, M. (1999). Springtime: Awakening of holism in our lives. *Beginnings, 19*(2), 1.

Garn, M. (1998). President's message. *Ohio State Homeopathic Medical Society Newsletter,* Fall/Winter, 1–2.

Gormley, J. (1998). A holiday message (to the NEJM). *Better Nutrition, 60*(12), 8.

Hammond, C. (1995). *The complete family guide to homeopathy.* New York: Penguin Studio.

Hufford, D.J. (1995). Cultural and social perspectives on alternative medicine: Background and assumptions. *Alternative Therapies in Health and Medicine, 1*(1), 53–60.

Kassin, S. (1998). *Psychology* (2nd ed.). Englewood Cliffs, NJ: Prentice Hall.

Lahey, B. (1998). *Psychology: An introduction* (6th ed.). New York: McGraw-Hill.

Landmark Healthcare and Interactive Solutions (1998). Landmark report on public perceptions of alternative care. Sacramento: Landmark Healthcare.

Loecher, B. (1997). *New choices for healing in women.* Emmaus, PA: Rodale Press.

Mayo Clinic Health Letter (1993, April). Alternative medicine: The scientific method separates help from hype, 6–7.

Moskowitz, R. (1980). Homeopathic reasoning. Paper presented at the symposium, "Homeopathy: the renaissance of cure," p. 2. San Francisco, CA.

Murray, M., & Pizzorno, J. (1998). *Encyclopedia of natural medicine* (2nd ed.). Rocklin, CA: Prima.

Patel, V. (1999). Advanced health and wellness pharmacy; Phoenix, AZ: *Natural Pharmacy, 3*(2), 13–14.

Prevention (1998). Alternative medicine gets big research bucks. *Prevention, 50*(11), 40.

Rew, L. (1999). Synthesizing philosophy, theory, and research in holistic nursing. *Journal of Holistic Nursing, 17*(1), 3–4.

Shealy, C. (1996). *The complete family guide to alternative medicine.* Rockport, Maine: Element Books.

Spencer, J., & Jacobs, J. (1999). *Complementary/alternative medicine: An evidence-based approach.* St. Louis: Mosby.

Stanford Center for Research in Disease Prevention (SCRDP) (1998). *The SCRDP's Health Improvement Program.* Paper presented at the meeting of Complementary and Alternative Medicine: Scientific evidence and steps toward integration. Stanford University, Stanford, CA.

Swackhamer, A.H. (1995). It's time to broaden our practice. *RN, 58*(1), 49–51.

CHAPTER 7

Psychological Approaches

Ellen Olshansky

Key Points

Variety of psychotherapeutic approaches
    Psychodynamic
    Psychoanalytic
    Cognitive-behavioral
    Interpersonal
    Strategic/solution-focused
    Crisis intervention
    Grief counseling
    Relational
Variety of complementary psychotherapeutic approaches
    Mind-body control strategies and the relaxation response
    Breath focus
    Body scan
    Progressive muscle relaxation
    Meditation
    Prayer
    Mindfulness
    Guided imagery
    Autogenic training and hypnosis
    Yoga

Women have played a specific role in male-led society in ways no other suppressed groups have done. They have been entwined with men in intimate and intense relationships, creating the milieu—the family—in which the human mind as we know it has been formed. Thus women's situation is a crucial key to understanding the psychological order.

—Miller, 1986, p. 1

One important way to assist women in achieving and maintaining a high level of wellness is through psychotherapy. Sometimes psychotherapy is initiated in crisis situations, but it is also often very useful as a health-promotion strategy. Various forms of psychotherapy exist, based on different underlying philosophical beliefs that guide these forms. The purpose of this chapter is to provide the reader with a very general overview of the large variety of approaches to psychotherapy. Such an overview is particularly important within our current context in which the meaning of the terms *therapist* and *therapy* are often quite confusing, as so many forms of therapy exist. This chapter presents an overview and description of psychotherapeutic approaches to women's wellness. It is important to note that the various psychological approaches were not developed for women specifically, but have been used with women as well as men. The one approach that has been developed through work with women and on behalf of women is that based on relational theory (Miller, 1986), although this approach likely is appropriate for men as well as for women.

Classic approaches include psychodynamic and psychoanalytic, cognitive-behavioral, interpersonal, strategic/solution-focused, crisis intervention, and grief counseling. The configurations of therapy include individual, family, and group. A newer approach to therapy developed by a group of women psychiatrists and psychologists, similar to an interpersonal and psychodynamic philosophy of therapy, is a relational approach based on relational theory.

In keeping with a holistic framework of women's health, several complementary forms of treatment for "mind-body" control and to elicit a "relaxation response" (Domar & Dreher, 1996) are described in this chapter. These complementary treatments may contribute to the achievement of an overall sense of wellness and well-being.

PSYCHOTHERAPEUTIC APPROACHES

Psychodynamic and Psychoanalytic Approaches

Psychodynamic therapy is based on the notion that individuals can benefit from understanding their own patterned defense mechanisms, which are cognitive and affective ways of managing situations and which are considered to be rooted in childhood. By elucidating them, a person develops an understanding of her existence and may be able to change those mechanisms that are no longer useful and, therefore, dysfunctional. The psychodynamic approach is also based on the notion that individuals can benefit from understanding their own conflicted relationships with significant persons in their lives, usually developed over time since childhood (Ursano, Sonnenberg, & Lazar, 1991). Psychodynamic therapy involves an ongoing psychotherapeutic relationship between the therapist and the woman, whereby the woman is able to work through these conflicted relationships from her past. This approach is less focused on alleviating specific current symptoms and more geared toward developing insight and understanding of one's self and one's responses to stressful situations. In the process of developing this insight, however, current symptoms are often alleviated.

This form of psychotherapy is founded on the psychoanalytic framework, with modifications from the classic, traditional psychoanalytic approach. For example, sometimes psychodynamic treatment can be accomplished within a brief rather than a long-term time frame. There are vast numbers of forms of brief psychotherapy (Applegarth, 1999). Regardless of the specific form, however, all of them include use of interpretation by the therapist, a clear focus for treatment, and support and reassurance (Cooper, 1995).

Cognitive-Behavioral Approach

The cognitive-behavioral psychotherapeutic approach is focused on attempting to alleviate specific current symptoms and problems. This approach is based on the notion that individuals interact with their environment and behave on the basis of their perceptions of that interaction. Applegarth (1999) explained that this interaction between the person and the environment is a major determinant of the person's behavior, cognitions, and affect, and is an underlying premise of the cognitive-behavioral approach.

Through the process of cognitive-behavioral psychotherapy, a woman is assisted in learning new skills for coping with problems.

This therapeutic process involves a strong collaboration between the therapist and the client, wherein they mutually decide upon goals for the treatment (Lehman & Salovey, 1990; Peake, Borduin, & Archer, 1988). Sometimes the client is given specific "homework" assignments as a strategy for learning to change one's behavioral and cognitive response to stressors in an effort to achieve these goals of learning new ways to cope with problems.

Interpersonal Approach

Klerman, Weissman, Rounsaville, and Chevron (1984) developed a psychotherapeutic method termed *interpersonal psychotherapy*. This method is based on many elements of the psychodynamic approach and has been used specifically for depression, in which it is termed *interpersonal psychotherapy for depression* (IPT). In this method, a brief therapy is used, consisting of a time-limited approach, in which the focus is on the interpersonal context, with the goal of alleviating current symptoms and improving interpersonal relationships. This method emphasizes the importance of one's interpersonal relationships as a central factor in contributing to one's psychological state of health.

Strategic/Solution-Focused Approach

A strategic therapeutic approach very specifically focuses on a person's psychological symptom(s). Through this approach, the therapist develops a strategy to address the specific symptom and, in so doing, assists the client in understanding why previous strategies did not work. The goal is to develop new strategies that are effective in alleviating the distressing symptoms. Aspects of both a systems approach and an interpersonal approach serve as foundations for this therapeutic modality. This kind of therapy is almost always brief and directly focused on the goal of specifically changing previously unsuccessfully attempted solutions to new strategic solutions to diminish the person's symptoms (Applegarth, 1999).

Solution-focused therapy is similar to strategic therapy. A major difference, however, is that instead of focusing on changing unsuccessful strategies that tend to make problems persist, solution-focused therapy seeks to find ways of solving the specific problem(s). There is less emphasis on understanding what was done in the past to attempt to solve the problems, and instead an immediate emphasis on developing effective solutions. These solutions are actually constructed by the therapist and the client together (Walter & Peller, 1992).

Crisis Intervention

Crisis intervention aims to relieve the client's current, usually transitory, difficulty that has occurred in relation to a specific event or situation. The goal of this approach is to help the client reclaim her previously stable adaptive coping skills by managing the immediate crisis situation. This approach, therefore, is very much focused on addressing immediate symptoms. After successfully alleviating the crisis situation, a client may then become involved in longer-term therapy to address underlying issues, depending upon the therapeutic orientation of the therapist, the nature of the crisis situation, and the desires of the client.

Grief Counseling

Grief counseling is an approach that assists clients to come to terms with losses, both expected and unexpected. From a wellness perspective, grief counseling is very important, as loss is part of everyone's life. Being able to confront one's losses in a healthy manner, resolving the grief surrounding them, contributes to general psychological wellness in the face of loss. A grief counseling approach focuses specifically on these losses in an effort to help the client move on in life, while also recognizing the profound loss experienced.

Relational Therapeutic Approach

The relational therapeutic approach to psychotherapy is based on the work of the Stone Center (discussed in Chapters 4 and 5). Therapists who use this mode of psychotherapy become active participants in the therapeutic process by virtue of their being part of an ongoing, therapeutic, mutually reciprocal, empathic relationship with the client. This approach is similar to and has part of its basis in elements of both a psychodynamic and an interpersonal approach, but it is founded on the specific concepts of relational theory (Miller, 1986).

According to relational theory, women (and men) develop healthy psychological selves through ongoing healthy relationships with others significant to them. For these relationships to be healthy, they must be mutually reciprocal and empathic. It is through such relationships that connections occur between individuals, with the result that these individuals develop a strong sense of themselves. This psychotherapeutic modality was developed originally to assist in women's psychological development and has particular relevance for women, with emphasis being on women in relationships and the notion that the relational selves of women are very significant in women's sense of themselves. Conversely, according to this theory, women who are in relationships that are unhealthy (i.e., are not mutually reciprocal nor empathic) have a higher risk of developing psychological problems, such as depression or low self-esteem. While this therapeutic approach has been developed for women, based on clinical work with women, its relevance for men is important as well.

Based on this underlying theory, a relational psychotherapeutic approach consists of an active interpersonal relationship between the therapist and the client (woman). This therapeutic relationship serves as a mode through which the woman can develop a healthy psychological self as the process of therapy and healthy, empathic interpersonal interaction progress. The woman is given an opportunity to develop a healthy, empathic relationship, whereby even the therapist may disclose, to an appropriate extent, some personal aspects of his or her own life, allowing for reciprocity. The mutuality, reciprocity, empathy, connectedness, and authenticity that eventually develop through this ongoing relationship play key roles in the therapy

COMPLEMENTARY PSYCHOTHERAPEUTIC APPROACHES

Domar and Dreher (1996) described various ways of achieving what they refer to as the "relaxation response" and gaining "mind-body control." This section briefly describes what is meant by the relaxation response and mind-body control. The various methods for achieving these goals are then described. As noted, these methods are not necessarily considered within the category of psychotherapy, but they do offer ways of assisting a woman to achieve a greater sense of well-being. By including these methods, a complementary, integrated, and comprehensive approach to women's wellness is possible.

Mind-Body Control and the Relaxation Response

Mind-body control refers to a holistic understanding of a person, whose physiological responses are highly interrelated with psychological responses. The concept of mind-body control is an essential aspect of the relaxation response. Domar and Dreher (1996) described the relaxation response as a way of gaining mind-body control.

When individuals are in a highly stressful situation, they often experience what is referred to as the "fight or flight" syndrome (Domar & Dreher, 1996) in which a distinct physiological response occurs. This response includes rapid heart and breathing rates, increased blood pressure, and muscle tension as a result of the secretion of hormones by the hypothalamus in response to the stressful situation. The relaxation response is a physiological response that counters the fight or flight response. When the relaxation response is elicited there is a slowing of both the heart and breathing rates, a decrease in blood pressure, and a relaxing of muscles (Domar & Dreher, 1996). There are several techniques described by Domar and Dreher (1996) for eliciting the relaxation response and these techniques are described in the following sections. Individual women may have differing responses to the usefulness of each of these methods and may or may not decide to try one or several of them. They are, however, useful and low-risk approaches to attempting to gain mind-body control and achieve the relaxation response.

Breath Focus

The idea behind breath focus is that if a person takes a long, slow, deep breath rather than the more common shallow breathing that most people do regularly and unconsciously, the relaxation response will be elicited. Breathing so that the diaphragm contracts is essential to the breath focus technique. Domar and Dreher (1966) noted that this technique is particularly useful for women with eating disorders.

Body Scan

The body scan technique is a mental exercise in which the person focuses on each part of her body in a systematic way, taking deep breaths as she focuses. The goal of this technique is to determine which parts of her body are carrying her tension. For example, she may become aware that her neck is very tense or that her abdomen is tense. Ultimately, by becoming aware of where the tension lies, she can focus on reducing this tension through deep breathing (breath focus)and eventually elicit the relaxation response. Domar and Dreher (1996) have found this technique useful in many situations, with one interesting and important one being infertility. They provided a description of a woman who was able to relax more effectively during a particular infertility procedure by engaging in body scan and breath focus, possibly influencing the success of the treatment.

Progressive Muscle Relaxation

The technique of progressive muscle relaxation is similar to the body scan approach. The difference, however, is that in progressive muscle relaxation the person tenses up each muscle group before relaxing. In this manner the person not only develops a greater awareness of where the tension exists in the body, but also learns how to relieve the tension with an increased awareness of the relief that can actually occur. Domar and Dreher (1996) noted that this technique is often very successful for women who have difficulty resting their minds from anxieties and worries and apprehensions.

Meditation

Meditation is an approach wherein the person focuses inwardly rather than externally by concentrating on breathing and on repeating a word or phrase or short prayer. In addition, the person allows any thoughts or feelings that occur and enter in consciousness to simply "float" along (Domar & Dreher, 1996). Meditation is used to achieve a sense of tranquility or calmness.

Prayer

Prayer is a specific example of meditation, where the phrase that is repeated is clearly related to a spiritual or personal meaning. Chapter 15 of this book (Spirituality and Women's Wellness) contains more detailed descriptions of various ways that spirituality influences wellness, with prayer being one way of practicing spirituality.

Mindfulness

Mindfulness is based on the philosophy of Buddhism from Tibet. The goal of mindfulness is to be present in the moment. By being able to be present in the moment, persons no longer take the present for granted. Rather, they are able to appreciate the moment and take greater advantage of the present instead of focusing on the past or the future.

Guided Imagery

Guided imagery consists of mentally focusing on images that are peaceful for an individual. Such images may be experiences or places or certain scenes that have evoked calmness. This technique can be used by women who are undergoing painful medical procedures as a way to help elicit the relaxation response and decrease the unpleasantness associated with the procedures.

Autogenic Training and Hypnosis

The technique referred to as autogenic training uses words that serve as an orientation, which help to calm down and relax the body. Domar and Dreher (1996) described autogenic training as a type of self-hypnosis, where the words or orientation directly influence the body. Hypnosis, which must be done under the guidance of a trained hypnotherapist, can also help to enhance one's mental capacities in the hopes of alleviating some symptoms (Domar & Dreher, 1996). Mehl (1988) reported that hypnotherapy can be used to help prevent premature birth.

Yoga

Yoga consists of attaining specific physical postures, deep breathing, and meditating. This approach to achieving relaxation is founded on Indian philosophy. The underlying premises are that breathing helps to purify the body by improving oxygen flow in the body, leading to increased energy. The postures, which require rhythmic breathing, increase the awareness and flexibility of the body and reduce muscle tensions. The meditating provides a way to become centered and calm.

REVIEW AND DISCUSSION

See boxes "Patient Education" and "Continuing Questions/Challenges" for discussion topics for this chapter.

Patient Education

Psychotherapy can help with
   Depression
   Anxiety
   Panic attacks
   Addictions
   Problems with relationships
There are many people who call themselves "therapists," so you need
to know from whom you are seeking help
   Psychiatrist
   Psychologist
   Psychiatric social worker
   Psychiatric nurse
   Other

Continuing Questions/Challenges

How can we help to decrease the "stigma" of mental health approaches
   to health promotion?
How can mental health approaches become part of "mainstream"
   health care?

REFERENCES

Applegarth, L.D. (1999). Individual counseling and psychotherapy. In *Infertility counseling: A comprehensive handbook for clinicians.* New York: Parthenon Books.

Cooper, J.F. (1995). *A primer of brief psychotherapy.* New York: Norton.

Domar, A.D., & Dreher, H. (1996). *Healing mind, healthy woman.* New York: Delta Publishing.

Klerman, G.L., Weissman, M.M., Rounsaville, V.J., & Chevron, E.S. (1984). *Interpersonal psychotherapy of depression.* New York: HarperCollins Publishers.

Lehman, A.K., & Salovey, P. (1990). An introduction to cognitive behavior therapy. In R.A. Wells, and V.J. Gianetti (Eds.), *Handbook of the brief psychotherapies* (3rd ed.). New York: Plenum Publishing.

Mehl, L.E. (1988). Hypnosis in preventing premature labor. *Journal of Prenatal and Perinatal Psychology, 8,* 234–240.

Miller, J.B. (1986). *Toward a new psychology of women* (2nd ed.). Boston: Beacon Press.

Peake, T.H., Borduin, C.M., & Archer, R.P. (1988). *Brief psychotherapies: Changing frames of mind.* Beverly Hills, CA: Sage Publications.

Ursano, R.J., Sonnenberg, S.M., & Lazar, S.G. (1991). *Psychodynamic psychotherapy.* Washington, D.C.: American Psychiatric Association Press.

Walter, J.L., & Peller, J.E. (1992). *Becoming solution-focused in brief therapy.* New York: Brunner/Mazel.

CHAPTER 8

Physical Activity/ Exercise

Brian Scott Austin

Key Points

Be aware of the female athletic triad.
  Disordered eating
  Amenorrhea
  Osteoporosis
Know the components of a healthy exercise program.
  Strength training
  Aerobics
  Stretching

Strengthening exercise prepares your body for a more active lifestyle. A big part is that you're getting stronger, but there's more: strength training also improves your balance and flexibility, reducing your risk of injury.

—Nelson, 1998, p. 39

Exercise has not been a traditional activity of women until recently. Only in the past 20 years have women participated in exercise programs in mass numbers on a regular basis. The main reason for this increase in participation has been the elimination of societal taboos that once frowned upon women engaging in exercise. Another reason for the increase in exercise participation is an increase in sports opportunities for young women at each level of growth. Many of these women continue to exercise once competitive playing days have ended. The third reason for an increase in exercise participation is the misguided belief that women should meet an inappropriate body type and size in order to gain social acceptance. It is this misguided belief that has some young women dying to be thin.

WHAT IS EXERCISE?

Exercise is defined as physical activity that is structured, planned, and repetitive for the purpose of enhancing or maintaining a level of physical fitness (Neiman,1995). Many daily activities are planned, structured, and repetitive, but may not enhance health or fitness. In order to enhance physical health, an exercise program must encompass strength training, aerobic exercise, and flexibility. Programs that incorporate all three of these facets will contribute to optimal fitness.

FACTORS LIMITING EXERCISE PARTICIPATION

Time is one of the biggest limiting factors to the success of any exercise program. The stresses of work, family, and other demands on available time limit the opportunities to incorporate the three facets that make up an exercise program. Appointments, work, and family often take a priority to the basic need for maintaining health and feeling good. When the stress of these factors becomes too great, good health can deteriorate into a medical problem. Medical problems often make exercise a necessity for managing the problem.

The biggest limiting psychological factor to exercise participation relates to fear and apprehension of the unknown. Each person is different and responds to different stimuli and stresses in unique ways. This is why a particular program will work for one person but fail to work for another. The mind has the ability to cripple the body from initiating action to make a change. Overcoming the doubts created by the mind is the first step to success in exercise. It may be necessary to create a support network to ensure that changes are implemented to ensure the success of the exercise program.

HEALTH PROMOTION THROUGH EXERCISE

Exercise is an opportunity to avert potential health problems or manage existing problems while accomplishing something physically and psychologically positive for the body. However, many people are unwilling or lack the knowledge to make the effort required to improve their physical condition.

A wealth of misinformation exists in the area of exercise and exercise technique. Many people fail to understand how exercise affects the physiological mechanisms that change and shape the body. Many women are under the misconception that lifting weights will cause them to "bulk up" like a man. While it is true that some growth will occur, the female body does not contain enough testosterone to create the growth occurring in men (Fleck, 1998). The growth occurring in a woman specifically relates to that individual's genetic potential. Muscular growth occurs when a muscle is required to work under varying degrees of stress, intensity, and frequency. The "bulking up" most women notice is often related to body composition.

Exercise is an essential component to feeling one's best. Exercise can help to strengthen the body and help ward off illnesses. A physically fit individual tends to have fewer absences and missed workdays than nonexercising individuals, resulting in lower health care costs for the person and a greater asset for the employer.

Exercise and proper nutrition are important elements in maintaining a healthy and properly functioning body. The cost of preventive care is small compared with the cost of heart bypass surgery. A sound exercise and nutritional program is nothing more than a preventive maintenance program for the body. There are many hospital-based wellness programs available to the public for a nominal cost. Other options include joining a YMCA or other health/fitness club. The key is to treat and care for the body in ways that facilitate attainment of optimal wellness.

The first step to obtaining peak fitness is the desire to improve one's health and well-being. Commitment to beginning and seeing the program through to success begins in the individual's mind and has to be something desired by that individual. Exercise requires a personal time commitment and investment.

RESEARCH SUPPORT FOR THE BENEFITS OF EXERCISE

An abundance of research indicates that exercise is beneficial to health. Many of the studies conducted have used the male population, but there is some ability to transfer the results to the female population. In the past 20 years, however, a concerted effort to increase the level and quality of health and health care among the female population has been one goal of the medical and research communities.

Beginning around age 30, the body goes through a deterioration process known as aging (Shepard, 1993). During this phase of life, the human body is more susceptible to the development of disease and medical problems than at any other point in the life span. The biggest contributing factor to the development of medical problems is lifestyle behavior (Neiman, 1995). A significant factor for women is the lack of structured exercise on a regular basis and a predominantly sedentary lifestyle.

Coronary Heart Disease

Coronary heart disease (CHD) is an equal opportunity killer in the United States. CHD accounts for nearly 250,000 deaths among women each year (Wenger, 1996). Among the female population, 40% of all coronary events result in the woman's death. In fact, in 67% of these cases, death occurs before there is an actual awareness of CHD. Symptoms are often ignored or misdiagnosed, resulting in the untimely death of the woman. Surgical procedures on women are less effective than those performed on men. Women have a greater tendency to develop postoperative complications than do men and women have twice the mortality rate from coronary artery bypass grafts than do men (Wenger, 1996).

The implications for women are clear. Heart disease strikes and harms women with an equal vengeance. Study data show that one fourth of the women in the United States have serum cholesterol levels greater than 240 mg/dL. One third suffer from hypertension, defined as values greater than 140 mm Hg systolic or 90 mm Hg diastolic. These factors are complicated by the fact that lifestyle behaviors such as smoking, being overweight, and being sedentary exacerbate the effects of the disease (Wenger, 1996).

Exercise is a key to reducing the potential risks of CHD. A single exercise session can result in a dramatic reduction in the resting blood pressure (Rueckert, Slane, Lillis, & Hansen, 1996). The results of the study by Rueckert et al. (1996) showed that blood pressure level would return to normal after a period of time, but subsequent exercise sessions work to lower blood pressure through the establishment of a training effect (Rueckert et al., 1996).

The heart is a fist-size muscle located in the chest; it is responsible for the delivery of oxygen-rich blood to the rest of the body. Contractions expel blood from the chambers of the heart to the working muscles via the systemic circuit. The blood returns to the heart and lungs for oxygen replenishment by way of the venous system. The heart is the direct beneficiary organ of aerobic or cardiovascular exercise. During exercise, the heart is required to work at a higher rate in order to meet the demands of increased need for oxygen-rich blood in the muscles performing the work. A heart muscle that is fit will be able to sustain higher-intensity workloads for greater periods before fatigue limits continued exercise at higher-intensity workloads. When the heart fails to receive stress at regular intervals, the ability to endure sustained workloads is limited.

Research shows that a strong cardiac muscle meets the demands for oxygen-rich blood by incrementally increasing the cardiac output (amount of blood pumped per minute) and stroke volume (amount of blood pumped per contraction) to meet the needs of the body (Durstine, Pate, & Branch, 1993). In a study conducted with patients suffering from peripheral arterial occlusive disease, oxygen uptake was reduced. Exercise rehabilitation has the potential to improve the walking economy of these patients. Results of the study found that patients with diagnosed arterial problems received benefits from exercise programs. This benefit is accomplished through the blunting of the slow component rise in oxygen uptake. This finding would suggest that restricted exercise ability due to advanced disease status makes physical activity a necessary component for the development of optimal fitness and health (Marks, Ward, Morris, Castellani, & Rippe, 1995).

Blood Lipid Levels

Exercise plays a significant role in the reduction of blood lipid levels, resulting in direct reduction in coronary disease risk factors. An average exercise participant will see a reduction in total cholesterol of 10 mg/dL over a sustained exercise program. Additionally, triglycerides circulating in the blood can be reduced by an average of 15 mg/dL. More specifically, the amount of high-density lipoprotein (HDL) cholesterol circulating in the blood stream will see an increase of 1.5 mg/dL, while the circulating amounts of low-density lipoprotein (LDL) cholesterol drops by an average of 5.1 mg/dL (Tran, Weltman, Glass, & Mood, 1983). A study conducted in Northern Ireland found that exercise history and physical fitness resulted in an improved transport of HDL cholesterol (McAuley et al., 1997). Additionally, it is widely accepted that exercise raises blood plasma HDL. Several studies have shown that persons with greater exercise participation show consistently healthier blood lipid profiles than do sedentary persons (Eaton et al., 1995). Leaf, Parker, and Schaad (1997) found that consistent exercise elicits changes in body fat composition, which favorably affects the levels of triglycerides circulating in the bloodstream. This finding is independent of changes in the person's capacity for aerobic work. This result shows chronic steady-state aerobic exercise at any intensity will affect adiposity, resulting in favorable triglyceride levels in blood plasma. Vigorous exercise has been shown to have a direct association with systolic blood pressure values in women (Menisink, Heerstrass, Neppelenbrock, Schuit, & Bellach, 1997). Additionally, this study revealed that frequency of exercise is an important dimension when considering the related health benefits of exercise. Murphy and Hardman (1998) examined the benefits of long and short bouts of walking. Their findings revealed that short bouts of brisk walking in previously sedentary women improved fitness. These results showed comparability to long bouts of walking at lesser intensities. Additionally it was found that short bouts were as effective as long bouts in reducing body fatness (Murphy and Hardman, 1998).

Obesity

The number of people diagnosed with clinical obesity has risen significantly in the United States over the past 20 years. The disease affects 33% of all females, and generates and sustains a $35 million weight-loss industry (McArdle, Katch, & Katch, 1996). Frequently, obesity begins in childhood and progresses throughout adult life. Between 1988 and 1991, one third of adults between 20 and 74 years of age were estimated to be obese (McArdle et al., 1996). Since this estimation was made, the criterion for determining clinical obesity has been redefined. The change in standards has increased the number of people classified as clinically obese.

Obesity is not the direct result of constantly overeating. Research into the causes of this affliction has shown the potential existence of a mutated gene, which may predispose some people to being overfat. Researchers have theorized that this gene may block signals from the brain that disrupt hormonal signals controlling metabolism. The disruption of signals from the brain may not be capable of ceasing the urge to eat after the requirement for food has been satisfied (McArdle et al., 1996).

The economic effect of obesity is tremendous. Annually, it is estimated that obesity-related illnesses cost $56.3 billion (Colditz, 1992). Cardiovascular problems account for $22.2 billion in medical expenses annually among the obese population. Additionally, musculoskeletal problems and non–insulin-dependent diabetes constitute the second and third most costly afflictions within this population. Obesity is chronic and degenerative in nature, and poses a serious threat to health at levels of 5 to 10 lb over ideal weight. The significance of the health threat rises drastically at higher levels of body fat and body weight (McArdle et al., 1996).

Regular exercise benefits the body by managing and controlling the true weight and body composition. Exercise, in conjunction with proper and sound nutritional management practices, reduces and maintains adequate body fat levels. Studies with animals have consistently shown that exercise and diet are significant factors in maintaining fat-free mass (McArdle et al., 1996). Animals placed in the sedentary control group exhibited higher levels of body fat than the experimental group. Other studies have shown that the development of fewer fat cells occurs when exercise begins at an earlier age. The results of animal studies have practical implications for humans. A Japanese study showed that exercise sessions reduced the amount of visceral fat in test subjects. The reduction of subcutaneous fat was not as significant. The reason for the lack of reduction in the subcutaneous fat level may be the result of differences in the lipolytic effect in relation to hormonal sensitivity. Previous investigations have displayed visceral fat as highly sensitive to hormonal influences, while this influence is intermediate in the subcutaneous abdominal region and low in the subcutaneous gluteal and hip region. A 15% reduction in caloric intake occurred in the two exercise groups, while caloric intake in the control group remained the same (Abe, Kawakami, Suqita, & Fukienaga, 1997). The main implication is that children and adults actively engaged in vigorous exercise display lower levels of body fat, when compared with sedentary individuals.

EXERCISE AND THE MIND

Humans possess the most complex and sophisticated computer. Known as the brain, it serves as the center of thought and control for the human body. Psychological benefits from exercise are far-reaching and substantial. Exercise plays a significant role in the measurable happiness and *sense of self* held by an individual. Success that occurs through exercise goal attainment serves to enhance self-esteem. Studies have shown that self-perceived success and value are directly attributable to a person's physical image (Douganis et al., 1991). A strong internal sense of control provides the impetus for *developing a physically healthy* body. Douganis, Theodorakis, and Bagiatis (1991) found that women possessing a strong sense of internal drive were able to lose more weight than were women lacking this drive. This results in a highly confident person more capable of meeting challenging tasks. Kamal, Blais, Kelly, and Ekstrand (1995) found that female athletes had higher levels of self-esteem than women who were sedentary.

Sensitivity to body image begins at an early age. Body image plays a significant role in the psychological development of adolescents (Dekel, Tanenbaum, & Kudar, 1996). In a study of Israeli youths suffering from scoliosis, the researchers found youths participating in regular physical activities scored higher on self-esteem questionnaires. Active females scored higher on the questionnaires than males who were not participating in regular physical activity.

Among females participating in sports, body image has greater importance in spotlight sports where physique receives subjective ratings. Physical appearance may mean the difference between winning and losing. Several studies have shown a great degree of aberrant eating behaviors in order to obtain the proper body image for competition. One study conducted with college-age female athletes found that 70% of the respondents were unhappy with their present body image. The survey also found that 90% of the respondents were or had engaged in unhealthy behaviors in an attempt to obtain a better body image (Davis, 1992).

SPECIAL CONCERNS FOR THE FEMALE POPULATION

Among the exercising population of females, there are several specific concerns that must be addressed. Known as the female athlete triad, these concerns make up a triple combination of disordered eating, amenorrhea, and osteoporosis. The true level of incidence of each component of this triad is unknown and cannot be attributed to any specific aspect of exercise. These three problems pose a serious threat to health, both long and short term. Women, regardless of activity, are candidates for the triad (Talbott, 1996). Ultimately death could be the result if left unchecked.

Disordered Eating

Disordered eating has long been a secret affliction of many women. It may be as simple as specific aversions to certain foods or as complex as anorexia nervosa or bulimia. It is and has been extremely difficult to diagnose the problems because of the shroud of secrecy surrounding these conditions. Disordered eating is treated as a mental disorder, which affects the functioning and health of the body.

Studies of female athletes have reported that rates as high as 62% of athletes surveyed practice or previously practiced some form of disordered eating (Smith, 1996). This figure may actually be higher for the nonathletic population. Outward appearances may or may not be visible, due to the highly secret nature of the affliction. Drummer, Rosen, Heusner, Roberts, and Counsilman (1987) found that junior high school aged swimmers were highly sensitive to body image. This study found that 40% of the young women questioned were very concerned with body image and weight as compared with the boys surveyed. Many of the young women surveyed reported previous experience with dieting to lose weight.

The two most serious forms of disordered eating are anorexia nervosa and bulimia. Both afflictions are mental disorders and carry serious health consequences if left untreated. Anorexia nervosa is defined as a morbid fear of fatness, distorted body image, refusal to maintain at least 85% of the body weight expected for height and weight, and the absence of three consecutive menstrual cycles (Smith, 1996). Anorexia is characterized by frequent trips to the bathroom during and shortly after eating a meal, complaints about being cold, repeated suggestions about being fat, eating alone, exercise beyond the normal training regimen, and secondary amenorrhea (Faigenbaum, Nye-McKeown, & Morilla, 1996). The woman will often try to hide the problem by wearing baggy clothes and frequently deny that a problem actually exists. Many anorexic women will suffer from moderate to severe depression (Faigenbaum et al., 1996).

Bulimia is an unnatural focus upon the body shape, manifested as displeasure or dissatisfaction. The most common behavioral problem is the necessity for a woman to binge and purge food from her system. Visual signs of manual purging are facial and peripheral edema, knuckle scarring, erosion of tooth enamel, bloodshot eyes, fatigue, swollen or sore throat, diarrhea or constipation, chest pains, and swollen parotid glands (Joy et al., 1997). Bulimic women will often deny that they have a problem, and signs are disguised or hidden. A common method of purging the system is using laxatives. Laxatives act to speed up the movement of food through the system. If the abuse of these drugs is prolonged, the intestinal system may become damaged.

Amenorrhea

The cessation of the menstrual cycle is usually due to pregnancy. However, studies have found that intense exercise and the curtailment of nutrients will result in the cessation of the normal cycle. Amenorrhea is a disruption of the normal reproductive function. The cause for the disruption needs further investigation. This disruption used to be considered a sign that an athlete was training at the right level of intensity and regular cyclic menses would return upon the end of intense training. Depending on the length of the disruption, however, this return to normal may or may not occur (Loucks & Horvath, 1984).

Amenorrhea is classified into two separate categories, primary and secondary. Primary amenorrhea is a delay of menarche beyond the age of 16. Secondary amenorrhea is the lack of consecutive menses after menarche. Within the adult and young adult population, oligomenorrhea, defined as having fewer than six menstrual cycles per year, is the most common affliction. Studies examining menstrual irregularities and exercise have been unable to pinpoint the exact cause. Intensity of exercise and hormonal imbalances are the primary focus of current research. The intensity of exercise bouts is believed to affect the brain-hypothalamic-pituitary-ovarian axis (Rogol, 1996). Intense exercise is believed to suppress the release of regulating hormones. Among competitive athletes, menstrual irregularities are reported to be as high as 50% (Loucks & Horvath, 1984; O'Connor, Lewis, & Kirschner, 1995; Fogelholm, Van Marken Lichtenbelt, Ottenheijm, & Westerterp, 1996). The level of irregularity among the noncompetitive athletic population is unknown.

The most common type of amenorrhea is hypothalamic chronic anovulation. Hypothalamic chronic anovulation results from a disruption of the central nervous system and hypothalamic area of the medulla. The reproductive system is still functional, but the hormonal influence is suppressed. The frequency of lutenizing hormone pulses directly affects the hypothalamus. The reduction in lutenizing hormone restricts the ovarian function. This restricted ovarian function is compounded by the abnormal secretion of gonadotropin-releasing hormone by the hypothalamus (Loucks & Horvath, 1984).

The effect of vigorous exercise and weight loss on reproductive function was reported in the *New England Journal of Medicine*. Untrained women were subjected to consecutive exercise periods of 4-week duration. The main purpose of the study was to attempt to disrupt the normal cycle (Bullen et al., 1985). Researchers were able to disrupt the normal cycle of all except four of the participants (N = 28 untrained college women). The women in the study were found to have a high incidence of anovulation and abnormal luteal function. During the course of the study, the women restricted their caloric intake, lending credibility to the theory that caloric intake and intense exercise disrupts the reproductive function (Bullen et al., 1985). Excessive restriction of calories during exercise may increase the loss of valuable minerals, nutrients, and circulating estrogen levels. These losses may predispose the person to the development of stress fractures and osteoporosis (Rochman, 1997).

Osteoporosis

The greatest long-term health risk to women is the development of inadequate bone density. Inadequate eating behaviors and amenorrhea are contributing factors to the development of osteoporosis. The restriction of calories and the low estrogen levels circulating in the body reduce the amount of calcium uptake. For a female, the peak years for bone mineral storage are between the onset of menarche and roughly 24 years of age, posing a serious problem for a young woman who is cutting nutrient intake in order to attain an unrealistic body image.

Osteoporosis is characterized by low bone-mass density accompanied by microarchitectural deterioration of the bone tissue (American College of Sports Medicine [ACSM], 1997). Deterioration of the bone tissues weakens the structural stability, increasing the potential for fractures resulting from skeletal fragility. Osteoporosis is classified into three categories. Osteopenia is diagnosed when the bone density falls between 1.0 and 2.5 standard deviations below the mean for young adults. Osteoporosis is considered a bone density mass of 2.5 standard deviations below the mean for women. Severe osteoporosis has the same standard deviations as osteoporosis in addition to one or more fragility fractures (ACSM, 1997). A key to preventing the development of osteoporosis is regular participation in exercise that incorporates load-bearing movements.

Extensive research has shown that the main reason for the development of osteoporosis in premenopausal women is chronic hypothalamic anovulation and hypoestrogenemia. Bone storage and density are formulated during the adolescent years and correspond to the linear growth phase of bones (Bailey, Faulkner, & McKay, 1996). Zernicke et al. (1995) found that bone mineral density of preadolescent gymnasts was highest in areas receiving the highest stress. This shows the extreme importance placed upon the uptake of minerals, especially calcium, during a young woman's life. Bone modeling occurs primarily during the adolescent years as a result of mechanical forces placed upon the bones. Mass is added to the bone internally and externally at the locations that received the highest loading forces. Modeling is a direct result of the growth phase of the bone (Bailey et al., 1996). Remodeling is the process that occurs during the majority of adult life. It is a maintenance process that acts to replace fatigued and damaged bone. It involves the reabsorption of calcium and results in the net loss of bone. If the bone mass and density are not adequate, then the remodeling process will put the woman in danger. Net bone loss is the result of inadequate and incomplete calcium replenishment (Bailey et al., 1996).

Amenorrheic and menopausal women are highly susceptible to bone losses higher than normal, due to the lower circulating levels of estrogen. Estrogen is a precursor for the uptake of calcium by the skeletal structure. Without adequate bone mineral uptake, the structural integrity of the skeleton is compromised. It should be pointed out that shear forces affect the storage of bone minerals at the points where the greatest loading occurs on the bone. Studies have shown that bone mineral density in athletes tends to be greater in the areas that are the most susceptible to fractures in old age (O'Connor et al., 1995). Basketball players, gymnasts, and volleyball players consistently show higher bone density values in the hips and upper femur than do nonathletes (Dyson, Blimkie, Davidson, Webber, & Adachi, 1997). Madsen, Adams, and Van Loan (1998) found that athletes in weight-bearing sports, when matched for age and height, showed higher bone density than sedentary and moderately active controls. This result supports the importance of exercise at sufficient intensities as necessary for adequate bone remodeling to occur.

In an examination of premenopausal women, a 1997 study of participants in the Australian Veterans Games found that bone density values were higher for participants involved in sports with high-impact forces than other sports. Participants received impact-force values based upon their individual sport. Players of basketball and netball received the highest values for impact. Running and field hockey received moderate impact-force value assignments, while swimming comprised the lowest group studied. A sedentary control group matched for age and height was also included in the study (Dook, James, Henderson, & Price, 1997). The results of the Australian study found that the high- and moderate-impact groups displayed the highest bone density values of the groups studied. Additionally, the exercising groups showed higher lean muscle tissue ratios than the nonexercising group. The exercise history of the participants was quite lengthy. The specific implications of this study are that lifetime exercise habits are important for the promotión of bone mass density values and muscular function. The study also supports the need for exercise routines or sports that incorporate loading forces in a controlled manner. This type of exercise is highly conducive to maintaining high bone density values in extremely critical skeletal areas, such as the hip and pelvic girdle.

An interesting point to the studies that have examined young women as research participants is the finding that despite eating problems and amenorrhea, bone mineral density values were higher in athletes than in nonathletes. It could be determined that the greatest risk to bone density values is the lack of exercise that incorporates jumping and loading forces. As barriers to sports and exercise participation are eliminated for young women, the greatest benefit to their health will be active participation in both. However, the adult female population must seek a more active lifestyle in order to diminish the risks of osteoporosis in their golden years.

EXERCISE: THE WAY TO BETTER HEALTH

A decision to begin an exercise program is made every day for the benefit of better health. A decision to quit exercising is made at just about the same rate. Exercise requires hard work and perseverance. Health benefits begin almost immediately, but they are not as noticeable or visible. Results do not materialize overnight and certainly not out of thin air. The achievement of good health is a result of a life-altering decision. The easy part of the process is *beginning an exercise program;* the hard work begins by trying to maintain what has been obtained.

COMPONENTS OF A SOUND EXERCISE PROGRAM

Several facets make up a sound exercise program. A total exercise program will incorporate the following modalities: **strength training, aerobic exercise**, and **flexibility**. Each facet is capable of standing alone, but only the benefits of that specific facet are received. The goal of any exercise routine should be to enhance the health and appearance of the body, mind, and soul. A total exercise program goes farther to meeting these goals than each individual facet alone.

Regardless of the modality chosen, frequency and intensity are two important factors necessary for success. Frequency of exercise is defined by the number of times per week that the routine is accomplished (Wathan, 1994a). Beginning exercise participants should begin slowly and refrain from the urge to attempt too much too soon. A good rule for beginners is three times per week. Following this recommendation will ensure a less painful transition from a sedentary life to a more active life. As the physical fitness improves, frequency of exercise can increase. Adequate rest and recovery are extremely important for the body and will reduce the potential development of overuse injuries. If the body is forced to withstand too much stress, then distribution of the stress lands on structures (bones) not designed to handle it. A prime example is the development of shin splints from running or walking. Shin splints result from the tibialis anterior being unable to absorb continued stresses incurred during running or walking. This inability to handle the repeated stress requires the tibia to absorb it. Bone is not designed to handle the repetitive stress, and the result is the development of a stress fracture. The pain associated with the injury affects walking and almost rules out continued running until the injury has healed. Rest from running is the general prescription for this type of injury. Interestingly, stress fractures may be a sign of larger problems, such as disordered eating and amenorrhea (Rochman, 1997).

Recommended frequency for specific modalities differs. Aerobic exercise can be performed every day. Stretching exercises should be done several times per day. Recommendations for strength training differ since there is some microscopic muscle damage that occurs with each session. Strength training guidelines entail a rest period for a specific muscle group of 36 to 48 hours. For instance, if the whole body is lifted on Monday, then the next strength training session should not occur until Wednesday. Without this interval, the muscles do not have the full benefit of adequate rest and the muscle breakdown process compounds (Wathan, 1994a).

Intensity of exercise is a reference to the level of difficulty required to complete the session or exercise. Exercise intensity is classified into low, moderate, and high categories (Wathan, 1994a). Intensity levels should vary from session to session, so that the body develops throughout a wide range of stress. If the body is forced to undergo high levels of constant stress, there will be a greater likelihood that exercise burnout or injury will result. A participant just starting out will inevitably encounter some soreness, but as exercise sessions become more regular, this soreness will disappear. The days of "no pain, no gain" are gone. Soreness should only result from changes in the level of intensity, and if a program is closely followed then soreness and pain should be minimal.

Other considerations for the beginning exercise participant concern the necessity of sound program development. In order to design and develop a sound exercise program, baseline physiological values should be gathered via an exercise testing session. A basic exercise testing session will include most of the following: health history screening, blood pressure measurement, heart rate check, aerobic capacity and recovery test, a muscular endurance test, body composition measurement, and an abdominal endurance test. With the results of these tests, the fitness specialist is capable of evaluating and determining the best modalities for use in improving the present fitness level. These results provide a beginning status of fitness, and subsequent tests will provide a tracking device for improvements in fitness (Semenick, 1994). Another consideration is the potential of hiring a personal trainer. This has the possibility of being a bonanza of information in helping to learn more about how the body works. A personal trainer is also a source of motivation for remaining fit through the tough times that are inevitable with any fitness program. This option, however, is not available to all women, as financial barriers clearly exist.

Strength Training

The weight room can be a formidable and daunting place, especially for women. Traditionally a domain for men, women are increasingly seeking the benefits of "pumping iron." One aspect that continues to plague women in the weight room is the fear of developing bulky muscles. For the most part, this fear is unfounded. While it is true that there will be some growth of the muscle, it will only be to the person's genetic potential (Fleck, 1998). There is no reason for a woman to shy away from heavy lifting as long as she is capable of lifting the weight with good form and technique.

The most common terms used in strength training are exercise, repetition, and set. Exercise is a body movement involving a group of muscles or a specific muscle. A repetition is one movement of the exercise and a set is a number of repetitions of the same movement. The maximum amount of weight lifted one time is called a one-repetition maximum. Most lifting programs are designed to use a percentage of the one-repetition weight maximum.

Depending on the goal of the program, a percentage range of the one-repetition maximum is used to assist in the achievement of the goals. Mass or size of a muscle increases through lifting 70% to 80% for six to eight repetitions. Lifting 80% to 100% for one to four repetitions will produce gains in strength. Repetitions of 12 to 20 with 50% to 70% will result in an increase in the definition of the musculature. A well-rounded lifting program will encompass specified periods of lifting to increase each of these areas. Known as periodization, it is an easy method to ensure that peak fitness becomes a reality (Wathan, 1994b). Each period usually consists of 4 to 6 weeks in each phase. Each phase is followed by a rest period of 1 week.

The first step in designing an exercise program is to determine the total available amount of time that can be used for completing the workout. The amount of time should be realistic, as most people are involved with jobs, children, and other responsibilities, limiting the amount of time available for exercise. A program should be easy to understand and afford the person the most expeditious means of accomplishing the complete workout. The easiest way to facilitate a complete total body workout is using one exercise per body part. Compound movements use several muscles to complete the exercise. Movements such as the squat, bench press, and shoulder press require the assistance from secondary smaller muscles. The direct stress is not placed upon the secondary muscles, but their assistance is called upon to finish the lift. Isolation movements such as the triceps pressdown isolate the triceps and require increased muscle fiber to complete the lift.

Safety when lifting weights is a prime consideration in strength training. Good form and technique are essential to lifting success and injury-free exercise. At no time should proper form and technique be sacrificed in order to lift a heavier weight or finish a specific number of repetitions. The use of proper spotting techniques will increase the level of safety when using free weights. Circuit machines provide the exerciser with a fixed range of motion and require the proper lifting technique in a safe and efficient manner. Barbells and dumbbells, known as free weights, require the lifter to use proper form and technique. Free weights are controlled only by the lifter and can be dangerous if misused or lifted improperly. Free weights require the recruitment of other muscles to assist in the stabilization of the weight, often requiring the use of a lighter weight in order to lift the weight safely. Apprehension over lifting free weights should be overcome with repeated lifting sessions.

Finally, strength training is the easiest way to sculpt the body. Diet and aerobic exercise will only serve to reduce the weight of the body. The improvement of fat-free mass is specifically enhanced through strength training (Yessis, 1994). A well-defined human physique is the result of time spent in the weight room. Research into maintenance of fat-free mass pinpoints strength training as highly important. Dieting research has shown that weight loss often includes the loss of lean muscle tissue, which is not conducive to body strength. Marks et al. (1995) examined the effects of caloric restriction of no less than 1,200 calories per day when combined with aerobic and strength training. Eighty women were split into four groups and tracked for fat loss on a restricted diet. Each of the four groups lost weight during the study. The group that incorporated dieting with cycling and resistance training significantly lowered body fat (−4.7%) as compared with any of the remaining three groups. Additionally, this group showed significant increases in strength for the chest press, arm curl, leg extension, and tricep extension. Both the diet-cycling group and the diet-cycling-resistance group showed significant increases in maximal oxygen uptake over the control group of dieting only (Marks et al., 1995). The implication of this study is that including a moderate restriction of calories with strength training and aerobic exercise will result in the loss of body fat while sparing muscle tissue. This study also shows that it is possible to gain strength and increase maximal oxygen uptake during the restriction of calories.

Aerobic Exercise: The Key to Weight Loss

Body fat is burned in the flame of carbohydrate. Most often, aerobic exercise is the only type of activity included in most programs. This form of exercise stresses the entire body, with the primary benefactors being the heart and lungs. Cardiac muscle becomes stronger through repeated bouts of exercise, increasing the efficiency of the heart by allowing it to beat fewer times when pumping blood and oxygen to the working muscles at work and rest.

Skeletal muscle undergoes specific adaptations with aerobic exercise. Muscle fiber becomes a more efficient extractor of oxygen from the blood (Terjung, 1995). These improvements result from the increase in the number of mitochondria found in the muscle fiber. The ability to use fatty acids and carbohydrate for fueling muscular contractions is enhanced significantly due to this increase in the number of mitochondria. Increased muscle capillary numbers significantly raise the ability to bathe the individual fiber in blood. This increase in capillary numbers assists the muscle fibers' ability to remove oxygen during intense exercise. During subsequent bouts of submaximal exercise, this benefit assists in the sparing of muscle glycogen. Aerobic endurance exercise increases the peak blood flow during extended bouts of training (Terjung, 1995).

Aerobic exercise is the most common form of exercise undertaken by the U.S. population. Running or jogging are the predominate forms of cardiovascular exercise, while walking and cycling are tremendously popular also. The key to any form of aerobic exercise is to ensure that the appropriate level of intensity is attained. Too often, there is a lack of fluctuation within the heart rate training zone to achieve significant benefits.

Finding the heart rate training zone is the best method to ensure that the proper intensity is achieved. In order to find the appropriate training zone, subtract the person's age from 220, which calculates the theoretical age-predicted maximum heart rate. Determining the zone is accomplished by multiplying a percentage of the age-predicted maximum. The lower percentage and the higher percentage establish the lower and upper portions of the heart rate training zone (Howley & Powers, 1994). The easiest method to count the heart rate is to purchase a heart rate monitor, which provides a digital display. The other method is via manual palpation of the carotid artery. Use of this method requires the person to stop exercising and place the middle and ring fingers on the left or right side of the neck. Using a watch, the person must count for 10 seconds the number of beats starting at 0. The total number of beats is multiplied by 6 in order to arrive at the current heart rate. This method requires the exercise session to halt temporarily so that the beat count is accurate.

Aerobic exercise can be done each day; however, it is very easy to develop burnout or overuse injuries. For the beginning exercise participant, 4 days per week at a light intensity is adequate to elicit health benefits. Aerobic exercise sessions should consist of at least 20 minutes of continuous movement. As fitness improves, sessions should increase up to 60 minutes. Exercise after 60 minutes will elicit a training effect, which reduces the amount of fat burned as the primary fuel for muscle contractions (Blair, 1990). Increased muscle efficiency is specifically the result of longer duration exercise. Intense sessions appear to be more beneficial in increasing mitochondrial content (Terjung, 1995).

Surface considerations should be considered in order to reduce the chance of impact injuries. The best surface for aerobic exercise is soft and stable. Knee injuries occur from constant pounding on hard surfaces such as concrete or asphalt. Gravel surfaces provide an unstable surface that could lead to potential ankle problems. Groomed walking trails provide a stable surface that is soft enough to protect the joints. In the event that exercise surfaces are limited, proper footwear is necessary to ameliorate the untoward effects of these surfaces.

Flexibility: The Key to a Pain-Free Exercise Experience

Increasing the range of motion in a specific joint is very possible with proper stretching techniques. Stretching should be an integral part of any exercise program. Flexibility is defined as the range of possible movement in a joint. Flexibility is affected by age and gender, mechanics, and structure. Flexibility can be improved with two sessions per week (Allerheiligen, 1994). There are three types of flexibility. Static flexibility relates to a range of motion that has no speed emphasis. Ballistic flexibility refers to bouncing or rhythmic movements. Dynamic flexibility is the ability to use a range of motion to enhance performance of activities at specific speed (Alter, 1996).

The range of motion in a joint relates directly to the structure of the joint in question, meaning that the range of motion found in a specific joint will not be comparable to the range of motion in another joint. Children are more flexible than adults, and women are more flexible than men. The primary reasons for gender differences are anatomical and types of activities undertaken (Allerheiligen, 1994). As the body ages, muscle tissue is lost and replaced with fibrous connective tissue.

Stretching is a planned and deliberate action taken to enhance the range of motion in a joint. Stretches are categorized as active or passive. Regardless of the type of stretching, it is vitally important that the person focus on the muscle receiving the stretch. It is important that consistency and relaxation become an integral part of the stretching program. Stretching is an individual activity that should not be a race with others. Animals instinctively stretch before initiating vigorous movements, although humans fail to stretch with any regularity.

The failure to stretch on a regular basis creates tight and awkward movements. Movement conducted in a limited range of motion is inefficient and affects proper biomechanics, which is a potential precursor to injury. The biggest asset to any exercise program is the ability to move through a large range of motion.

The first step is to warm the muscle by exercising lightly for 5 to 10 minutes (Anderson, 1980; Allerheiligen, 1994; Alter 1996; Mattes, 1990; McAtee, 1993). This light preexercise raises the temperature of the muscle and assists in making the muscle more compliant. In stretching a muscle, a slight discomfort should be felt which should disappear when the stretch is released. A muscle should not be forced beyond the current range of motion. A consistent stretching program will facilitate an increase in the range of motion over a period of time (Allerheiligen, 1994).

CONCLUSION

Women need exercise to diminish the potential risks associated with inactivity and to promote health benefits associated with exercise. The present and future health status will dramatically improve with consistent exercise. Research has shown that exercise is beneficial in reducing the many conditions that are harming the female population. Strength training, aerobic exercise, and stretching provide unique benefits that serve to enhance optimal wellness.

REVIEW AND DISCUSSION

See boxes "Patient Education" and "Continuing Questions/Challenges" for discussion topics for this chapter.

Patient Education

Benefits of exercise
  Decreases risk for coronary heart disease.
    Lowers blood pressure.
    Strengthens cardiac muscle.
    Lowers blood LDL lipid levels.
    Raises blood HDL lipid levels.
    Controls body weight.
  Provides psychological benefits.
    Increases self-esteem.
    Improves body image.
  Decreases bone loss.
Cautions with exercise
  Don't overdo it.
  Make sure that *all three components* of healthy exercise program are
    included.

Continuing Questions/Challenges

How can patients be motivated to initiate and maintain a regular
  exercise program?
How can health care providers help to prevent the female athletic
  triad?

REFERENCES

Abe, T., Kawakami, Y., Sugita, M., & Fukunaga, T. (1997). Relationship between training frequency and subcutaneous and visceral fat in women. *Medicine and Science in Sports and Exercise, 29,* 1243–1251.

Allerheiligen, B. (1994). Stretching and warm-up. In T. R. Baechle (ed.), *Essentials of strength training and conditioning* (pp. 289–298). Champaign, IL: Human Kinetics.

Alter, M. J. (1996). *Science of flexibility* (2nd ed.). Champaign, IL: Human Kinetics.

American College of Sports Medicine. (1997). Position stand on osteoporosis and exercise. *Medicine and Science in Sports and Exercise, 29,* I–VII.

Anderson, R. A. (1980). *Stretching.* Bolinas, CA: Shelter.

Bailey, D., Faulkner, R., & McKay, H. (1996). Growth, physical activity, and bone mineral acquisition. In J.O. Holloszy (Ed.), *Exercise and sports science reviews* (pp. 233–267). Baltimore: Williams & Wilkins.

Blair, S.N. (1990). Exercise and health. *Sports Science Exchange, 3,* 1–5.

Bullen, B. Skrinar, G., Beitins, I., von Mering, G., Turnbull, B., & McArthur, J. (1985). Induction of menstrual disorders by strenuous exercise in untrained women. *New England Journal of Medicine, 312,* 1349–1353.

Colditz, G.A. (1992). Economic costs of obesity. *American Journal of Clinical Nutrition, 55,* 503s.

Davis, C. (1992). Body image, dieting behaviors, and personality factors: A study of high performance athletes. *International Journal of Sports Psychology, 23,* 179–192.

Dekel, Y., Tenenbaum, G., & Kudar, K. (1996). An exploratory study on the relationship between postural deformities and body image and self-esteem in adolescents: The mediating role of physical activities. *International Journal of Sports Psychology, 27,* 183–196.

Dook, J., James, C., Henderson, N., & Price, R. (1997). Exercise and bone mineral density in mature female athlete. *Medicine and Science in Sports and Exercise, 29,* 291–296.

Douganis, G., Theodorakis, Y., & Bagiatis, K. (1991). Self-esteem and locus of control in adult female fitness participants. *International Journal of Sports Psychology, 22,* 154–164.

Drummer, G., Rosen, L., Heusner, W., Roberts, P., & Counsilman, J. (1987). Pathogenic behaviors: Weight-control behaviors in competitive swimmers. *Physician and Sports Medicine, 15,* 75–79.

Durstine, J.L., Pate, R.R., & Branch, J.D. (1993). Cardiorespiratory responses to acute exercise. In Steven J Blair (ed.), *Resource manual for guidelines for exercise testing and prescription* (2nd ed.) (pp. 66–77). Baltimore: Williams & Wilkins.

Dyson, K., Blimkie, C., Davison, K., Webber, C., & Adachi, J. (1997). Gymnastic training and bone density in pre-adolesecent females. *Medicine and Science in Sports and Exercise, 29,* 443–450.

Eaton, C.B., Lapane, K.L., Garber, C.A., Assaf, A.R., Lasater, T.M., & Carelton, R.A. (1995). Sedentary lifestyle and risk of coronary heart disease in women. *Medicine and Science in Sports and Exercise, 27,* 1535–1539.

Faigenbaum, A., Nye-McKeown, J., & Morilla, C. (1996). Coaching athletes with eating disorders. *Journal of Strength and Conditioning, 18,* 22–30.

Fleck, S.J. (1998). Strong evidence. *Athletic Business, 22*(8), 52–56.

Fogelholm, M., Van Marken Lichtenbelt, W., Ottenheijm, R., & Westerterp, K. (1996). Amenorrhea in ballet dancers in the Netherlands. *Medicine and Science in Sports and Exercise, 28,* 545–550.

Howley, E.T., & Powers, S.K. (1994). *Exercise physiology: Theory and application to fitness and performance.* Dubuque, IA: Brown and Benchmark.

Joy, E., Clark, N., Ireland, M., Matire, J., Nattiv, A., & Varechok, S. (1997). Team management of the female athlete triad: Part 1. *Physician and Sports Medicine, 25,* 95–110.

Kamal, A.F., Blais, C., Kelly, P., & Ekstrand, K. (1995). Self–esteem attributional components of athletes and non-athletes. *International Journal of Sports Psychology, 26,* 189–195.

Leaf, D.A., Parker, D.L., & Schaad, D. (1997). Changes in VO2 max, physical activity, and body fat with chronic exercise: Effects on plasma lipids. *Medicine and Science in Sports and Exercise, 29,* 1152–1159.

Loucks, A., & Horvath, S. (1984). Athletic amenorrhea: A review. *Medicine and Science in Sports and Exercise, 17,* 56–72.

Madsen, K., Adams, W., & Van Loan, M. (1998). Effects of physical activity, body weight and composition, and muscular strength on bone density in young women. *Medicine and Science in Sports and Exercise, 30,* 114–120.

Marks, B.L., Ward, A., Morris, D.H., Castellani, J., & Rippe, J.M. (1995). Fat-free mass is maintained in women following a moderate diet and exercise program. *Medicine and Science in Sports and Exercise, 27,* 1243–1251.

Mattes, A. L. (1990). *Flexibility: Active and assisted stretching.* Sarasota, FL: Aaron Mattes.

McArdle, W.M., Katch, F.I., & Katch, V.L. (1996). *Exercise physiology: Energy, nutrition, and human performance* (4th ed.) (pp. 603–630). Baltimore: Williams & Wilkins.

McAtee, R.E. (1993). *Facilitated stretching.* Champaign, IL: Human Kinetics.

McAuley, D., McCrum, E.E., Stott, G., Evans, A.E., Duly, E., Trinik, T.R., Sweeney, K., & Boreham, C.A.G. (1997). Physical fitness, lipids, and apolipoproteins in the Northern Ireland Health and Activity Survey. *Medicine and Science in Sports and Exercise, 29,* 1187–1191.

Menisink, G.B.M., Heerstrass, D.W., Neppelenbroek, S.E., Schuit, A.J., & Bellach, B. (1997). Intensity, duration, and frequency of physical activity and coronary risk factors. *Medicine and Science in Sports and Exercise, 29,* 1192–1198.

Murphy, M.H., & Hardman, A.E. (1998). Training effects of short and long bouts of brisk walking in sedentary women. *Medicine and Science in Sports and Exercise, 30,* 152–157.

Neiman, D.C. (1995). *Fitness and sports medicine: A health-related approach* (3rd ed.). Palo Alto, CA: Bull Publishing.

Nelson, M.E. (1998). *Strong women stay slim.* New York: Bantam Books.

O'Connor, P., Lewis, R., & Kirschner, E. (1995). Eating disorders symptoms in female college gymnasts. *Medicine and Science in Sports and Exercise, 27,* 550–555.

Rochman, S. (1997) The stress before the fracture. *Training and Conditioning, 6,* 13–21.

Rogol, A. (1996). Delayed puberty in girls and primary and secondary amenorrhea. In O. Bar-Or (ed.), *The child and adolescent athlete* (pp.304–317). London: Blackwell Scientific Publications.

Rueckert, P.A., Slane, P.R., Lillis, D.L., & Hansen. P. (1996). Hemodynamic patterns and duration of post-dynamic exercise hypotension hypertensive humans. *Medicine and Science in Sports and Exercise, 28,* 24–32.

Semenick, D. (1994). Selecting appropriate tests. In T. R. Baechle (Ed.), *Essentials of strength training and conditioning* (pp. 250–253). Champaign, IL: Human Kinetics.

Shepard, R.J. (1993). Physiologic changes over the years. In S.J. Blair (Ed.), *Resource manual for guidelines for exercise testing and prescription* (2nd ed.) (pp. 397–408). Baltimore: Williams & Wilkins.

Smith, A. (1996). The female athlete triad. *Physician and Sports Medicine, 24,* 67–86.

Talbott, S. (1996). Female athlete triad: Not just for athletes. *Journal of Strength and Conditioning, 18,* 12–16.

Terjung, R. L. (1995). Muscle adaptions to aerobic exercise. *Sports Science Exchange, 8,* 1–4.

Tran, Z.V., Weltman, A., Glass, G.V., & Mood, D.P. (1983). The effects of exercise on blood lipids and lipoprotiens: A meta-analysis. *Medicine and Science in Sports and Exercise, 15,* 393–402.

Wathan, D. (1994a). Training frequency. In T. R. Baechle (Ed.), *Essentials of strength training and conditioning* (pp. 455–458). Champaign, IL: Human Kinetics.

Wathan, D. (1994b). Periodization: Concepts and applications. In T.R. Baechle (Ed.), *Essentials of strength training and conditioning* (pp. 459–472). Champaign, IL: Human Kinetics.

Wenger, N. K. (1996). Preventive coronary interventions for women. *Medicine and Science in Sports and Exercise, 28,* 3–6.

Yessis, M. (1994). *Body shaping.* Emmaus, PA: Rodale Press.

Zernicke, R., Salem, G., Barnard, J., Woodward, J., Jr., Meduski, J.W., & Meduski, J.D. (1995). Adaptions to immature traebecular bone to exercise and augmentary dietary protein. *Medicine and Science in Sports and Exericse, 27,* 1486–1493.

CHAPTER 9

Nutrition

Leslie Bonci

Key Points

- Develop good food habits early in life (if possible).
- Eat a balanced diet that includes a variety of macro and micro nutrients.
- Make healthy nutrition a priority.
- Develop a healthy and realistic body image.
- If modifications in nutrition are needed, make them gradually and over time.
- Use dietary supplements in an informed way and for realistic reasons.
- Assess current nutritional status.
- Assess risk factors for disordered eating.
- Educate regarding a healthy, balanced diet.
- Assist in making healthy nutrition a priority.
- Address any unrealistic issues related to body image.
- Assist in improving nutritional intake.
  —Educate.
  —Motivate.
  —Encourage.
- Develop short-term and long-term goals.
- Work over time to continue to encourage healthy dietary modifications.
- Refer for nutrition counseling if needed.

Food does far more for your body than satisfy hunger. It supplies fuel for energy, protects against disease, and plays an essential role in overall health and vitality.

—Judelson & Dell, 1998, p. 146

This chapter addresses the latest research on nutrition for women, including weight management, osteoporosis prevention, and nutrition strategies for decreasing the risk of cancer and heart disease. The specific issues surrounding gender and food are explored, as well as the cultural aspects of food, and the role of women as caregivers in relationship to food. Age-specific nutrient requirements are highlighted, as well as the increased prevalence of body image disturbance and disordered eating patterns that affect women of all ages. Current research programs addressing women's health are highlighted.

THE FOOD MESSAGE GIVEN TO WOMEN

When it comes to eating, discussing diet strategies, or conversation in any weight support group, one of the most prevalent underlying themes is that a woman should nurture others, but not necessarily herself. Although women are more apt to respond favorably to public health messages and nutritional strategies to improve health, the message is processed differently, and in some cases presented differently, via media; as a result, nutrition needs are not always met. Unfortunately, too many women pursue the restrictive or denial approach to eating, thus shortchanging themselves nutritionally, as well as denying themselves the pleasurable, enjoyable, and social aspects of eating. Women are living longer, but by the time a woman starts to take care of her own body, after years of taking care of others, some of the long-term nutritional damage may have already occurred. Another point of consideration is the fact that more women are joining the work force, which can influence food preparation in the home with regard to time and food choices.

NUTRITIONAL WELLNESS AND WELL-BEING

Do women eat in a nutritionally "well" way? In a recent American Dietetic Association survey (1997), women were more apt than men to be interested in health and wellness and in following nutrition guidelines, but do not necessarily put these guidelines into practice. Many women do not have a healthy relationship with their own bodies, and food becomes an enemy or obstacle, rather than a benefit or necessity. Mothers are quick to stress the importance of breakfast for their children, or to ensure that lunch is packed or obtained in school. Wives may pack lunches for their spouses and provide a nourishing evening meal for the family, yet may think nothing of skipping meals all day and nibbling on a salad at dinner in the hopes of losing a few pounds. The deleterious effect on energy, mood, and physical well-being negates the temporary benefits of a few lost pounds of water weight.

PLANTING THE SEEDS

The ultimate goal of nutrition education should be to plant the seeds early, with a more aggressive campaign on the benefits of food for both men and women. Certain sports companies have taken this message to heart with brilliant ad campaigns aimed at encouraging young women to participate in sports. Kudos to Nike, Adidas, and Reebok for their educational programs for young women. The same approach needs to filter down to fashion magazines, television, and the movie screen. The messages need to be reinforced at very young ages. Jenny and Johnny both need to be fueled optimally. Young women should not be encouraged to "eat like a lady." Eating is a basic survival skill , and is not supposed to be a feminine trait. When young women are queried as to eating habits of their male peers, they respond with amazement and some degree of jealousy regarding the amount of food consumed and eating habits of young men. The question, "Why is it OK for him and not for me?" is frequently echoed in schools across the United States. It is not OK, it is not right, and it may be harmful in the long run for women to have such food phobia. Women also need to learn to be self-caring and self-nurturing regarding body image. Women of all ages do display such empathy to friends, but they can be so cruel to themselves, with self-disparaging remarks about their own bodies. Are self-starvation and self-loathing a nurturing response?

NUTRITIONAL BALANCE

As defined previously, balance refers to equilibrium, stability, and harmony. The word *balance* has been applied to nutrition in terms of nitrogen balance or fluid balance. More globally, many women are out of balance when it comes to eating. Calorie level may be too low or too high, or the diet may not be balanced with regards to macro nutrient intake. Stability in diet is often lacking as well. Adolescent girls are greatly influenced by peers when it comes to food acceptability and selection (Story, 1984). Women are more prone to fluctuations in eating, in part internally due to the menstrual cycle, and externally through media messages, peers, and environmental influences. Women often lack harmony when it comes to their own eating issues and nourishment. Many women do not have a harmonious or healthy relationship with food. Even in women who are making an earnest attempt to modify diet in a healthy way, the focus is more on what one should not eat, rather than on what one can.

PRIORITIZING NUTRITIONAL NEEDS

When it comes to one's own nutritional goals as compared with those of the family, the priority is everyone else first. As a result, nutritional needs may be shortchanged or forgotten. Women need to place nutritional goals on the same pedestal as work, family, and fun. Only the woman can fuel herself; no one else can assume that responsibility. To be functional, productive, healthy and energized, women need to be able to prioritize by scheduling self-nurturing time, including fueling and exercise. Attending to everyone else's needs at the dinner table, and then sitting down or standing at the kitchen sink to hurriedly eat cold food is unappealing and not a pleasurable eating experience. In the ideal world mealtimes would be pleasant, relaxing, and stress-free. Even with busy lifestyles, however, an adjustment in meals, by having a sandwich and fruit before rushing off to a soccer game or board meeting, and even ordering take-out for a later evening meal, can be less stress producing, and do more to nourish, than leaving the house on empty.

DEVELOPING A HEALTHY BODY IMAGE

The notion of an "ideal" body has invaded all ages. Young girls are confronted with Pocahontas and Ariel, slim, beautiful cartoon characters. School-age children often chastise or distance themselves from heavier peers. Preadolescent and adolescent girls are increasingly susceptible to disordered eating behaviors in the attempt to emulate a fashion model, television or movie actress, or music star. Eating disorder estimates for young women in the United States now approach 1% of the population (Fukagawa, 1992). Bulimia currently affects 4% to 10% of adolescent women. (Drewnowski, Yees, & Krahn 1988;

Fukagawa, 1992; Halmi, Falk, & Schwartz, 1981). Adult women often fall prey to these insidious messages with constant comparing and self-ridicule. The message is always on what a woman can change rather than liking herself the way she is. Children model their parents' behavior. A young woman who has grown up in the home of a dieting mother is much more likely to have a negative self-body image (Waterhouse, 1997). The positive message needs to begin at an early age. Children's television programs need to include cartoon characters in a range of shapes, sizes, and ethnicities. Boosting body image in the classroom, by encouraging discussion and productive critique of the media messages is extremely important. Daily affirmation of one's self-worth, and even a positive comment on some aspect of one's physical appearance can be tremendously worthwhile. It is also crucial that cultural differences be addressed when discussing body image. The ideal body type in one culture may be considered to be a sign of illness in another culture. The fashion model, although hardly an ideal for anyone, may send an entirely different message to an African American teen than to a Caucasian teen. Emphasis on some other aspect of self, not just the physical, whether it be academic, athletic, or professional, can enable a woman to achieve a better view of self.

Sound nutrition practices contribute to a healthy body image. A body that is well fueled will think more clearly and perform more efficiently than a body that is continuously depleted or deprived. Being empowered and enabled imply that the body must be functioning optimally. Women need to strive for and are entitled to physical well-being (through nourishment, physical activity, and good health practices); mental well-being, which includes being properly fueled for maximal cognitive functioning; and emotional well-being, through a well-established support system, as well as fostering a positive self-image and healthy body image.

ACHIEVING AND MAINTAINING A HEALTHY BODY

Nutrition is one of the few things in life over which an individual has total control. Very young children express the desire to self-feed, and very quickly manifest eating personalities. Children have an innate sense of hunger and satiety, which unfortunately is ignored with age. One of the key components of attaining a healthy physical body is to pay attention to one's internal cues when it comes to eating. Most people eat in response to external signals, such as time, smell, and visual stimuli (known as appetite), and not in response to physical hunger. Emotional triggers can be another cue to eat, and women tend to eat more in response to emotional cues, such as boredom, stress, anxiety, or grief than men. By rediscovering one's hunger cues and eating to satisfy hunger when the body is hungry, not several hours later, a women can fuel her body optimally with regard to quantity. Eating should not be a uninutrient approach. The body will function best when fueled by a variety of macro nutrients, including carbohydrate, protein, and fat, as well as the micro nutrients (vitamins and minerals).

Much has been written regarding calorie requirements for women, and many women focus solely on calories without the composition of the diet. A disease risk-reducing, health-promoting eating plan should consist of the following:

> Calories: Resting energy expenditure = 10 × weight (kg) + 6.25 × height (cm) – 5 × age (yr) – 161 (Mifflin et al., 1990)
> Carbohydrate requirements: 55% of total calories
> Protein requirements: 15% of total calories
> Fat requirements: up to 30% of total calories

Women have been bombarded with the message of consuming a low-fat or fat-free diet. Even though countries of the world that traditionally consume a low-fat diet have lower rates of certain chronic diseases than the U.S. population, it is important to look at the composition of the entire diet, which places a greater emphasis on plant foods than does the Western diet. It is not a question of substituting fat-modified foods in other countries of the world, because they consume foods that are naturally lower in fat. In the United States, the trend is toward the purchase of lower-fat foods, which are not always nutritionally dense. Fruits, vegetables, whole grains, and legumes are naturally low-fat foods, but these items are not purchased with the same degree of zeal and frequency as reduced-fat snack and dessert items, which are nutritionally void. The focus needs to be on the entire plate, with the emphasis on what people can eat, not what they should avoid. An excellent resource is the Daily Food Guide for Women, developed by the California Department of Health Services (Newman & Lee, 1991).

Eating should be a multisensory experience. Food should look appealing, smell appetizing, and taste great. Many women adopt the belief that if it tastes good, it can't be good for you, or that dieting implies a boring, devoid-of-taste meal plan. On the contrary, women who consume a more varied diet feel more satisfied, and are more adherent with regards to the dietary modifications. Eating should also include culturally appropriate foods. Most dietary guidelines, whether they are written for hypertension, hyperlipidemia, or diabetes, do not include enough traditional foods of different nationalities and geographic regions. The American Dietetic Association has released a series of culturally specific books that can serve as an excellent resource (www.eatright.org or Sales@eatright.org).

NUTRITION FOR THE LONG HAUL

Disease prevention and health promotion are not quickly attained. Lifestyle practices followed over the course of a woman's lifecycle may be somewhat predictive of outcome, with the goal being to encourage positive, realistically achievable, health-promoting behaviors. Nutrition is involved in the etiology of or as part of treatment for most of the leading causes of death in women. Many eating plans for chronic diseases or weight management demand such drastic changes in the individual's baseline diet that adherence diminishes rapidly. The weight management plan illustrates dramatic evidence that the all-or-none approach is too extreme to follow for any extended period of time, with the endpoint being weight regain. Whatever dietary modifications a woman decides to implement, whether to lower risk of breast cancer or heart disease or to lose weight, they should be modifications that she can adhere to 6 months down the road. Small, gradual changes that are manageable, not life altering, and are outcome focused will be much more effective than sweeping modifications in diet. The box "Dietary Strategies" lists examples of realistic dietary strategies.

If a woman adopts a new eating plan for health benefits, she needs to be able to see results. Cholesterol and glucose levels, blood pressure, and body weight do not change rapidly in response to dietary modifications. Other positive outcomes that are more subjective and have a quicker response will encourage a woman to stick with her new eating plan. The box "Positive Outcomes of Improved Nutritional Intake" outlines positive outcomes associated with dietary modification.

DIETARY RECOMMENDATIONS FOR SPECIFIC DISEASES

One of the most exciting aspects of nutrition and disease is the new emphasis on what **should** be included, in contrast to the former **choose-and-avoid** approach to nutrition counseling. In June 1999, the American Dietetic Association and Dietitians of Canada released a

---

Dietary Strategies

- To increase fiber, add 5 g a week—achievable through a piece of fruit or a softball-sized vegetable serving.
- To increase water, add one glass a day, working up to eight or more glasses over an 8-week period of time.
- To decrease sweets, try to cut the portion down, not eliminate!
- To decrease sodium, choose to salt food in cooking only, not at the table.
- To increase meal frequency, try to include something every 3 to 4 hours, to get the habit established.
- If evening eating is a major problem, try to include a substantial snack midafternoon.
- To cut portions at dinner, cut the usual portion in half, and then go back for seconds.

---

position paper on women's health and nutrition. For dietary modification to be effective, however, it needs to be viewed as therapy and used daily, just as a medication would be prescribed. Many people find it far easier to take a pill rather than change diet. Effects of medication are very specific to the disease process, whereas diet is more general, not only for the purpose of managing an existing disease or condition, but also for lowering the risk for other diseases as well. Nutrition is a critical component of risk reduction and disease management, and should be a cornerstone of treatment and prevention. Results of the Dietary Approaches to Stop Hypertension (DASH) study have demonstrated the benefits of dietary modification for lowering blood pressure as effectively as antihypertensive medications (Appel et al., 1997). The

---

Positive Outcomes of Improved Nutritional Intake

- Improved energy
- Better coordination
- Less anxiety or irritability
- Better sleep patterns
- Easier walking up stairs
- Better bowel habits
- Sense of accomplishment for doing something good for the body

---

DASH diet recommends a daily intake of 8 to 10 servings of fruits and vegetables and 2 or 3 servings of low-fat dairy products daily. Recommendations for hyperlipidemia include the use of soy products, anthocyanins, (in fruits and vegetables), tea, and omega-3 fatty acids (fatty fish) for the antiatherogenic and antithrombotic effect. Results of the Nurses' Health Study have suggested that decreasing *trans*-fatty acids and saturated fatty acids with unhydrogenated monounsaturated and polyunsaturated fats may be more effective at preventing heart disease than decreasing total fat intake (Hu et al., 1997). Daily inclusion of whole grains (Jacobs et al., 1998) and soy protein may improve the lipid profile (Potter et al., 1998). Newer guidelines for diabetes management focus on the individualization of the overall amount of dietary carbohydrate and fat requirements to optimize blood glucose and lipid concentrations, instead of eliminating certain foods items (American Diabetes Association, 1998). Promoting optimal bone health is now a multifaceted nutrient approach, including protein, calcium, and vitamins D and K. Decreasing sodium intake and moderating protein intake may also prevent urinary calcium losses (National Institutes of Health [NIH] Consensus Conference, 1994). The high-protein diets, which are currently quite popular, may be detrimental to bone health. Preliminary research on phytoestrogens, especially the isoflavones in soy, has demonstrated a potentially positive effect in protecting bone mineral density in postmenopausal women (Potter et al., 1998).

Dietary modifications for cancer are focusing more on lowering the risk. Earlier research, suggesting that dietary fat should be greatly decreased, has not been shown to decrease the risk of breast cancer. Newer studies, focusing on the use of phytoestrogen-containing foods, flaxseed, sulforaphanes in cruciferous vegetables, and the flavonols in tea, foster a less guilt-producing, more inclusive approach to nutritional well-being. The most protective diet is one that includes a variety of foods, not a reliance upon a multitude of supplements. The phytochemicals are best obtained from food sources, not isolated substances sold in a health food store. The guidelines set forth by the U.S. National Cancer Institute and the Canadian Cancer Institute encourage a high-fiber, moderate-fat approach to eating, with an emphasis on fruit, vegetables, and whole grains instead of the "good-bad" approach to eating (American Institute for Cancer Research, 1997).

AGE-SPECIFIC NUTRITION REQUIREMENTS

It is imperative that the positive aspects of eating be stressed at a very early age. Everyone is entitled to be well nourished. In 1999, the

American Dietetic Association released a revised position paper on dietary guidance for healthy children aged 2 to 11 years. General guidelines recommend an eating plan with 20% to 30% of calories from fat, no more than 300 mg of cholesterol daily, less than 10% of calories from saturated fat (American Academy of Pediatrics Committee on Nutrition, 1998), and a fiber intake of age plus 5 g/day (Williams, 1995). In addition, young children should be trying to increase fruit and vegetable intake to reach at last five servings per day. The Dole Company has several innovative and interactive teaching tools (www.dole5aday.com). The 1997 dietary reference intakes (DRI) for calcium recommends an intake of 1,300 mg/day for children aged 9 to 10 (Food and Nutrition Board, 1997). The messages of strong bones and healthy hearts need to be reinforced during the formative growth years. Parents function as mentors, food providers, and role models. If the message given to young children is the importance of breakfast, parents need to be eating breakfast as well. Adequate calories and macro and micro nutrients will result in optimal physical development. National surveys have documented inadequate intakes of certain key micronutrients in adolescents, including iron, calcium, zinc, magnesium, phosphorus, folate, and vitamins A, E, and B6. (Alaimo et al., 1994; Johnson et al., 1994; National Center for Health Statistics, 1983; Wright et al., 1991). Concurrent intakes of fat, total fat, saturated fat, cholesterol, and sugar remain above recommended levels. The importance of calcium, fruits and vegetables, and protein and carbohydrates should be part of the school curricula, the playing field, and the dining room table. Recently analyzed data from the Child and Adolescent Trial for Cardiovascular Health (CATCH) study has demonstrated the positive effects of diet and exercise intervention in schools (Nader, Stone, Lytle et al., 1999).

The adolescent years can be traumatic to a young woman's physical and emotional well-being. Availability and accessibility to healthy foods, as well as a source of factual and reliable nutrition information can be quite helpful. Calorie needs go down in this age group, compared with younger females. The recommended dietary allowance (RDA) for calories for young women aged 11 to 24 years is 2,200 kcal/day, compared to 2,400 kcal/day for young girls aged 7 to 10 years (National Academy of Sciences, 1989), but the overall macro nutrient and micro nutrient composition remains the same. Teens often want to experiment with different eating patterns, such as vegetarianism, and need resources to educate them with proper strategies (Story, 1984). The Vegetarian Nutrition Practice Group of the American Dietetic Association (www.eatright.org) and the Vegetarian Resource

Group are excellent resources for reliable vegetarian nutrition information (www.vrg.org). At this age, calcium needs are the highest, and the RDA for calcium increases from 800 mg/day as a young girl to 1,200 mg/day for young women aged 11 to 24 years (National Academy of Sciences, 1989). The 1994 NIH Consensus Development Conference on Optimal Calcium Intake (1994) recommended a daily calcium intake of 1,500 mg/day for young women aged 11 to 24 years. Most adolescent girls consume only two thirds of the recommended calcium intake daily (Alaimo et al., 1994). The ads of the now-famous "milk mustache" as well as an array of calcium-fortified foods, including orange juice, cereal and rice, and more palatable calcium supplements, can do a lot to boost the bone health of young women. Other issues of concern include obtaining adequate dietary iron. This can be accomplished through inclusion of fortified cereals, lean red meat or dark meat of poultry, and consuming a food high in vitamin C at meal or snacks to enhance iron absorption. Optimal folate status is critical for DNA and RNA synthesis and amino acid metabolism. Food manufacturers have started to fortify breads and cereal with folate, and orange juice is often fortified as well. The young woman who skips breakfast is most often the one with suboptimal folate levels, as the high-folate foods are often consumed at the breakfast meal.

Dieting is quite prevalent in the adolescent female population. Studies have demonstrated a dieting prevalence in this population ranging from 44% to 61% of the population (American School Health Association, 1988; Maloney, McGuire, Daniels, & Specker, 1989; Serdula et al., 1998), with fasting, diet pills, self-induced vomiting, and laxative use being the most frequently employed means of weight control (American School Health Association, 1988). According to the latest analysis of the third National Health and Nutrition Examination Survey conducted from 1988 to 1994, 11% of adolescent females were considered to be overweight (Morbidity and Mortality Weekly Report [MMWR], 1997). As young women make the transition from teen to adult, activity level typically lessens, and weight can become more of an issue. Strategies for maintaining good nutrition with a small amount of fewer calories can be helpful for weight maintenance. As a young woman approaches the childbearing years, prepregnancy dietary modifications include an increased need for folic acid to decrease the incidence of neural tube defects in the developing fetus. Pregnancy and lactation increase requirements for calories and protein (RDA) as well as calcium, iron, and, in high-risk pregnancies, other micro nutrients (Institute of Medicine, 1991; Institute of Medicine, 1990). Following the Food Guide pyramid recommendations will enable a woman to be adequately nourished during her pregnancy and through lactation. Weight goals for pregnancy should be based on the body mass index (Institute of Medicine, 1990).

Adult women tend to focus more on disease prevention and may try to modify diet in a healthy way to lower their disease risk. Currently, 35% of women aged 20 to 74 are considered to be overweight (Kuczmarski, Flegal, Campbell, & Johnson, 1994). Weight is a risk factor for many of the chronic diseases that affect women. It is critical that the dietary strategies are not so extreme, time consuming, or different from the rest of the family that adherence becomes impossible.

As a woman approaches menopause, dietary requirements start to change again in response to hormonal fluctuations. The emphasis is placed on strategies to lower the risk of heart disease and cancer and to maintain weight and bone health. The most fragile population is the older woman, in part due to physical problems and economic hardships. Dietary requirements are often not met, especially for calcium and magnesium. Energy needs decline with advancing age, but the macro and micro nutrient profile does not change. Protein requirements may not be met in the older women, and the RDA may be insufficient to achieve optimal protein nutrients (Gersovitz, Motil, Munro, et al., 1982). Fluid intake may be inadequate in older women. The recommendations are for 30 mL/kg of body weight with a minimum of 1,500 mL for small women (U.S. Department of Agriculture, 1993). Consumption of fruits and vegetables can help to prevent micro nutrient deficiencies as well as bowel regulation. Although many older women choose to take supplements, the issue of cost and high dosages of particular nutrients is a great concern. The emphasis needs to be placed on foods that supply a range of nutrients in addition to phytochemicals. The concepts of balance and variety are critical to achieving optimal nutrition. For the older adult, supermarkets are not always user-friendly, nor are they geared to the single person. Small cans, bulk produce, and asking the butcher to split meat packages are ways to cut cost and quantity. Small changes in diet are far easier and less stressful. It is not necessary to purchase special items, such as low-sodium canned vegetables, but instead to use frozen vegetables without added salt. Non-fat dry milk powder is an excellent and inexpensive way to boost protein and calcium and is very shelf stable. Recent recommendations for calcium range from 1,000 mg/day for women on hormone replacement therapy (HRT) (Food & Nutrition Board, 1997) to 1,200 mg/day (DRIs) to 1,500 mg/day for women not on HRT (NIH Consensus Development on Optimal Calcium Intakes, 1994).

Nutrition education programs targeted to older women, which include creative strategies for cooking for one and shopping tips with an emphasis on health promotion instead of dietary restriction, may be quite helpful. Table 9–1 summarizes the age-specific nutrition recommendations for women based on the Food Guide Pyramid.

THE SUPPLEMENT GAME

Nutritional supplements are big business and are continuing to grow. Many products are marketed exclusively to woman, from the Mega-Woman vitamin to Venastat for varicose veins. Some of these products may be helpful, and some may be harmful. Certain herbs must be used with caution in a woman contemplating pregnancy. An older woman taking Prozac for depression may experience an adverse reaction if she takes St. John's wort concurrently. A teenaged girl, hop-

Table 9–1 Food Guide for Young Children and Adolescents, Adult, and Older Women

Nutrient	Young Children, 2–6	Children, Teen Girls, Active Women	Less Active Women, Older
Grains	6	9–11	6
Vegetables	3	4	3
Fruit	2	3	2
Milk	2	2–3*	2–3*
Meat	2	2 (6 oz)	2 (5 oz)

*Women who are pregnant or breast-feeding, teenagers, and young adults to age 24 need three servings daily.

Sources: Data from The Food Guide Pyramid, *Home and Garden Bulletin No. 252* (HG-249), 1992, U.S. Department of Agriculture; and The Food Guide Pyramid for Young Children, (HG-252), 1999, U.S. Department of Agriculture.

ing to drop a few pounds before the prom, may choose one of the many products designated as fat burners, and experience adverse effects from the diuretic, laxative, or stimulatory nature of the ingredients. Supplements are heavily marketed to the female population, but with an emphasis on what is wrong and how the supplement can fix the problem, rather than a preventive emphasis. Eating and food are much more holistic concepts that are nurturing, sense-appealing and energy-yielding. Supplements can be an enhancement to a varied, healthy eating plan, but will not be the panacea for a suboptimal diet, nor a replacement for food. Women need to be educated about appropriate supplement use, as well as adverse effects. Health care practitioners need to be familiar with supplements, or have access to resources in order to better educate patients and consumers (FDA Web site: http://vm.cfsan.fda.gov/~dms/aems.html; NIH National Center for Complementary and Alternative Medicine Web site: http://nccam.hin.gov; NIH Office of Dietary Supplements and IBIDS Dietary Supplements Reference Database Web site: http://dietary-supplements.info.nih.gov).

LOOKING AHEAD

The Women's Health Initiative Study Group, which began recruitment in 1993, is the largest study of women's health designed to answer, among other questions, the role of diet in the treatment and prevention of heart disease, osteoporosis, and breast and colon cancer. The dietary intervention stresses a low-fat diet (20% of total calories) with at least five servings of fruits/vegetables per day and six servings of grains daily. The goals of the dietary intervention are to develop new eating patterns and assist dietary change with regard to food selection, food purchasing, food preparation, dining out, and dealing with high-risk situations (Women's Health Initiative Study Group, 1998). It is hoped that this study will be the template for future nutrition studies for women to accomplish the goals of health promotion and disease prevention in an empowering, realistic manner.

REVIEW AND DISCUSSION

See boxes "Patient Education" and "Continuing Questions/Challenges" for discussion topics for this chapter.

Patient Education

- Emphasize what you should eat rather than what you should not eat.
- Emphasize that the DASH diet is effective for lowering blood pressure.
- Decrease *trans*-fatty acid and saturated fat intake to prevent heart disease.
- Emphasize individualization of dietary carbohydrate and fat intake.
- Emphasize adequate intake of protein, calcium, and vitamins D and K to promote bone health.
- Focus on benefits of phytoestrogen-containing foods, flaxseed, sulforaphanes in cruciferous vegetables, and flavonols in tea.
- Emphasize high-fiber, moderate-fat intake.

Continuing Questions/Challenges

- How do we motivate women to develop and maintain healthy nutritional habits?
- How can we decrease the incidence of disordered eating?
- In what ways can the health care system foster healthy eating habits for all persons at all ages?

REFERENCES

Alaimo, K. et al. (1994). *Dietary intakes of vitamins, minerals and fiber of persons ages 2 months and over in the United States: Third national health and nutrition examination survey, phase I, 1988-91.* Hyattsville, MD: National Center for Health Statistics. Advance data from Vital and Health Statistics; no. 258.

American Academy of Pediatrics Committee on Nutrition. (1998). Cholesterol in children. *Pediatrics, 101,* 141–147.

American Diabetes Association. (1998). Nutritional principles for individuals with diabetes mellitus. *Diabetes Care, 21*(1 Suppl), S32–35.

American Dietetic Association. (1999). Dietary guidance for healthy children aged 2–11 year (position of the American Dietetic Association). *Journal of the American Dietetic Association, 99,* 93–101.

American Dietetic Association's Nutrition Trends Survey. (1997, August).

American Dietetic Association and Dietitians of Canada. (1999). Position of the American Dietetic Association and Dietitians of Canada: Women's health and nutrition. *Journal of the American Dietetic Association, 99,* 738–751.

American Institute for Cancer Research/World Cancer Research Fund. (1997). *Food, nutrition and the prevention of cancer: A global perspective*. Washington, DC: Author.

American School Health Association. Association for the Advancement of Health Education, Society for Public Health Education. (1988). The National Adolescent Student Health Survey. *A report on the health of America's youth*, 1–178. Oakland, CA: Third Party Publication Company.

Appel, L.J. et al. (1997). A clinical trial of the effects of dietary patterns on blood pressure. *New England Journal of Medicine, 336*, 1117–1124.

Drewnowski, A., Yee, D., & Krahn, D. (1988). Bulimia in college women. *American Journal of Psychiatry, 145*, 753–755.

Food and Nutrition Board. (1997). *Dietary reference intakes for calcium, phosphorus, magnesium, vitamin D, and fluoride*. Washington, DC: National Academy Press.

Fukagawa, N. (1992). Eating disorders: Diagnosis and management. *Seminars in Pediatric Gastroenterology and Nutrition, 3*, 1–2.

Gersovitz, M., Motil, K., Munro, H.N., et al. (1982). Human protein requirements: Assessment of the adequacy of the current recommended allowance for dietary protein in elderly men and women. *American Journal of Clinical Nutrition, 35*, 6–14.

Halmi, K., Falk, J., & Schwartz, E. (1981). Binge-eating and vomiting: A survey of a college population. *Psychological Medicine, 11*, 697–706.

Hu, F.B., et al. (1997). Dietary fat intake and the risk of coronary heart disease in women. *New England Journal of Medicine, 337*, 1491–1499.

Institute of Medicine (1991). *Nutrition during lactation*. Washington, DC: National Academy Press.

Institute of Medicine. (1990). *Nutrition during pregnancy*. Washington, DC: National Academy Press.

Jacobs, D.R., et al. (1998). Whole-grain intake may reduce the risk of ischemic heart disease in postmenopausal women: The Iowa Women's Health Study. *American Journal of Clinical Nutrition, 68*, 248–257.

Johnson, R.K., et al. (1994). Characterizing nutrient intakes of adolescents by sociodemographic factors. *Journal of Adolescent Health, 15*, 149–154.

Judelson, Dd.R., & Dell, D.L. (1998). *The women's complete wellness book*. New York: Golden Books.

Kuczmarski, R.J., Flegal, K.M., Campbell, S.M., & Johnson, C.L. (1994). Increasing prevalence of overweight among U.S. Adults: The National Health and Examination Surveys, 1960–1991. *Journal of the American Medical Association, 272*, 205–211.

Maloney, M.J., McGuire, J., Daniels, S.R., & Specker, B. (1989). Dieting behavior and eating attitudes in children. *Pediatrics, 84*, 482–489.

Mifflin, M.D., St. Jeor, S.T., Hill, L.A., Scott, B.J., Daugherty, S.A., & Koh, Y.O. (1990). A new predictive equation for resting energy expenditure in healthy individuals. *American Journal of Clinical Nutrition, 51*, 241–247.

Morbidity and Mortality Weekly Report. (1997). Update: Prevalence of overweight among children, adolescents and adults—United States, 1988–1994. *MMWR, 46*(9), 199–202.

Nader, P.R., Stone, E.J., Lytle, I.A., et al. (1999). Three year maintenance of improved diet and physical activity: The CATCH cohort. *Archives of Pediatric and Adolescent Medicine, 153*, 695–704.

National Academy of Sciences, National Research Council (1989). *Recommended dietary allowances* (10th ed.). Washington, DC: National Academy Press.

National Center for Health Statistics. (1983). *Dietary intake source data, United States 1976–80,* Vital and Health Statistics , series 11, no. 231. Hyattsville, MD: U.S. Department of Health & Human Services.

National Institutes of Health Consensus Conference. Consensus Development on Optimal Calcium Intake. (1994). Optimal calcium intake. *Journal of the American Medical Association, 272,* 1942–1948.

Newman, V., & Lee, D. (1991). Developing a daily food guide for women. *Journal of Nutrition Education, 23,* 76–82.

Potter, S.M., et al. (1998). Soy protein and isoflavones: Their effects on blood lipids and bone density in postmenopausal women. *American Journal of Clinical Nutrition, 68*(6 Suppl), 1375S–1379S.

Serdula, M.K., et al. (1998). Weight control practices of US adolescents and adults. *Annals of Internal Medicine, 119,* 667–671.

Story, M. (1984). Adolescent life-style and eating behavior. In L.K. Mahan, & J.M. Rees (Eds.), *Nutrition in adolescence* (pp. 77–103). St. Louis, MO: Mosby.

U.S. Department of Agriculture Human Nutrition Information Service. (1993). *Food facts for older adults.* Home and Garden Bulletin No. 251. Washington, DC: U.S. Government Printing Office.

Waterhouse, D. (1997). *Like mother, like daughter.* New York: Hyperion.

Williams, C.L. (1995). Importance of dietary fiber in childhood. *Journal of the American Dietetic Assocation, 95,* 1140–1146.

The Women's Health Initiative Study Group. (1998). Design of the women's health initiative clinical trial and observational study. *Controlled Clinical Trials, 19,* 61–109.

Wright, H.S., et al. (1991). The 1987–88 nationwide food consumption survey: An update on the nutrient intake of respondents. *Nutrition Today, 26,* 21–27.

APPENDIX 9–A

Internet Resources

American Dietetic Association. Ethnic and Regional Food Practices: A Series. www.eatright.org or Sales@eatright.org, or phone: (800) 877-1600 x 5000. Internet resource.

American Dietetic Association, 216 West Jackson Boulevard, Chicago, IL 60606-6995, phone 1-800-366-1655. E-mail: www.eatright.org

Dole Company Web site: http://www.dole5aday.com. Internet resource.

Food and Drug Administration's Web site: http://vm.cfsan.fda.gov/~dms/aems.html

National Institutes of Health National Center for Complementary and Alternative Medicine: http://nccam.hin.gov

National Institutes of Health Office of Dietary Supplements and IBIDS Dietary Supplements Reference Database: http://dietary-supplements.info.nih.gov

Vegetarian Resource Group/Vegetarian Journal, PO Box 1463, Baltimore MD, 21203. E-mail: www.vrg.org

CHAPTER 10

Traditional Pharmacological Approaches to Women's Wellness

Carol Patton

Key Points

Goal of pharmacotherapy is to produce maximum benefits with minimal toxicity.

Must consider individual health history, including allergies, current use of medication(s).

Must consider implications of medication for individual's partner (if she has a partner).

Must make sure patient is fully informed regarding the medication.

Must consider pharmacotherapy within the context of all other possible treatment approaches.

Health care practitioners frequently neglect the crucial step of finding out what medications a woman is taking, including over-the-counter drugs, before prescribing others.

—Boston Women's Health Book Collective, 1998, p. 569

The focus of this chapter is on pharmacological approaches to selected women's health issues. This chapter describes and discusses common issues with respect to women's well-being and selected pharmacological approaches. This chapter also describes and discusses other selected issues with respect to pharmacological choice, potential side effects, long-term implications, and efficacy of the medications.

Annually, in the United States prescriptions are written for more than 40,000 pharmaceutical products. In addition, it is reported that the consumer purchases more than 100,000 nonprescription products over the counter. There have been more than 70 new prescription medications introduced to the market over the past 2 years (Physician's Desk Reference, 1999).

Consumers of health care are now more conscientious than ever about pharmacological therapies, whether prescribed by a health care provider or are over-the-counter purchases. It is difficult to pass a newsstand and not see a leading journal article dealing with women's health and pharmacological information. Health care providers typically are confronted on a daily basis with women's preventive health care issues and are very much involved in developing treatment and health-promotion plans that involve pharmacological agents. Consumers are developing highly sophisticated knowledge with regard to over-the-counter medications as well. For these reasons, it is imperative that those health care providers interacting with women be knowledgeable and informed about the most common traditional pharmacological therapies dealing with women's health and wellness.

Pharmacology is one way the health care provider can assist women in restoring and/or maintaining health. Several factors must be considered in selecting therapies for common women's health issues. Involving the woman in the decision-making process regarding which medications to take will empower her and provide her with information necessary to facilitate safe, efficient, and effective use of pharmacotherapeutics as one part of her health promotion plan.

IMPORTANT ISSUES IN PHARMACOLOGICAL THERAPY

The ultimate goal of any pharmacotherapeutic regimen is to produce maximum benefit with minimal toxicity. Each woman is different with respect to her physiochemical body. It is important to discuss with the woman previous experience with medications, assessing her medication history with great detail and specificity. It is critical to ascertain whether or not she has had success with a particular drug line or had untoward symptoms.

Another essential area to assess is whether or not the woman has prescription coverage for medications. This is a very important factor, which will and often does limit access to the therapy due to cost. To date, there are approximately 9 million women of childbearing age in the United States who do not have any type of health insurance (U.S.

Preventive Health Services Task Force, 1996). Women are more likely to earn less and work in jobs that do not provide health care benefits. Some women have partners who work but do not have benefit coverage for the spouse or significant other. Women aged 45 and older are reported to be unemployed more often than their male counterparts, work on a part-time basis without health care benefits, or lose health care coverage if they divorce or become widowed. Elderly women comprise a majority of the long-term care facility residents because they are known to outlive their male counterparts and have a greater incidence of chronic diseases (Vela, 1996). The ability of women to pay for medications is often a critical issue in determining a health promotion plan. Some drug companies have need-based programs available to assist persons with limited or no ability to pay for essential medications, and these resources should be used to provide much-needed services to uninsured or underinsured women in need of prescription drugs.

It is critical to involve the woman in the decision-making process when selecting a medication. She may have a preference of dosing schedules or method of medication administration. The "fit" must be a good one in order to maximize adherence and integration of the therapies into her lifestyle.

Some women prefer to have a second opinion from another health care provider prior to initiation of a drug therapy. This is not something that should be perceived as negative or adversarial by the health care provider. Again, the focus of holistic care is to empower the woman to make choices that will be consistent with her values and beliefs. Some providers offer this choice of seeking a second opinion on a regular basis.

The role of the woman's partner, if she has one, is also important to consider with respect to selection of pharmacotherapeutics. It is important to ask the woman for input as to how the medications she will now be taking will affect her relationship with her partner. While women are often empowered to maximize self-care, it is important to offer the opportunity to discuss the various treatment plans with the partner. For example, antihypertensive medications can cause tiredness and affect libido. It is important to help the partner understand the implications in order to create a supportive role for him or her. Many factors limit the ability for this type of discussion and exchange in office environments today, but it is essential that this atmosphere be created in an effort to achieve holistic health care.

The consumer must be fully informed as to the importance of the therapy as well as potential implications on her lifestyle and well-being. Oftentimes the health care provider can offer sample trial therapies in order to prevent unnecessary expenditures on medications that may not be a good fit with the woman.

Clinical knowledge of the drug, including overt side effects, expected effects, the precise mechanism of action, drug elimination, and potential toxicity, is a must for all who prescribe traditional pharmacological therapies. The health care provider must have an understanding of how the drugs affect the entire body, both physically and psychologically. It is assumed that health care providers providing traditional pharmacological therapies to women have knowledge and understanding of the molecular mechanisms of drug action, clinical guidelines with respect to dosing and safe administration, use of traditional medications in preventive aspects of care, potential signs and symptoms, and actions to take in the event of an untoward outcome. The dosing pattern and frequency must be considered in order to fit into the woman's work schedule and lifestyle.

TRADITIONAL CLINICAL PHARMACOLOGICAL THERAPIES FOR SELECTED WOMEN'S HEALTH ISSUES

Osteoporosis

Incidence and Prevalence

The United States Preventive Services Task Force Report (1996) indicated that the annual cost of fractures sustained by women who have osteoporosis is approximately $8 billion a year. This figure includes both the estimated direct and indirect costs of care. It has been estimated that there are approximately 1.3 million osteoporotic-related fractures annually in the United States. Osteoporotic fractures are more likely to occur in postmenopausal women after the age of 45, and the primary sites for fractures are the proximal femur, distal forearm, and the vertebral bodies. Osteoporotic fractures occur as a result of low bone mass. There are numerous risk factors for osteoporosis that can be identified and modified. Health-promotion education, early recognition of modifiable risk factors, and pharmacological interventions can significantly improve client outcome with respect to osteoporosis.

Pathophysiology of Osteoporosis

Osteoporosis is a disorder resulting from a reduction in actual bone mass and associated structures of the bone (Kumar, Cotran, & Robbins,

1997). As a result of the decreased bone mass and structural changes, there is an increase in the fragility of the bones. In osteoporosis the bone mass per volume is decreased, leading to increased susceptibility for fracture (Brody, Larner, & Minneman, 1998).

The human bone is composed of trabecular and cortical components. The trabecular bone is also referred to as "spongy bone" or "callous bone" and is the center of the bone (Goss, 1998). The trabecular component of the bones is very sensitive to metabolic and hormonal influences and makes up approximately 20% of the skeleton. The cortical component of the bone is the outside portion of the bone and makes up about 80% of the human skeleton.

In osteoporosis there is an imbalance between bone resorption and bone formation. Bone formation occurs through a delicate balance between osteoclast activity and osteoblast production. Osteoblasts are the bone-forming cells and osteoclasts are the cells that break down and reabsorb previously formed bone. Approximately 99% of all body calcium is stored in bone (Vander, Sherman, & Luciano, 1998). Total bone mass is a very important determinant of the risk of osteoporosis (Kumar et al., 1997). The total bone mass is determined by several factors, including but not limited to, physical activity, diet, and hormone status, as well as age and gender. Men have a higher bone density than women and blacks have a higher bone density than whites. Other predictors reported to be associated with a higher incidence of osteoporosis include, but are not limited to, Caucasian women, increased age (greater than 45), women who have undergone removal of their ovaries prior to natural menopause, parity, and lactation history, as well as a history of cigarette smoking. (U.S. Preventive Health Services Task Force, 1996; Berarducci & Lengacher, 1998).

Maximum bone growth is usually achieved by epiphyseal closure, occurring at about age 17. After this time, a process of new bone tissue regeneration known as "remodeling" occurs (Goss, 1998). In osteoporosis, this remodeling process is altered.

Pharmacological Recommendations for Osteoporosis

Calcium Therapy. The usual dietary intake of calcium after the age of 50 is not sufficient to sustain adequate bone mass, requiring the addition of calcium supplements. The daily recommended dosages are 1,000 mg of calcium if the woman is currently on estrogen replacement therapy. If the woman is not on estrogen replacement, the calcium supplementation should be 1,500 mg/day, or estrogen supplementation may be added. In order for calcium absorption to occur, the woman's body must have adequate amounts of vitamin D. Women who do not eat dairy products should have daily supplementation of vitamin D 400 IU (10 µg). Any daily intake of vitamin D greater than 800 IU (20 µg) is not recommended and can actually lead to vitamin D toxicity. These larger doses have not proven beneficial in prevention or treatment of osteoporosis (Goss, 1998). Calcium does not prevent loss of estrogen-dependent bone immediately after the onset of menopause but it does affect the peak bone mass over time. It is reported that calcium potentiates the effect of estrogen and calcitonin on actual bone mass (Peters, 1998). Calcium supplements should be administered in three or four daily divided dosages and ingested with food for maximum absorption. Absorption of calcium maleate is reported to be slightly better than that of calcium carbonate (Burki, 1998).

Calcitriol. While the larger doses of vitamin D supplementation have not proved beneficial in prevention or treatment of osteoporosis and have the potential for toxicity, there has been documentation that calcitriol (1,25-hydroxyvitamin D_3) in a dose of 0.25 µg twice daily decreases the incidence of vertebral and appendicular fractures in women ages 50 to 80. Other studies reported that dosages of 0.43 to 0.8 µg/day occasionally result in hypercalcemia. Current calcitriol medications include Rocaltrol and an injectable form called Calcijex (Nurse Practitioner's Prescribing Reference, 1999).

Hormone Replacement Therapy. Estrogen replacement therapy decreases the incidence of fractures in postmenopausal women by 25% to 90%; when estrogen therapy is withdrawn, there is an increase in the loss of estrogen-dependent bone. For this reason, estrogen replacement therapy must be long-term therapy. It is preferable that women begin estrogen supplementation within the 3 to 5 years of beginning natural menopause and within 6 to 12 months following surgically induced menopause. The initial dose of estrogen replacement should be 0.625 mg/day of conjugated estrogen, 1 mg/day of 17 β-estradiol or 50 to 100 mg/day of transdermal estrogen. Estrogen replacement therapy and its relationship to osteoporosis are discussed later in the section dealing with menopause. It is important to note that estrogen is usually administered in conjunction with progesterone; therefore, the term *hormone replacement therapy* rather than *estrogen replacement therapy* better represents this form of treatment.

Calcitonin. Calcitonin is documented to be effective in inhibition of osteoclastic activity of the bone; however, calcitonin must be administered in frequent injections consisting of 50 to 100 IU on alternating days. Calcitonin supplementation has recently become available in the form of intranasal spray, with dosing consisting of one spray intranasally into alternating nostrils daily. The treatment periods for calcitonin supplementation are 2 months on and 3 months off. Potential side effects from calcitonin administration can be gastrointestinal upset and dermatological reaction. Miacalcin nasal spray is administered once each day in alternating nostrils.

Bisphosphonates. The use of bisphosphonates in osteoporosis has been demonstrated to inhibit bone turnover. Bisphosphonates directly affect bone and calcium metabolism. The bisphosphonates inhibit osteoclasts but have no documented effect on osteoblasts. Alendronate sodium (Fosamax) has been documented to inhibit bone resorption without causing osteomalacia, a defective mineralization of the bone (Kumar, 1997).

Fosamax is the first documented drug actually to reverse bone loss associated with osteoporosis in postmenopausal women. Because of its amino group's properties, Fosamax actually works by attaching to the bone. More specifically, Fosamax significantly increases bone density in the hip and vertebrae. Fosamax has also been documented to decrease the incidence of vertebral and appendicular fractures, although the long-term effects of the drug have not been documented due to its relative newness to the market. Fosamax can be administered on a continuous, ongoing basis. In women who have diagnosed osteoporosis, the dose of Fosamax is 10 mg daily. Only 1% of the drug is absorbed, and gastrointestinal side effects are common. The drug must be taken first thing in the morning upon arising, with at least 6 to 8 ounces of water, and the woman must remain in an upright position for at least 30 minutes (Physician's Desk Reference, 1999).

Selective Estrogen Receptor Modulators (SERMs). SERMs are the newest class of pharmacological therapy to be initiated in the treatment of osteoporosis. SERMs are reported to be estrogenic (act like estrogen in some tissues) and antiestrogenic (block estrogen receptors in other tissues) (Jordan, 1998). SERMs are also referred to in contemporary literature as "designer estrogens."

Two SERMs currently in use are tamoxifen and raloxifene. A 4-year study (Physician's Desk Reference, 1999) reported that tamoxifen was significant in treating women with breast cancer. This is a new area being investigated by pharmaceutical companies to develop products specifically aimed at certain estrogen receptors. Raloxifene hydrochloride (Evista) reduced the incidence of breast cancer in more than 50% of the women enrolled in osteoporosis trials (Physician's Desk Reference, 1999). Raloxifene was used to treat women with breast cancer, and a secondary finding was that the women who were treated had an actual increase in bone mass, lower low-density lipoprotein levels (LDL), and no stimulatory effect on the endometrium. Raloxifene is administered in a dose of 30 to 150 mg daily, with a usual dose of 60 mg. Evista can be taken anytime during the day, with or without food.

SERMs are still being studied clinically and appear to have promise and potential for maintaining bone integrity (Goss, 1998). Because of the relative newness of these drugs to the market, there are no conclusive studies to date about long-term effects. The short-term effects of Evista are reported to be mild and include hot flashes and leg cramps. Evista is contraindicated for women who are currently pregnant or planning pregnancy and women who have a history of blood clots in the veins, including deep vein thrombosis, pulmonary embolism, or retinal vein thrombosis. These side effects have been rarely reported but are serious potential side effects of Evista. The reporting rate of blood clots in the veins is similar to that reported for women on estrogen replacement (Peters, 1998).

Hormones and the Menstrual Cycle

In order to fully understand hormone replacement therapy (HRT), it is essential to understand the normal menstrual cycle and the fluctuating hormone levels associated with it. When a woman reaches puberty, each of her ovaries will contain approximately 300,000 ova. Each month the ovaries will increase secretion of estradiol, which is the most active form of estrogen. This increase in estradiol will facilitate the maturity of approximately 20 egg follicles. Usually, only one of the ova will fully mature and be released by the ovary in a process known as ovulation. When the follicle ruptures it will produce another hormone, progesterone. The hormone levels of estradiol and progesterone will fluctuate throughout the woman's menstrual cycle. Estrogen will steadily increase during the first 21 days of the cycle; it will reach a plateau at ovulation, and decrease during menstruation. On the other hand, progesterone levels will increase at the time of ovulation, peak after the egg is shed and decrease if pregnancy does not occur. Over time, the ovaries actually shrink and dwindle in size, leaving only a few ova at the time of menopause.

Menopause

It is reported that there are more than 40 million American women over the age of 50 (National Women's Health Resource Center, 1995). The majority of these women will experience menopause at the mean age of 51 (Realini, 1998). Menopause is a naturally occurring phenomenon. Menopause is the actual cessation of menstrual periods. Menopause can only be determined after the woman has had no menstrual period for 12 consecutive months. During menopause the woman no longer produces an egg each month and will no longer shed the endometrium in the form of a menstrual period. *Climacteric* is another term given to the period of transition from reproductive years to postreproductive years. This term can be perceived by the woman as negative and stigmatizing. The cessation of menstruation signifies the end to the childbearing years and is received in a variety of ways by women, depending on their sense of self and orientation. Others welcome the cessation of menses with delight.

In order to prepare for menopause, the woman's body begins to produce less and less of the hormones estrogen and progesterone. The ovaries can and usually do begin to produce less and less estrogen and progesterone as early as the mid- to late-30s. As a result of these changes in hormone levels there is a change in the menstrual pattern, including flow and length of menses. Perimenopause usually begins 3 to 5 years before menopause. This is a time that is signified by even more decreases in hormone levels and is usually accompanied by an increase in symptoms. The changes in hormone levels tend to cause symptoms such as hot flashes, insomnia, fatigue, headache, irritability, depression, inability to focus or concentrate, irregular eating patterns, and premenstrual syndrome. Oftentimes perimenopause is confused with menopause because of the symptoms the woman experiences.

Surgical Menopause. A hysterectomy is the surgical removal of the uterus. A total hysterectomy is the removal of the uterus and the cervix, and these women no longer have menstrual periods because of the absence of a uterus. Since the ovaries are not removed, they will continue to function and produce hormones estrogen and progesterone as in a normal cycle. Usually even one ovary can produce estrogen and progesterone. These women will most likely experience menopausal symptoms in the same fashion and at about the same time as women with an intact uterus.

Oopherectomy is the surgical removal of one or both ovaries. If both ovaries are removed, the woman will have sudden cessation of production of estrogen and progesterone and she will experience an abrupt menopause. This will occur whether or not the woman has an intact uterus. This is known as surgical menopause, and the woman may experience sudden, abrupt onset of menopausal symptoms. Without estrogen replacement therapy, these women are at increased risk for developing heart disease and osteoporosis.

Hormone Replacement Therapy

Early initiatives for HRT came from much controversy over use of estrogen therapy in treating symptoms of menopause in the 1960s (National Women's Health Resource Center, 1995). Dr. Robert A. Wilson believed that women who were on estrogen replacement therapy appeared to have less heart disease, fewer vertebral fractures, less vaginal dryness, and appeared more youthful in the postmenopausal years (National Women's Health Resource Center, 1995). Studies were then undertaken in clinical trials to study the specific effects of estrogen replacement therapy in the prevention of heart disease.

Prior to initiating HRT, it is important to rule out other potential underlying causes of the patient's symptomatology. For example, hypothyroidism can cause a person to have insomnia and hyperthyroidism can cause hot flashes. A serum sample for follicle-stimulating hormone (FSH) can be drawn for measurement of FSH level; a high level indicates that the woman is approaching or has gone through menopause. While the FSH level will be elevated and can be useful in the treatment of menopause, it does not provide any marker by which to gauge hormone replacement dosages (Realini, 1998). Often, however, the woman may experience signs and symptoms of menopause before the FSH level is elevated, indicating that it is important to treat the woman rather than the laboratory values presented on paper. Symptoms commonly reported by women are hot flashes, vaginal symptoms, abnormal bleeding, urinary symptoms, depression, and insomnia. Another key consideration with respect to ordering such diagnostic laboratory tests is whether or not this value will affect the treatment of the patient. If this value is critical to making the treatment decision then it should be ordered; however, if the woman is symptomatic the test may offer little benefit at the cost of an expensive test.

The current recommendation is that HRT should begin within the first 3 years of menopause to achieve maximum benefit. The most common HRT regimen consists of 21 to 23 days of estrogen alone and then adding progestin to the remaining 10 to 13 days of that cycle (National Women's Health Resource Center, 1995). The woman is then off the therapy for approximately 1 week, during which time she will experience uterine bleeding. This cyclical replacement therapy closely approximates what would naturally be occurring in the body in a regular menstrual cycle. It has also been reported that the woman can be taught to rotate the days she chooses to use progesterone in her cycle in order to control the times that she experiences bleeding. While bleeding on cyclical HRT is expected, there are indications for diagnostic work-up to rule out other potential problems, particularly uterine cancer. If bleeding occurs during cyclical therapy before day 10 or is heavy or prolonged, it should be explored.

Another method of HRT administration is known as the "continuous" combined hormone regimen. In continuous combined therapy women take doses of both estrogen and progesterone each day of the month. The woman may experience breakthrough bleeding when higher estrogen doses and lower doses of progestin are used (National Women's Health Resource Center, 1995). With continuous therapy, the occurrence of bleeding will be less predictable and usually subsides after 6 to 10 months (Realini, Taylor, 1998). There should be an investigation if the woman on continuous therapy continues to have heavy or prolonged bleeding after 6 to 10 months.

The method of administration for estrogen replacement, whether topical or oral or injection, is really a matter of personal preference of the woman. It is documented that there is no advantage to the woman with one particular form unless she has a documented history with absorption problems (Burki, 1998). There is also no documented difference between continuous combined regimens and sequential HRT other than the women's feelings about experiencing bleeding.

For women who have an intact uterus, administration of estrogen in combination with progestins is important to reduce the risk of endometrial neoplasia. A woman with an intact uterus should be given combination estrogen and progestin therapy because of the increased incidence of endometrial hyperplasia and potential for endometrial cancer unless contraindicated for another reason (Realini, 1998). Women who have had hysterectomies should be given continuous estrogen replacement only.

HRT has been found to decrease osteoporosis, decrease LDL, increase high-density lipoproteins (HDL), decrease cholesterol and fibrinogen, and decrease overall risk factors for cardiovascular disease. (D'Epiro, 1998, December).

Estrogens are rapidly absorbed in the gastrointestinal tract, skin, and mucous membranes. Estrogen dosing should be determined by using the smallest possible dose to relieve associated symptoms. Estrogens can be natural or synthetic. HRT usually consists of synthetic estrogens while oral contraceptives are natural estrogen derivatives (Lucas, 1998, October). In the United States, the most common form of estrogen is oral conjugated equine estrogens (CEE; Premarin). Progesterone is naturally produced in the body by the ovaries and it is the most important progestin. Progesterone is rapidly absorbed when administered by any route, is rapidly metabolized in the liver, and is not effective when administered orally (Katsung, 1997). Because natural progesterone is not effective when administered orally, synthetic forms have been developed. These synthetic progesterones are called progestins. Progestational hormones are commonly used in oral hormonal contraception. Recommended progesterone dosage for women with a uterus is medroxyprogesterone acetate (MPA) 5 to 10 mg either days 13 to 25 every month or 7 days of personal preference. Another option is to administer MPA 2.5 to 5 mg with estrogen 0.625 mg every day.

The patient usually takes estrogen for the first 21 to 25 days of the month. The recommended dose is 0.3 to 1.25 mg/day of CEE or 0.01 to 0.02 mg/day of ethinyl estradiol. The most often prescribed estrogen is 0.625 mg of CEE or its equivalent once daily. The cyclical variation would include adding progestin in the form of medroxyprogesterone acetate from 5 to 10 mg/day or its equivalent, usually on the first 10 to 14 days of the month. Patients who have only local vaginal symptoms such as vaginal dryness can use a topical preparation administered locally. It is important to keep in mind that topical administration of estrogens results in almost complete absorption into the systemic circulation, and these products need to be administered cyclically (Brody et al., 1998).

The continuous therapy consists of daily doses of estrogen (0.625 mg of CEE) plus medroxyprogesterone acetate 2.5 to 5.0 mg/day every day of the month. The cyclical regimen is currently prepackaged for cyclical therapy as Premphase and for the continuous combined as Prempro. It has been documented that other estrogen and progesterone combinations can be used, but data regarding systemic side effects are not currently available.

Health care providers must be prepared to respond to the informed consumer and her partner with respect to benefits and risks of HRT. It is clear that there is still much-needed outcome research in the area of HRT and discussion and clarity as to the risks and benefits of HRT.

The PEPI (Postmenopausal Estrogen/Progestin Interventions) trials report that there was an increased incidence of uterine cancer, particularly adenomatous or atypical endometrial hyperplasia, in women who received unopposed estrogen replacement. There was no increase in uterine cancer in women who received combination, or opposed, HRT (Cumming & Cumming, 1998). Combination therapy was the standard regimen for women who had not had a hysterectomy.

Studies are currently being conducted to explore the effects and outcomes of HRT with respect to women's health. While many of these studies are inconclusive, there are data to indicate the benefits of HRT in postmenopausal women. There have been several studies to date that explored the relationship of estrogen and lipid levels. It is documented that the use of unopposed estrogen elevates HDL cholesterol levels and more specifically the subfraction of HDL, the HDL_2 cholesterol. It is also documented that estrogen increases uptake of LDL in the liver and actually decreases the size of these molecules, making the molecules less atherosclerogenic (D'Epiro, 1998, December).

It appears that the benefits of HRT on lipid levels alone provide improved cardiac benefit, but it is also documented in the literature that estrogen also has an effect on the arterial walls. More specifically, estrogen interferes with the vascular responses to catecholamines, thereby decreasing cardiac workload with exercise and improving myocardial contractility. Based on these findings, it was reported that women should therefore receive progestin at night when myocardial demands were less and estrogen in the morning when myocardial demands increase. It is suggested that use of HRT in women could significantly reduce cardiac risk factors, particularly those associated with high lipid levels (McBride & Underbakke, 1998). Observational studies have revealed a 40% to 50% reduction in coronary events in women who were on HRT (Cumming & Cumming, 1998).

Studies are also currently underway to investigate the relationship of HRT with neuronal functioning, an area that warrants further investigation through larger clinical trials. Estrogen replacement and osteoporosis have been discussed earlier in this chapter. Many women express concern over increased risk of breast cancer with HRT. A meta-analysis was conducted in 1997 on this subject by the Collaborative Group on Hormone Factors in Breast Cancer (Lazzaro et al., 1998). This analysis did confirm the linear relationship between estrogen replacement therapy and length of time for the therapy as related to an increased incidence of breast cancer, although the risk was small. It is of importance to note that the studies included in this analysis were conducted in the 1980s, when higher dosages of estrogen were used. There is currently great interest in designing new drugs that are synthetic estrogenlike agents. These are referred to in the literature as "designer estrogens." The ultimate goal is to have a drug that provides the benefits of estrogen without increasing risk of cancer. Other potential risks of HRT include increased risk of deep vein thrombosis, pulmonary embolism, and gallbladder disease. Table 10–1 lists commonly prescribed hormone replacement products.

Depression

An estimated 23 million noninstitutionalized adults in the United States suffer from a cognitive, emotional, or behavioral disorder (U.S. Preventive Services Task Force, 1996). These statistics do not include adults who abuse alcohol and other substances. Depression is a common disorder that affects all ages across the pouplation.

In 1990, the direct costs of depression in the United States were estimated to be $30.4 billion and in 1996 this figure rose to $44 billion annu-

Table 10–1 Hormone Replacement Products Commonly Used*

Menopausal State	Hormone Replacement
Perimenopausal (with intact uterus)	Norethindrone acetate and ethinyl estradiol (Loestrin 21 1/20)
Postmenopausal (with intact uterus)	Conjugated equine estrogen 0.625 mg days 1–25 and Medroxyprogesterone acetate 5–10 mg either days 13–25 every month or 7 days of personal preference, or MPA 2.5 to 5 mg with estrogen 0.625 mg every day
Postmenopausal (without uterus)	Conjugated equine estrogen 0.625 mg daily

*While these are the most common estrogen replacements and dosages, it should be noted that there is a multiplicity of estrogen and progesterone preparations available, with new ones being developed frequently. It is the woman's personal preference, in collaboration with the health care provider, in deciding the combination of therapies and the route of administration (e.g., creams, topical patches, or oral preparations).

ally (U.S. Preventive Services Task Force, 1996). Not only is the direct care ticket for depression high, but the care which results as sequelae to undiagnosed or untreated depression renders the costs even higher. It has been documented that the suicide rate is at least 8 times greater in the depressed population than in the general population. No documented figures exist for the indirect costs measuring the oftentimes far-reaching impact of depression. *Healthy People 2000* (U.S. Department of Health and Human Services, 1992), a document that reflects objectives for disease prevention and health promotion in the United States, specifically sets forth the goal of increasing to at least 45% the proportion of people with major depressive disorders who obtain treatment (the baseline for this particular objective was 31% in 1982).

It is also clearly evident in *Healthy People 2000* that a sequela to major depressive disorders is approximately 30,000 completed suicides annually. Many persons presenting with depression symptomatology never receive treatment. From a public health and preventive health perspective, suicide is a serious potential outcome of mental disorders, including depression. In order to treat depressive disorders successfully they must be first and foremost accurately diagnosed. It is critical to more concisely and accurately diagnose and treat depression in women earlier. It is evident in the literature that women experience acute exacerbations as well as chronic episodes of depression, which require pharmacotherapeutic intervention.

Pharmacological Agents Used in Treatment of Common Depressive Disorders

For purposes of this section it is assumed that prior to the initiation of pharmacological therapy, all aspects of mental health have been assessed and addressed, including the assessment that a patient would not commit harm to self or others. When a woman is clinically depressed and all other pathologies have been ruled out, it is appropriate to introduce pharmacological treatment plans. There are several drug classifications to choose from in treatment of depressive and anxiety-related disorders.

Women have many roles that they must play on a daily basis. Often the roles conflict, creating stress that is manifested in ways such as sleep disorders, inadequate coping, frequent arguments with children and partners, and difficulties in the workplace. Common signs and symptoms often include insomnia, stomach upset, either increased or decreased appetite, feeling tired, sleeping more, low level of energy, and generally not being able to "feel happy." In an acute condition or an acute exacerbation of a chronic depressive disorder, use of pharmacotherapy can be implemented.

Prior to the development and use of benzodiazepines in the 1960s, women usually dealt with anxiety and depressive symptoms with alcohol, opiates, cigarettes, barbiturates, and sedative-hypnotics. Women still experience the same anxieties and symptoms they have always had, but now there are more effective ways to treat them clinically.

It is particularly helpful to use benzodiazepines in combination with other drug classifications in treatment of depressive disorders. Benzodiazepines are often referred to as "anxiolytics" because of their ability to reduce anxiety. These medications are very lipid soluble and are absorbed within minutes after oral administration. Intramuscular administration is often slower and less predictable than the oral route (Brody et al., 1998).

There has been much controversy among health care providers over use of the benzodiazepines in the treatment of depressive and anxiety disorders. Some providers will not prescribe them because of their potential for addiction. Close counsel with the patient and her partner helps to lay the groundwork for this concern as well as bring clarity to the treatment plan. They can know what to expect with the treatment and they can be counseled by the health care provider so that he or she will know if the patient is improving with the therapy.

Once it has been determined by the health care provider that the patient is stable, it is appropriate to begin medications that may help the person regain self-control and mobilize resources to deal with stressors. The use of short-term therapy often is enough to stabilize the patient, to help her sleep for longer periods and gain control of her situation. Usually 3 or 4 days is enough to get the patient through the crisis.

While other drug levels are being titrated to therapeutic levels, the benzodiazepines provide short-term stability and patient control. While the benzodiazepines are for short-term use, they do have an addictive potential over the long term, but data indicate that patients have a much lower tendency for abuse of these medications than was previously assumed (Brody et al.,1998). Short-term use of the benzodiazepines (4 to 8 weeks) in the event of recurrent symptomatology is also quite effective and appropriate. It is reported that these medications actually help in the prevention of a secondary disorder while the primary one is being addressed and treated. Overdose with benzodiazepines alone is rare, but danger exists when these drugs are taken in combination with alcohol and/or other central nervous system depressants. Table 10–2 lists the common forms of benzodiazepines used for the treatment of depression.

Assessing for other medications that the woman is taking is critical. This is particularly true with respect to other medications that are highly protein bound as well as the monoamine oxidase inhibitors (MAOs). In particular, the most significant drug interactions, which can be lethal, occur between MAOs and selective serotonin reuptake inhibitors (SSRIs).

MAOs interact in an adverse manner with other medications, including over-the-counter sympathomimetic medications. They also interact significantly with and potentiate the effects of alcohol, barbiturates, and narcotic analgesics. The most significant interaction with MAOs is with SSRIs. In this case, the combination can actually produce a "serotonin syndrome" which manifests in hyperthermia, shivering, myoclonus, agitation, increased aggressiveness, hypomania, tremors, nausea, and even coma (Brody et al., 1998).

Another drug classification that is successful in the treatment of depressive disorders are the SSRIs. Fluoxetine (Prozac) is the prototype SSRI. While Prozac has been useful as an antidepressant, it has also been reported to have positive treatment outcomes with anxiety disorders, including but not limited to, panic attacks and obsessive compulsive disorders as well as premenstrual syndrome.

Certain antihistamines such as diphenhydramine (Benadryl) and hydroxyzine (Atarax, Vistaril) can be used effectively to treat and help establish control in acute and chronic depressive episodes as well. These tend to be particularly helpful if taken as needed when acute exacerbations of depressive disorders occur. They are also helpful when taken in combination with certain other depressive medications and when administered at bedtime. Antihistamines can be purchased over the counter in generic form, at a relatively low cost.

Table 10–2 Benzodiazepine Drugs

Benzodiazepines Commonly Used	Daily Dose	Onset of Action
Lorazepam (Ativan)	2–6 mg	Intermediate
Diazepam (Valium)	2–60 mg	Rapid
Clonazepam (Klonopin)	1–10 mg	Intermediate
Alprazolam (Xanax)	0.25–4.0 mg	Intermediate

Preventive Prenatal Pharmacological Therapies

The area of preconception and prenatal counseling requires providing information to the woman on special supplemental needs. This is particularly true with respect to iron, folate (folic acid), and calcium supplementation. Folate or folic acid is important in DNA synthesis and in normal growth as well as protein metabolism. Iron promotes hemoglobin formation and production of energy. A folate deficiency has been associated with the increased incidence of neural tubal defects in infants. Calcium is essential in pregnancy for bone and teeth formation, blood clotting, and myocardial functioning and neuronal transmission. Calcium supplementation is recommended, at least 1,200 mg/day. Iron is recommended at 30 to 60 mg/day, and folate is recommended at 1 mg/day. The daily recommended folic acid dose during pregnancy is variable from 1 mg to 5 mg, depending on the patient's history. If there is a known reported history of neural tubal defects the dose will be higher; if there is no known history of defect the dosage is usually 1 mg/day. The actual physiological dose of folic acid is 0.4 mg/day, but most of the prenatal vitamins contain at least 1 mg of folic acid supplementation. It should also be noted that daily intake of vitamin A in excess doses during pregnancy has been linked to birth defects; therefore, pregnant women should be advised not to exceed the multivitamin dose of vitamin A (*Physicians' Desk Reference,* 1999). Some of the common prenatal vitamin supplements and their components are listed in Table 10–3.

Use of Medications during Pregnancy

There are five categories to which medications are assigned in relation to effects during pregnancy. These Food and Drug Administration (FDA) pregnancy categories assist the health care provider in identification of those medications that have known teratogenic effects on the fetus, those suspected to have teratogenic effects, medications that to date have not been demonstrated to have teratogenic effects on the fetus, and medications that have nonteratogenic effects during pregnancy. Each medication should be individually reviewed by the health care provider with respect to the pregnancy categories. Table 10–4 lists these categories.

Cardiovascular Health for Women

There are over 490,000 deaths associated with coronary heart disease each year in the United States (U.S. Preventive Health Services Task

Table 10–3 Prenatal Supplements

Common Prenatal Supplements	Dose	Content
Fero-Folic-500	1 daily	Iron (sulfate) 105 mg Folic acid 0.8 mg Vitamin C 500 mg
Zenate Advanced Formula	1 tablet daily (before breakfast)	Vitamin A 3,000 U Thiamine 1.5 mg Riboflavin 1.6 mg Niacinamide 17 mg Pyridoxine 2.2 mg Vitamin B_{12} 2.2 µg Folic acid 1 mg Vitamin C 70 mg Vitamin D 400 units Vitamin E 10 units Calcium (as carbonate) 200 mg Iron (as fumarate) 65 mg Iodine (as potassium) 175 µg Magnesium (as oxide) 100 mg Zinc (as oxide) 15 mg
Stuartnatal Plus	1 tablet daily	Vitamin A 4,000 U Thiamine 1.5 mg Riboflavin 3 mg Niacinamide 20 mg Pyridoxine 10 mg Vitamin B_{12} 12 µg Folic acid 1 mg Vitamin C 120 mg Vitamin D 400 IU Vitamin E 22 mg Calcium (as sulfate) 200 mg Iron (as fumarate) 65 mg Copper 2 mg Zinc 25 mg
Prenate Ultra	1 tablet daily	Vitamin A 2,700 U Thiamine 3 mg Riboflavin 3.4 mg Niacinamide 20 mg

continues

Table 10–3 continued

Common Prenatal Supplements	Dose	Content
		Pyroxidine 20 mg
		Vitamin B_{12} 12 μg
		Folic acid 1 mg
		Vitamin C 120 mg
		Vitamin D 400 U
		Vitamin E 30 U
		Calcium (as citrate) 200 mg
		Copper 2 mg
		Iodine 150 μg
		Iron (elemental) 90 mg (as carbonyl)
		Zinc 25 mg
		Docusate sodium 50 mg
Prenate 90	1 tablet daily	Vitamin A 4,000 U
		Thiamine 3 mg
		Riboflavin 3.4 mg
		Niacinamide 20 mg
		Pyridoxine 20 mg
		Vitamin B_{12} 12 μg
		Folic acid 1 mg
		Vitamin C 120 mg
		Vitamin D_3 400 U
		Vitamin E 30 U
		Calcium (as carbonate) 250 mg
		Copper 2 mg
Niferex-PN	1 tablet daily	Iron (elemental) 90 mg as slow-release ferrous fumarate 270 mg)
		Zinc 25 mg
		Docusate sodium 50 mg
		Vitamin A 4000 U
		Thiamine 3 mg
		Riboflavin 3 mg
		Niacinamide 10 mg
		Pyridoxine 2 mg
		Cyanocobalamine 3 μg
		Vitamin C 50 mg
		Vitamin D 400 IU

continues

Table 10–3 continued

Common Prenatal Supplements	Dose	Content
		Calcium (as carbonate) 125 mg Folic acid 1 mg Iron (polysaccharide iron complex) 60 mg Zinc (as sulfate) 18 mg
Niferex-PN Forte	1 tablet daily	Vitamin A 500 IU Thiamine 3 mg Riboflavin 3.4 mg Niacinamide 20 mg Pyridoxine 4 mg Cyanocobalamin 12 μg Vitamin C 80 mg Vitamin D 400 IU Vitamin E 30 IU Calcium(as carbonate) 250 mg Copper 2 mg Folic acid 1 mg Iodine 0.2 mg (iron polysaccharide complex) 60 mg Magnesium 10 mg Zinc (as sulfate) 25 mg
Natalins RX	1 tablet daily	Vitamin A 4,000 U Thiamine 1.5 mg Riboflavin 1.6 mg Niacin 17 mg Pantothenic acid (as calcium) 7 mg Pyridoxine 4 mg Vitamin B_{12} 2.5 μg Biotin 0.03 mg Folic acid 1 mg Vitamin C 80 mg Vitamin D 400 U Vitamin E 15 U Calcium (as carbonate) 200 mg Iron (as fumarate) 60 mg Copper (as oxide) 3 mg Magnesium (as hydroxide) 100 mg Zinc (as oxide) 25 mg

continues

Table 10–3 continued

Common Prenatal Supplements	Dose	Content
Materna	1 tablet daily	Vitamin A 5,000 U
		Thiamine 3 mg
		Riboflavin 3.4 mg
		Niacinamide 20 mg
		Pantothenic acid 10 mg
		Pyridoxine 10 mg
		Vitamin B_{12} 12 µg
		Biotin 30 µg
		Folic acid 1 mg
		Vitamin C 100 mg
		Vitamin D 400 U
		Vitamin E 30 U
		Calcium (as carbonate) 250 mg
		Iron (as fumarate) 60 mg
		Chromium 25 µg
		Copper (as oxide) 2 mg
		Iodine (as potassium) 0.15 mg
		Magnesium (as oxide) 25 mg
		Manganese 5 mg
		Molybdenum 25 µg
		Zinc (as oxide) 25 mg

Source: Data from *The Nurse Practitioner's Prescribing Reference,* © Prescribing References, Inc.

Force, 1996). The projected cost estimates of coronary heart disease were greater than $60 billion in 1995 in the United States. These estimates were based on lost income and incurred medical expenses. While these statistics are staggering, there are clearly some modifiable risk factors. Prior to menopause women typically have better cardiovascular health status than their male counterparts; however, after menopause there is an increase in cardiovascular risk factors that makes the woman at significantly increased risk for cardiovascular disorders.

After menopause, coronary heart disease becomes the leading cause of death in women (Foody & Sprecher, 1998). It is reported that a woman has a lifetime risk greater than 30% of developing coronary heart disease and that this number increases each decade over the age of 50 (Brunton & Edwards, 1998). It is also reported that 36% of

Table 10–4 FDA Pregnancy Safety Categories of Medications

Category	Safety Findings
A	Adequate studies in pregnant women have failed to show a risk to the fetus in the first trimester, and there is no evidence of risk in later trimesters.
B	Animal studies have failed to show a risk to the fetus, but there are no adequate studies in pregnant women; or animal studies have shown an adverse effect but human studies have not shown a risk to the fetus in the first trimester and there is no evidence of risk in later trimesters.
C	Animal studies have shown an adverse effect on the fetus but there are no adequate studies in humans, but the benefits may outweigh the risks; or there are no animal studies and no adequate human studies.
D	There is positive evidence of human fetal risk but the benefits may outweigh the risks.
X	Animal or human studies have shown fetal abnormalities or toxicity, and the risk outweighs the benefits.

Source: Reprinted with permisison from *The Nurse Practitioner's Prescribing Reference,* © Prescribing References, Inc.

women between the ages of 55 and 64 have increased incidence of coronary heart disease, and 55% of women over age 75 have such a risk. Females are more likely than their male counterparts to die within the first year of a myocardial infarction.

The risk for cardiovascular disease among women is primarily due to lowered estrogen levels, which affect changes in lipoprotein levels, specifically creating an increase in serum cholesterol levels and LDL levels. In turn, the HDL levels tend to fall, creating greater risk for cardiovascular disease. The decreased estrogen levels result in physiological changes in the vasculature, including an increased likelihood of clotting and fibrinolysis. The numbers of massive thrombi in a small vessel are actually smaller arteriosclerotic plaques that have ruptured or broken loose and subsequently resulted in clot formation and blockage in a major vessel.

It is estimated that estrogen replacement therapy can reduce cardiovascular risk in the menopausal woman by as much as 35 to 50% (Brunton & Edwards, 1998). One of the major modifiable cardiac risk factors is elevated blood cholesterol levels. High or elevated blood cholesterol is a serum cholesterol level greater than 240 mg/dL and is termed *hypercholesterolemia.* The normal range for cholesterol is 160 to

200 mg/dL. It is not enough to look at the total cholesterol level alone, but also to evaluate levels of HDL and LDL when considering pharmacological intervention. The higher the cholesterol and lipid levels, the greater the likelihood of an embolic event resulting in sudden death or major disability.

It does appear that women have approximately a 10-year delay in the onset of coronary heart disease when compared with their male counterparts and it is believed to be due to the protective effects of estrogen. It is also known that additional risk factors exist for persons who have a familial history of inherited lipid disorders such as hypercholestrolemia and in familial combined hyperlipidemia (U.S. Preventive Services Task Force, 1996). After menopause, the risk of cardiovascular disease increases exponentially for women as compared with their male counterparts.

Cholesterol and Lipids

With respect to LDL the first line of therapy should be diet; however, if diet alone has not resulted in lower LDL levels after 6 months, there is a clear need and indication to begin pharmacological therapy. The goal with elevated LDL is to have it be ≤100 mg/dL.

The more risk factors the woman has, the more aggressive the treatment must be. Women with evidence of coronary heart disease would need to have prompt lipoprotein analysis and require a very aggressive intervention. The desirable total cholesterol level should be less than 200 mg/dL, and the HDL should be ≥35 mg/dL. Borderline high cholesterol is 200 to 239 mg/dL and high is ≥240 mg/dL. The LDL cholesterol ideally should be <130 mg/dL. Borderline high-risk is considered 130 to 159 mg/dL and high risk is ≥160 mg/dL. These numbers alone should not be the deciding factor for pharmacological intervention, but rather there should be a holistic assessment of the woman, her lifestyle, and other significant indicators for determining intervention based on risk factor identification and analysis.

Initiation of pharmacological therapy should be based on reliable indices, including the laboratory results. Of particular importance is the need to make certain that serum samples should be fasting samples for more accurate reflection of the woman's serum levels; the lipoprotein sample for analysis should be taken 9 to 12 hours postprandially. Clinical decisions to initiate therapy should not be based on a one-time lab value but rather based on an arithmetic mean or average of two separate readings approximately 1 to 8 hours apart. If these serial values differ by greater than 30 mg/dL, a third result should be obtained and the arithmetic mean of the three readings should be used for decision making. In evaluating lipid levels, it is important to note a range rather than one exact number.

Drug therapies currently used for lowering cholesterol and lipid levels have potential side effects and can affect liver function and renal function, and have been known and reported to produce rhabdomyolysis. These medications also have the potential to interact with other medications, and careful, deliberate decisions to use them should be based on a thorough assessment of the patient for underlying pathologies that would increase the potential side effects.

Hypertension

Hypertension is defined as a systolic blood pressure ≥140 mm Hg and a diastolic blood pressure ≥90 mm Hg. It was once believed that only the diastolic was the important one in hypertension. It is now known, however, that an elevated systolic is of great concern as well because of the increased systemic vascular resistance and the increased demands on the myocardium as well as the increased likelihood of dislodging a thrombus or arterial insufficiency under increased pressure. A vessel wall with years of plaque formation under high pressure sustained over long periods of time can result in plaque rupture and clot formation in a major cardiac vessel, resulting in sudden death or major disability. The vessel may only be partially occluded, but with the plaque rupture total occlusion can result, a situation even more common when the woman also has hypertension.

Hypertension is a risk factor for a multiplicity of other pathologies, including but not limited to coronary heart disease, congestive heart failure, cerebrovascular accident, ruptured aortic aneurysm, renal dysfunction, and retinopathies (U.S. Preventive Services Task Force, 1996). It has been documented that there is less control of hypertension in the United States than previously (Cutler, Willett, & Simons-Morton, 1998). Table 10–5 provides the classification for blood pressure levels.

Hypertension is another modifiable risk factor in women's health with early detection and intervention. With respect to pharmacological interventions, there are several drug classifications that can be implemented quite successfully in the control of hypertension.

Recommended follow-up for persons with normal blood pressure is a check every 2 years. For high normal, the person should be rechecked in 1 year. With stage I (mild) it is recommended that this be confirmed in 2 months. With stage 2 (moderate) the blood pressure should be reevaluated every month, and with stage 3 (severe) the pressure should be evalu-

Table 10–5 Blood Pressure Classification

Blood Pressure Reading	Systolic (mm Hg)	Diastolic (mm HG)
Normal	< 130	< 85
High Normal	130–139	85–89
Hypertension		
Stage 1 (mild)	140–159	90–99
Stage 2 (moderate)	160–179	100–109
Stage 3 (severe)	180–209	110–119
Stage 4 (very severe)	≥ 210	≥ 120

Source: Data from *Fifth Report of the Joint Committee on Detection, Evaluation, and Treatment of High Blood Pressure Education,* NIH Publication No. 93–1088, 1993, National Heart, Lung, and Blood Institute, National Institutes of Health.

ated every week until the stable point is achieved. The goal of antihypertensive therapy is to maintain the blood pressure around 140/90, with the number modified depending on each individual patient.

The implicit underlying assumption in this chapter is that prior to initiating pharmacological therapy, the health care provider has ruled out any other underlying pathophysiological or psychological cause for the hypertension. There is still controversy in the literature as to when the individual should be treated. A holistic and comprehensive assessment should be completed prior to the initiation of any therapy.

The health care provider is challenged to find the "right fit" of medication for the woman. It is not enough to tell her to take the medication and come back for a recheck of her blood pressure in 2 months. What is clear is that, again, not one size fits all with respect to antihypertensive medications. Many of the medications alter the woman's level of functioning. It is important to keep in mind that when a woman's "set point" pressure is lowered through pharmacological therapies, the woman often anecdotally reports feeling tired, reports decreased libido and inability to concentrate. At the outset of antihypertensive therapy it is important to explain to the woman what she may experience. It is even better if her partner can be present for this discussion, as oftentimes the woman will stop taking her medication because she has had decreased libido and is experiencing difficulties in her relationship. It is important that this be a unified effort to provide the support and environment conducive to helping control the blood pressure.

The cost of antihypertensive medication varies. Many women may not have adequate insurance to cover the costs of prescription medications, which can be quite costly. When the woman is faced with the choice of feeding her family or purchasing medications, she will often forego the medication in order to provide for her family. It is often helpful if the health care provider can obtain samples from drug representatives and a trial therapy can be initiated. Some drug companies have patient programs in which the health care provider can complete an application in collaboration with the patient and free medications can be received for certain medications for a designated period of time. This is of great benefit to many women, and the health care provider should always explore this option with the pharmacy representatives. It is helpful if the woman has access to a blood pressure monitoring device and records her pressure at a given time so that the health care provider can assess patterns and trends in the readings over time. It is often not feasible, however, to ask the woman to return to the setting too frequently, creating an economic burden for her and a prime reason for her to discontinue her own therapy.

One of the challenges in treating hypertension is that it is often asymptomatic. In other words, hypertension usually does not hurt. On the other hand, if a person complains of a headache and it is known that there is a history of hypertension either in the family or for this particular patient, the health care provider must consider hypertension in this person.

One of the common errors of health care providers, however, is to initiate therapy for hypertension on a patient who does not actually need it. A person may have what is referred to as "labile hypertension," which means the pressure fluctuates and does not stay consistent. It is because of this lability that at least three readings are encouraged before a decision to treat with medications is made, unless the patient is experiencing symptoms or the blood pressure is dangerously high.

Hypertensive emergencies are cases in which the person requires immediate blood pressure reduction not necessarily to normotensive states, but to lower the pressure in order that end target organs, such as the kidneys, are not damaged. Specific examples of hypertensive emergencies include hypertensive encephalopathy, unstable angina, acute myocardial infarction, acute left ventricular failure, dissecting aortic aneurysm, eclampsia, or intracranial hemorrhage. Hypertensive urgencies would be situations in which the blood pressure must be reduced within a few hours, including stage 3, in which the systolic is ≥ 180 and the diastolic is ≥ 110 mm Hg. These would include situations such as severe perioperative hypertension, target organ complications such as renal failure, and optic disc edema.

The person should be instructed in how to accurately take and record her blood pressure over a specified time period, usually 2 to 3 weeks. Again, it should be noted that the person might need treatment if she becomes symptomatic during this time. The rationale for this is that many people experience "white coat phenomenon" and they can exhibit as much as 20 to 30 mm Hg higher in blood pressure systolically or diastolically just because they have had to come to the office to get their pressure checked. They become anxious and nervous and the result is an elevated pressure. If antihypertensive therapy is initiated on this reading alone, it will be inaccurate and once the person begins the recommended therapy she will become hypotensive and symptomatic. It is clear that serial readings are essential in identifying blood pressure patterns and trends before initiating therapy.

There are several classifications of drugs that are effective in hypertension. There have been clinical trials to study efficacy and benefit of several drug classifications. These clinical trials are ongoing and the clinical databases are ever expanding. Once again, the goal for the health care provider to keep in mind with respect to pharmacological treatment of hypertension is to choose the most effective, best-tolerated medication that is the least expensive and has a conducive dosing regimen.

The preferred therapy is to maintain blood pressure preferably less than 140/90. It is also preferred to choose monotherapy with one medication that will accomplish this goal. It should still be emphasized that there is no one best fit for all patients, and what works well for one may be completely ineffective in another. There will always be patient outliers who need to have different medication protocols and perhaps polytherapy, depending on their individual circumstances and underlying comorbid conditions or disease states.

First-line drug therapy in treatment of hypertension is usually considered to be use of a diuretic, particularly thiazide diuretics. Diuretics offer the opportunity for monotherapy, are relatively inexpensive, and most often lower the pressure enough to maintain control. The health care provider must be knowledgeable as to the type of diuretic and appropriate monitoring of laboratory values, particularly with respect to loop diuretics that are potassium depleting.

It has been documented in the literature that diuretics and β-blockers actually reduce mortality and morbidity secondary to hypertension. After diuretics, the next preferred line of drug therapy indicated in hypertension would be from β-blockers, angiotensin-converting enzyme (ACE) inhibitors, calcium channel blockers, α-blockers, and/or αβ-blockers.

If a person does not then achieve control of hypertension, the drug dosage can be titrated up to achieve control, or a second drug can be added and those dosages can be titrated upward to achieve control. If the particular drug line chosen has not resulted in control, it is then appropriate to change the drug line. It is for this reason that monotherapy and assessment of control is critical before initiating many drug lines and not being able to ascertain which one or ones need to be replaced. In this case, the patient may need a "drug holiday" and the initial therapy protocol reinstituted. The titration of drug dosages should be added in slow, gradual increments with the patient performing home monitoring and recording of pressures for determination of serial trends and patterns.

There are now on the market several combination drugs, which are combinations, for example, of ACE inhibitors and diuretics, or β-blockers and diuretics, providing choice for the provider and also enhancing likelihood of patient adherence. It is difficult to remember to take medication at different times during the day, and the more times of administration the greater there is likelihood of forgetting to take it. Combination drug therapies may be used in initial treatment of hypertension; however, the basic underlying concepts for initiation of therapy should be considered, which are to begin with the lowest possible dose and monitor with slow incremental titration upward.

The most frequently encountered side effects of tne antihypertensive medications, according to drug classification, are listed in the box "Side Effects of Various Classifications of Antihypertensive Medications."

Monitoring of blood pressure should routinely be done on the hypertensive patient every 3 to 6 months unless otherwise indicated.

Premenstrual Syndrome

Premenstrual syndrome (PMS) is the name that has been given to a phenomenon related to a group of symptoms associated with menstruation. The symptoms include, but are not limited to, cravings for food, breast tenderness, water retention, mood swings, depression, headache, and anxiety. Premenstrual symptoms may occur days prior to the onset of menstruation each month during the luteal phase of the menstrual cycle (usually 5 to 11 days before onset of menses) and subsequently resolve with end of menses (Brown, Freeman, & Ling, 1998). It is believed that PMS is associated with alterations in neuro-hormones and neurotransmitters and will vary in individual women (Brown et al., 1998).

There is currently no laboratory test with which to diagnose premenstrual syndrome; however, treatment of the woman should be based on her presenting symptomatology and clinical presentation. It is impor-

---

Side Effects of Various Classifications of Antihypertensive Medications

- Thiazide diuretics—potassium depletion
- β-Blockers—contraindicated in patients with a known history of bronchospasm; mask signs and symptoms of hypoglycemia in diabetics; increase triglycerides and decrease HDL
- α-Blockers—orthostatic hypotension, dizziness, weakness, and syncope
- ACE inhibitors—cough, rash, elevated serum potassium levels, angioedema, and renal insufficiency
- Calcium antagonists—headache, dizziness, edema (dihydropyridines), constipation, atrioventricular block, bradycardia; may exacerbate congestive heart failure
- Central α-2 agonists—sedation, dry mouth, fatigue, rebound hypertension
- Peripheral adrenergic antagonists—orthostatic hypotension, sedation, and depression
- Direct vasodilators—edema, tachycardia, positive antinuclear antibodies (hydralazine), hypertrichosis (minoxidil)

---

tant with PMS, as it is with all conditions, to elicit a thorough history and a physical exam, including a gynecological exam if the woman has not had one recently or there is an index of suspicion for other underlying pathology. It is important to ascertain the onset and duration of symptoms in order to provide holistic, comprehensive care.

It is important to assess the woman's level of functioning and how PMS symptoms are affecting her in daily activities. Many women believe that there are no helpful interventions and deal with the symptoms on a monthly basis. Many women feel hopeless with respect to the symptoms and do not ask for help unless the health care provider offers the suggestion.

There is no one best therapy for all women with regard to PMS. Again, each woman is an individual with a unique body chemistry and lifestyle, and this should be factored into any decision with regard to treatment. Pharmacological therapy usually consists of drugs from several classifications. The most frequently used medications are diuretics, nonsteroidal anti-inflammatory drugs (NSAIDs), SSRIs, anxiolytics, and oral contraceptives. These drug classifications may be utilized as monotherapy or in combination therapy.

NSAIDs inhibit synthesis of prostaglandins at the cellular level, thereby reducing inflammation and discomfort. NSAIDs should not be prescribed for a woman with a known or documented history of gastric or peptic ulcer disease. The NSAIDs help some women, but not all, to produce relief of many PMS symptoms. This is particularly true if the NSAIDs are started 3 to 5 days (sometimes as many as 7 days) prior to the onset of monthly menstruation. NSAIDS are utilized in pain control associated with PMS primarily by inhibiting prostaglandin synthesis The uterus has multiple receptor sites that are believed to affect uterine contraction. Anti-prostaglandins inhibit edema, cellular exudate, and pain at the cellular level. The NSAIDs also inhibit cyclooxygenase. Cyclooxygenase is the enzyme responsible for the conversion of arachidonic acid to prostaglandins. It should be noted that there are many NSAIDs available on the market and, once again, individualism of the patient must be stressed. For example, one patient may do very well with high-dose Motrin while another experiences gastrointestinal upset from the same dose. It is important to trial the patient with a medication to find the best individual fit and dosing. NSAIDs can range from inexpensive over-the-counter to quite costly prescriptions. These variables must be factored in when considering therapy. NSAIDs are contraindicated in persons with a known history of gastrointestinal bleeding and are contraindicated in persons who are currently on anticoagulation therapy. The box "Common Nonsteroidal Anti-inflammatory Drugs" lists commonly used NSAIDS.

Oral contraceptives have also been documented to have benefit in treatment of PMS symptoms. Particularly progesterone has been used in the treatment of PMS symptoms. It has been documented that oral contraceptives containing progesterone may provide stabilization of neurohormones, thereby resulting in decreased symptoms (Lucas, 1998). The health care provider should prescribe low-dose estrogen with progesterone or progesterone-only as therapy. It should be noted, however, that to date this therapy remains controversial and there are conflicting reports in the literature with regard to effects of estrogen on PMS symptomatology.

There have also been reports in the literature regarding clinical studies examining the effects of antidepressants such as Xanax and Prozac on PMS symptoms. It appears that Xanax offers some relief, but that cost benefit must certainly be considered; however, Xanax does have chemically addictive potential if taken over time.

Prozac has also been studied over the last 5 years as to its potential in treating PMS symptoms. Prozac use has resulted in some positive effects in treating PMS depression and associated anxiety. Successes have been reported in using Prozac in interrupted cycles for relief of PMS symptoms prior to the menstrual period, as well.

Common Nonsteroidal Anti-inflammatory Drugs

Salicylates
  Acetylsalicylic acid (Ecotrin, aspirin, Bufferin, Ascriptin)
  Salsalate (Dilsalcid, Salsitab)
  Diflunisal (Dolobid)
  Choline magnesium trisalicylate (Trilisate)

Oxicams
  Piroxicam (Feldene)

Acetic Acids
  Diclofenac potassium (Cataflam)
  Diclofenac sodium (Votaren)
  Indomethacin (Indocin)
  Tolmetin sodium (Tolectin)
  Sulindac (Clinoril)
  Etodolac (Lodine)
  Nabumetone (Relafen)

Fenamates
  Meclofenamate sodium (Meclomen)
  Mefenamic acid (Ponstel)

Proprionic Acids
  Ibuprofen (Advil, Nuprin, Rufen, Advil, Motrin, Motrin IB)
  Fenoprofen calcium (Nalfon)
  Naproxen sodium (Aleve, Anaprox, Naprelan)
  Oxaprozin (Daypro)
  Flurbiprofen (Ansaid)
  Ketoprofen (Actron, Orudis, Orudis KT, Oruvail)
  Naproxen (Anaprox)

Source: Data from *The Nurse Practitioner's Prescribing Reference,* © Prescribing References, Inc.

The ultimate role of the health care provider with respect to PMS is to treat each woman as an individual from a holistic perspective. Only that individual can describe and relate her symptomatology. It is critical to listen to and recognize the myriad of symptoms that can result from PMS and to trial therapeutic pharmacological modalities to find the best fit for the individual.

Pain Management in Women's Health

There are several pharmacological therapies available to the health care provider with respect to management of pain. It is important to determine whether or not this is an acute versus chronic pain prior to initiation of drug therapy. It is also crucial to rule out any other underlying comorbid conditions that may be causing or in some cases exacerbating the painful condition. Another important consideration with respect to pain medications is that there are now many different preparations and forms of pain medications, including topical creams or lotions as well as oral preparations.

Pain, whether acute or chronic in nature, can interfere with the very essence of one's being. It interferes with sense of self and relationships as well as ability to carry out activities of daily living. In these cases it is important to begin therapies that are well tolerated, efficacious, and have the least side effects at the least expense to the woman. Another important factor to consider is the degree of pain the woman is experiencing. This emphasizes the need for the health care provider to become comfortable with an operational definition of pain. Pain is quantifiable only by the person experiencing it; personal and professional judgments of the health care provider can result in inadequate doses of pain medications to effect adequate pain control. Anecdotally, pain is the main reason patients present to primary care practices and emergency departments. In other words, when something hurts enough, the person seeks care.

Common first-line pain medications may be acetominophen (Tylenol) over the counter. There are many strengths for Tylenol and there are very few side effects from Tylenol if the person has no underlying medical condition. It has recently been noted, however, that harm can come to the liver if the person has more than two alcoholic drinks per day and takes Tylenol.

Aspirin and aspirin-containing products have been a good first-line drug therapy in the treatment of pain for quite some time. There are numerous preparations available for pain control when taken for a short while; however, caution should certainly be exercised in use of aspirin and aspirin-containing products with flu-like symptoms and also if the person is on anticoagulation therapy. In some special circumstances the physician may order aspirin daily in addition to anticoagulation therapy. Aspirin has also been documented to erode the stomach lining and cause gastritis. Aspirin or salycilate overdose is a serious threat to a patient and this is particularly a concern for women who may be on fixed incomes and taking large quantities of aspirin for pain control.

Corticosteroids is another classification of medications which act in a natural way in the body to decrease inflammation in cases where often other medication modalities have not proven beneficial or effective. A short course such as 40 mg/day of oral prednisone can be quite effective in decreasing inflammation and discomfort. It is essential to educate the woman about the potential drug interactions while taking prednisone and that it must be taken with food. In some instances it can be caustic to the gastric surface. Two other key factors to keep in mind with administration of oral steroids is that long-term use can affect bone integrity and that it can mask signs and symptoms of underlying infectious processes that may be occurring simultaneously in the body.

The nonsterioidal anti-inflammatories (NSAIDs) are a drug classification that inhibits prostaglandin synthesis and decreases edema and release of endotoxins at the cellular level. NSAIDs work locally at the site of the inflammation and should be administered regularly during an acute episodic event or an exacerbation of a chronic event. High dose NSAIDs taken regularly for three days will usually help decrease local inflammation and get the pain under control. Long term use of NSAIDs has been linked to the formation of stomach ulcerations and gastritis associated with gastrointestinal bleeds over time. Patients must be cautioned on dosing regimens and length of the therapy as well the potential side effects when taking these medications. Patients taking the NSAIDs must be properly educated in their use and potential side effects. If patients do not understand how the drug works, they are more likely to take it only when they experience the pain event as opposed to taking it regularly over the short run to lessen local inflammation. Women experiencing arthritis pain can benefit tremendously with NSAIDs because the arthritis and associated disorders cause production and release of prostaglandins from the cell membrane. The NSAIDs inhibit this release when given in regular maintenance dosages.

Narcotic analgesics are another classification of drugs that can be used to control acute episodic pain or an acute exacerbation of chronic pain. Some of these preparations are opioid analgesics and others are combination opioids and salycilates. These medications are often useful in combination therapy with the NSAIDs.

It is important that the health care provider provide the woman with the medications that will deal with the problem and educate her accordingly. In some cases, it is important to include the significant other in the treatment plan because he or she too needs to understand the importance of pain control and its implications. Society is often judgmental, as can be health care providers when patients truly require narcotic analgesics. The literature is reflective of concerns with use of narcotic analgesics; however, there is abundant evidence in the literature to support appropriate drug selection in managing both acute and chronic pain events. The health care provider must be knowledgeable of the acceptable dosages and implications for the narcotic analgesics either as monotherapy or in combination therapies. It is essential to educate the woman and her significant other as to the effects of the medication, the dosing regimens, and the safety issues that may arise as a result of the medication regimen. This is particularly true when pain medications are prescribed for the elderly female.

REVIEW AND DISCUSSION

See boxes "Patient Education" and "Continuing Questions/Challenges" for discussion topics for this chapter.

Patient Education

Patients must be informed about medication, including
- Medication's mechanism of action
- Medication's side effects
- Method of elimination of medication
- Potential toxicity of medication
- How medication interacts with other drugs/therapies

Continuing Questions/Challenges

How can health care providers be sure that the patient is disclosing all medications/treatments currently being taken (to prevent any untoward interactions)?
What issues arise with the use of "experimental drugs?"

REFERENCES

Berarducci, A., & Lengacher, C.A. (1998). Osteoporosis in perimenopausal women. *American Journal for Nurse Practitioners, 2*(9), 9–14.

Boston Women's Health Book Collective. (1998). *Our bodies, ourselves for the new century.* New York: Touchstone.

Brody, T.M., Larner, J.L., & Minneman, K.P. (1998). *Human pharmacology: Molecular to clinical.* St. Louis, MO: Mosby.

Brown, C.S., Freeman, E.W., & Ling, F.W. (1998). An update on the treatment of premenstrual syndrome. *American Journal of Managed Care, 4*(2), 266–274, 277–278.

Brunton, A.B., & Edwards, R.K. (1998). Hypertension. In R.B.Taylor (Ed.), *Family medicine: Principles and practice* (pp. 640–649). New York: Springer-Verlag.

Burki, R.E. (1998, February). Keeping pace with osteoporosis. *Clinical Advisor,* 22–29.

Cumming, D.C., & Cumming, C.E. (1998). Hormone replacement therapy: should your patient do with—or without—it? *Consultant, 38*(10), 2417–2432.

Cutler, J.A., Willett, W., & Simons-Morton, D.G. (1998, May). Preventing hypertension: a new urgency. *Patient Care Nurse Practitioner,* 38–46.

D'Epiro, N.W. (1998, December). HRT: new data, continuing controversies. *Patient Care Nurse Practitioner,* 18–34.

Foody, J., & Sprecher, D. (1998, June). Current concepts in preventive cardiology. *The Clinical Advisor,* 56–62.

Goss, G.L. (1998). Osteoporosis in women. *Nursing Clinics of North America, 3*(4), 573–578.

Jordan, V.C. (1998, October). Designer estrogens. *Scientific American,* 60–67.

Katsung, B.G. (1997). *Basic and clinical pharmacology.* Norwalk, CT: McGraw Hill.

Kumar, V., Cotran, R.S., & Robbins, S.L. (1997). *Basic pathology.* Philadelphia: W.B. Saunders Company.

Lazzaro, M., Mizell, V., Thompson, M., & Weber, D. (1998). Chemoprevention trends in breast cancer. *Advance for Nurse Practitioners, 6*(11), 26–74.

Lucas, B.D. (1998, October). A practical update of contraceptive options. *Patient Care,* 63–92.

McBride, P.E., & Underbakke, G. (1998). Dyslipidemias. In R.B. Taylor (Ed.), *Family medicine: Principles and practice* (pp. 1056–1063). New York: Springer-Verlag.

National Women's Health Resource Center. (1995, July/August). *The menopause and hormone therapy.*

Nurse Practitioner's Prescribing Reference. (1999, Fall). *Clinical Management of Dyslipidemia.* New York: Prescribing References, Inc.

Peters, S. (1998). Menopause: A new era. *Advance for Nurse Practitioners, 6*(7), 61–64.

Physician's Desk Reference. (1999). 53rd Edition. Montvale, NJ: Medical Economics Co.

Realini, J.P. (1998). Menopause. In R.B. Taylor (Ed.), *Family medicine: Principles and practice* (pp. 909–915). New York: Springer-Verlag.

U.S. Department of Health & Human Services. (1992). *Healthy people 2000: Summary report.* Sudbury, MA: Author.

U.S. Preventive Health Services Task Force. (1996). *Guide to clinical preventive services* (2nd ed.). Baltimore: Williams & Wilkins.

Vander, A., Sherman, J., & Luciano, D. (1998). *Human physiology: The mechanisms of body function.* Boston: McGraw-Hill.

Vela, S.B. (1996). Hyperlipidemia. In R. Rubin (Ed.), *Medicine: A primary care approach* (pp. 295–298). Philadelphia: W.B. Saunders Company.

CHAPTER 11

Herbal Remedies for Women's Wellness

Natalie Pavlovich

Key Points

Herbal remedies are made from various components of plants:

Roots	Flowers
Leaves	Seeds
Stems	Fruit
Bark	

Each herbal remedy has a specific effect on an organ or system of the body. Herbs come in various forms:

Tinctures	Fresh
Tablets	Dried
Extracts	

Classification system for assessment of safety developed by the American Herbal Products Association (AHPA):

Class 1: Safe when used appropriately.

Class 2: Specific restrictions noted (external use only; not to be used during pregnancy; not to be used during lactation; other specific restriction [such as not to be taken with other drugs, foods]).

Class 3: To be used under the supervision of an expert qualified in appropriate use of herbs.

Class 4: Insufficient data exist for correct classification.

What is a medicinal herb? Simply, any plant whose seeds, berries, roots, leaves, bark or flowers are used for medicinal purposes.

—Loecher & O'Donnell, 1997

Herbal therapy is one of the world's oldest complementary modalities. Traditionally herbs have been used as medicine throughout human existence, beginning with the Stone Age, continuing during Egyptian, Grecian, and Roman civilizations, extending through the Middle Ages, and entering modern-day civilization. Throughout the ages, herbs usually became associated with folk healers in the various cultural groups. Specific herbs (also known as "home remedies") have been effective in helping individuals with specific problems. More than 75% of the world population uses herbal medicines as a major form of therapy for ailments (Spencer & Jacobs, 1999). In America today, the rediscovery of the healing power of plants is apparent (Natural Pharmacy, 1998; Brevoort, 1998; Greenwalk, 1998; Emerich, 1999).

GENERAL USE OF HERBS

Although herbal remedies are usually taken for a specific condition or symptom, the herbs generally support and aid the whole body. Each herbal remedy has a specific effect on the different organs and systems in the body. The symptoms experienced by an individual are viewed as signs of distress or adjustment within the body. In herbology, the remedy aims to eliminate the causative factor of the problem; in so doing, the distressing symptoms then begin to diminish.

The various components of the plant, including the root, leaves, stem, bark, flowers, seeds, or fruit, are used in the preparation of herbal remedies. Recently the World Health Organization (WHO) published the first set of 25 monographs, which included 13 herbs prepared from the plant roots. Some of the best-known herbs are actually roots. These herbs are listed in Table 11–1.

Herbs come in various forms, including tinctures, tablets, or extracts. Gardner (1999) recommended that herbal tinctures be used whenever possible, rather than dried or capsulated ones. Herbal tinctures are liquid preparations made by steeping a dried herb in vinegar, glycerin, or alcohol. This tincture may be taken straight, in juice or as a tea. Dried herbs, which are only about 20% water, are more potent

Table 11–1 Summary of Herbs Made from Plants That Are Roots

Common Name	Botanical Name
Asian ginseng	Panax ginseng
Astragalus	Astragalus membranaceus
Bulpleurum	Bupleurum falcatum
Garlic	Allium sativum
Ginger	Zingiber officinale
Goldthread	Coptis supp.
Indian snakeroot	Rauvolfia serpentina
Licorice	Glycyrrhiza supp.
Onion	Allium cepa
Platycodon/balloonflower	Platycodon grandiflorum
Rhubarb root	Rheum supp.
Turmeric	Curcuma longa
Valerian	Valeriana officinalis

Source: Adapted with permission from M. Blumenthal, The Roots of Herbal Medicine, *Natural Pharmacy*, Vol. 3, No. 2, pp. 16–19, © 1999, Mary Ann Liebert, Inc.

and more concentrated than fresh herbs, which are the least concentrated, consisting of about 80% water. Fresh herbs are usually made into a tea or sprinkled on foods. Dried herbs, also, are frequently used as a tea or mixed in foods. Dried herbs have a longer shelf life than the fresh herbs. The herbal extract is a liquid or dry concentrated form of the natural plant, usually taken as a liquid, capsule or tablet (Dickstein, 1999).

To address any issues or questions about the safety of herbs, the American Herbal Products Association (AHPA) has established a classification system. These categories are listed in the box "Safety Classification of Herbs."

COMMON HERBAL REMEDIES FOR SPECIFIC WOMEN'S HEALTH CONDITIONS

There are several commonly used herbal remedies for women's conditions. The next section of this chapter describes briefly certain common hormonal and/or reproductive health conditions experienced by most women, with suggestions for herbal remedies for these conditions. These include cystitis, cysts and fibroids, endometriosis, menstrual difficulties and irregularities, premenstrual syndrome, vaginitis,

---

Safety Classification of Herbs

Class 1—Herbs can be taken safely when used appropriately.

Class 2—Herbs to be used with specific restrictions for one of four reasons:
1. for external use only
2. not to be used during pregnancy
3. not to be used while breast-feeding
4. other specific use restrictions as noted, such as not to be taken with specific drugs or ailments

Class 3—Herbs for which significant data exist to recommend the following labeling: "To be used only under the supervision of an expert qualified in the appropriate use of this substance." The labeling must include information related to proper use, dosage, contraindications, potential adverse effects and drug interactions, and any other relevant information related to the safe use of this substance.

Class 4—Herbs for which insufficient data are available for classification.

Source: Data from *Natural Pharmacy,* Vol. 2, No. 12, pp. 20–21, © 1998, Liebert Publishing Group, Inc.

---

infertility, pregnancy, childbirth, breast-feeding, menopause, hormone replacement therapy, and depression. In the last section of this chapter, suggested herbal remedies for additional symptoms and conditions common to women that are beyond the category of reproductive health are described.

Each condition or symptom is described briefly. The common herbal alternatives to allopathic drugs for the particular symptom or condition are identified and discussed. For each herb mentioned, the common name and the botanical name, which consists of at least two names, with the first representing the genus and the second the species, are included (Blumenthal, 1998). This herbal identification then is followed by a brief description of the herb's properties and actions, including possible adverse reactions.

Cystitis

Cystitis, a bacterial bladder infection that may be acute or chronic, is a common occurrence among 10% to 20% of women (Murray & Pizzorno, 1998). Cystitis is more common in women because they have a shorter urine passage (urethra) which transports the urine from the bladder than do men. Acute cystitis occurs with a sudden onset and is associated with typical symptoms that include painful burning urination; increased urinary frequency, especially at night; a feeling that the bladder still needs to be emptied after the woman has tried to urinate; lower abdominal pain; and a strong, cloudy, foul-smelling or dark urine (Murray & Pizzorno, 1998).

Cranberry (*Vaccinium macrocarpon* or *Vaccinium oxycoccos*), goldenseal (*Hydrastis canadensis*), and **uva ursi** (*Arctostaphylos*) comprise the three major herbal remedies for cystitis. Cranberry, in particular, has been known to inhibit the growth of bacteria in the bladder and urinary tract (Challem & Berkson, 1999; Elias & Masline, 1995; Mindell & Colman, 1992). Cranberry is often taken as juice. **Goldenseal** is helpful in the treatment of bladder infections, due to its antimicrobial properties, but it is not recommended during pregnancy. Also, the fresh plant of goldenseal can cause itching or a skin rash in a sensitive individual (Keville, 1996; Murray & Pizzorno, 1998). Uva ursi, also known as bearberry or upland cranberry, is most useful in the treatment of urinary tract infections as it contains an antiseptic component that is effective against *Escherichia coli*. Uva ursi promotes urination due to its diuretic property (Murray & Pizzorno, 1998). This remedy is not tolerated well over an extended period of time because it irritates the stomach. Also, it is not recommended for pregnant women (Murray & Pizzorno, 1998).

Additional herbs are also recommended for alleviating the symptoms of cystitis. **Celery** (*Apisum graveolens*) is considered an excellent natural diuretic that promotes the flow of urine through the kidneys. It is important to note that celery juice should not be used during pregnancy because it contains a strong abortive property, stimulating uterine contractions (Mindell & Colman, 1992). **Gotu kola** (*Centella asiatica*), also known as sheep rot, Indian pennywort, water pennywort, and marsh pennywort, is effective in helping to eliminate chronic interstitial cystitis due to its diuretic action. It also acts as a circulatory and tissue toner (Mindell & Colman, 1992). This remedy should not be taken in combination with Ginger. Gotu kola also may aggravate itching. If large doses are taken over a period of time, it may cause headaches or unconsciousness (Mindell & Colman, 1992). **Juniper berry** (*Juniperus communis*) is famous for its effectiveness in relieving urinary tract problems, including urinary retention. Women should avoid the use of juniper berries during pregnancy because it can stimulate the uterus, causing abortion. Also, it is recommended that this herb not be taken for more than 6 consecutive weeks at a time (Mindell & Colman, 1992). **Licorice** (*Glycyrrhiza glabra*) has a soothing effect on bladder ailments as well as related kidney ailments. Women with edema, high blood pressure, slow heart rate, or who are pregnant are advised not to use this remedy (Mindell and Colman, 1992).

Some women develop chronic interstitial cystitis, which is a persistent form of bladder irritation not due to an infection. The two significant herbal remedies for this condition are gotu kola, described above, and **horsetail** (*Equisetum arvense*). This herb is also known as bottlebrush and shave grass, and is a well-known genitourinary astringent for chronic interstitial cystitis.

Cysts and Fibroids

Fibrocystic Breast Disease

Fibrocystic breast disease (FBD) occurs in approximately one third of women living in the United States who are of reproductive age, whereas this condition is not as prevalent among European women (Keville, 1996). Women often experience pain and swelling of the breasts shortly before their menstruation. **Evening primrose oil** (*Oenothera biennis*), in capsule form, is often used to treat symptoms of breast tenderness (Mindell & Colman, 1992). It is recommended that this herb be taken with vitamin E. Vitamin E has the ability to detoxify and to increase circulation, thus encouraging the cysts to drain and help the blood and lymph system to carry excess fluids away from the cysts (Keville, 1996). **Prickly ash bark** (*Xanthoxylum americanum*) is recommended for severe cases of FBD. Its primary action is to increase the blood circulation and improve lymph drainage (Keville, 1996). Keville (1996) recommends additional herbs to assist with encouraging lymph drainage. **Burdock root** (*Arctium lappa*) is recommended for its action on lymphatic congestion, and it also acts as a blood purifier. **Calendula** (*Calendula officinalis*), often known as marigold, is also helpful in reducing inflamed lymph nodes. This remedy is not recommended for pregnant women or for women with heavy menstrual flow. **Cleavers** (*Galium aparine*) is useful when cystic growths are apparent. **Dandelion root** (*Taraxacum officinale*) acts as an effective and safe medicinal remedy that also serves as a blood cleaner. **Mullein** (*Verbascum thapsus*) is known for its use in lymphatic congestion. It is important to note that the fresh plant of this remedy can cause itching or a skin rash in a sensitive individual (Keville, 1996; Murray and Pizzorno, 1998).

Ovarian Cysts

The cysts that develop on the ovary are usually filled sacs that may become enlarged, causing pressure on nearby organs. As a result, the woman experiences painful or impaired circulation. The herbal remedies recommended for ovarian cysts are the same as for FBD (Keville, 1996).

Uterine Fibroids

Fibroids are nonmalignant tumors that develop within the uterine wall and are common in women. The symptoms vary depending on the location of the fibroids in the uterus. For instance, if the fibroids put pressure on the bladder region, women will experience frequency of urination. If the tumors exert pressure on the endometrium, women may experience menorrhagia and dysmenorrhea. If these uterine fibroids are discovered early, herbal therapy has been found to be effective (Marti & Hine, 1998).

The three herbs strongly recommended for fibroids are **chaste berry** (*Vitex agnus-castus*), **raspberry leaf** (*Rubus idaeus*), and **wild yam root** (*Dioscorea villosa*). Chaste berry is well known for regulating female hormonal action and is effective in reducing symptoms of dysmenorrhea (Herbal Research Publications, 1995). Raspberry leaf works as a uterine tonic. It is important to note, however, that if taken with allopathic drugs, raspberry leaf reduces the absorption ability of the drugs (Hardy, 1998). Wild yam root has antispasmodic effects and is therefore useful in relieving dysmenorrhea and ovarian or uterine pain (Herbal Research Publications, 1995; Keville, 1996).

Endometriosis

As with FBD, endometriosis is less common among European women than among women in the United States. Endometriosis occurs in approximately 10% to 25% of women living in the United States who are of reproductive age (Keville, 1996; Pillitteri, 1995; Youngkin & Davis, 1994). In endometriosis, tissue from the lining of the uterus attaches itself outside the endometrial cavity. Endometriosis may produce discomfort, although the severity of symptoms does not always correlate with severity of the endometriosis. Some of the symptoms include dysmenorrhea, menorrhagia, sensation of heaviness in the pelvic area, low back and low abdominal pain, flatulence, and constipation, sometimes accompanied by depression and insomnia.

Although herbal remedies have helped women with endometriosis, this approach can often take several months to be effective. **Burdock**

(*Arctium lappa*), **chaste berry** (*Vitex agnus castus*), and **milk thistle** (*Silybum marianum*) are recommended for endometriosis. Burdock is recommended in combination with chaste berry, assisting the liver to clear estrogen from the body (Keville, 1996). Chaste berry assists in decreasing the overabundance of estrogen, a major factor contributing to endometriosis. Milk thistle, also known as Mary thistle and wild artichoke, is a liver tonic, which is important, as the liver is essential in excretion of waste from the body. This remedy is useful in clearing the liver of toxins. The active ingredient is silymarin, a unique type of flavonoid with antioxidant ability (Elias & Masline, 1995; Gottlieb, 1995; Keville, 1996).

Women with endometriosis often experience cramping, inflammation, bleeding, and pain. Two remedies recommended for these major symptoms are **cramp bark** (*Viburnum opulus*) and **wild yam root** (*Dioscorea villosa*) (Dale, 1997). Dale (1997) recommended that wild yam root be applied topically and mixed with natural progesterone.

Evening primrose oil (*Oenothera biennis*) and **ginger** (*Zingiber officinale*) are helpful in relieving cramping and other related menstrual pain (Keville, 1996). Evening primrose oil, also known as sundrops, contains high levels of γ-linolenic acid (GLA). Once GLA enters the body it is converted into prostaglandins, which are fatty acids that produce effects on the body. These effects include causing inflammation (Keville, 1996, p. 35) as a result of trauma, wounds, or surgery (Keville, 1996, p. 46); cramping pain of dysmenorrhea (Copstead & Banasik, 2000, p. 764; Keville, 1996, p. 171); and increasing hyperactivity (Keville, 1996, p. 230). This herb is effective in alleviating many symptoms, including inflammatory conditions and bloating (Elias & Masline, 1995). In particular, it has antispasmodic qualities that are helpful in relieving menstrual pain (Elias & Masline, 1995).

Horsetail (*Equisetum arvense*) and **red raspberry** (*Rubus idaeus*) are helpful in controlling uterine bleeding (Elias & Masline, 1995). Horsetail is also known as bottlebrush, shave grass, scouring rush, and pewterwort. Red raspberry is a uterine tonic that helps to reduce bleeding as well as to strengthen the uterus (Elias & Masline, 1995).

Echinacea (*Echinacea angustifolia, Echinacea pallida, Echinacea purpurea*), **motherwort** (*Leonurus cardiaca*), **nettles** (*Urtica dioica*), and **passion flower** (*Passiflora incarnata*) are suggested for relief of uterine cramping. Echinacea, also known as purple coneflower, strengthens the immune system (Keville, 1996) and repairs connective tissues and fibers. (Gottlieb, 1995). A recent survey indicated that at least 7% of Americans have used this remedy (Dickstein, 1999). Echinacea should not be used for more than 8 weeks to treat systemic diseases or by individuals with autoimmune disorders (Toscano, 1998). Motherwort is helpful in relaxing the uterine muscle and, with consistent use for at least 3 to 4 months, the amount of bleeding begins to decrease with a concurrent noticeable decrease in cramping (Gottlieb, 1995). The fresh plant of motherwort can cause itching or a skin rash in a sensitive individual (Keville, 1996; Murray & Pizzorno, 1998). Nettles, also referred to as stinging nettle, contains calcium, chlorophyll, iodine, iron, magnesium, potassium, silicon, sodium, sulfur, tannin, and vitamins A and C, which are helpful in alleviating the condition of endometriosis (Keville, 1996). Passion flower has an antispasmodic effect that assists in relaxing smooth muscle (Keville, 1996).

Menstrual Difficulties/Irregularities

Women experience a variety of menstrual difficulties, including menstrual cramps (dysmernorrhea), irregular periods, scanty periods, or abnormal menstrual bleeding. Amenorrhea is an absence of flow when it is normally expected. Menorrhagia is excessive loss of blood. Metrorrhagia is loss of blood between periods, also known commonly as "spotting." Oligomenorrhea is scanty and less frequent menstrual flow. The various herbal remedies for these menstrual conditions are described in this chapter.

For overall menstrual difficulties and irregularities, six common remedies are considered to be helpful. **Black cohosh** (*Cimicifuga racemosa*) should be avoided in lactating women and which may cause an upset stomach (Foster, 1996). **Blue cohosh** (*Caulophyllum thalictroides*) (Foster, 1996) can cause itching or a skin rash in a sensitive person (Keville, 1996; Murray & Pizzorno, 1998). **Chaste berry** (*Vitex agnus-castus*) should be avoided by a woman who is breast-feeding (Foster, 1996). **Dong quai** (*Angelica sinensis, Angelica polymorpha, Angelica dahurica,* or *Angelica atropurpurea*) helps because of its vasodilatory and antispasmodic effects as well as combating other menopausal symptoms including vaginal dryness. Dong quai should not be used in pregnant women because it stimulates labor (Keville, 1996). Lactating women should avoid this remedy. Also, this herb has a demonstrated potential drug interaction with blood-thinning agents (Keville, 1996). **Motherwort** (*Leonurus cardiaca*) is used for all menstrual difficulties, especially for abdominal spasms. Although it is known that the herb affects the uterus, Foster (1996) claims that there have been no toxicity studies reported. However, Keville (1996) stated that the motherwort from a fresh plant can cause itching or a skin rash in a sensitive individual (Murray & Pizzorno, 1998). **Parsley** (*Petroselinum crispum, Petroselinum sativum*) is effective in alleviating painful menstruation as well as for producing diuresis. Also, it may induce menstruation (Foster, 1996; Mindell & Colman, 1992). Several precautions with parsley have been recommended. Parsley should be avoided during pregnancy because it may cause an abortion (Mindell & Colman, 1992). It should be avoided in women with kidney inflammation. The seeds of parsley may cause bleeding and inflammation of mucosal lining of the gastrointestinal tract. It is also reported that light-skinned individuals may experience photodermatitis, and it can cause itching or a skin rash in a sensitive individual (Foster, 1996; Keville, 1996).

Amenorrhea

Three broad types of amenorrhea have been identified. If menstruation has not started in a woman by the age of 16, this is referred to as primary amenorrhea. If menstruation stops after at least one period has occurred, this is referred to as secondary amenorrhea. Women frequently experience this second type of amenorrhea due to stress, loss or gain of weight, breast-feeding, excessive exercise, change in lifestyle, or physical ailments, and may be due to menopause. The third type of amenorrhea is known as irregular or erratic menstruation. In this case, menstruation may occur a few times a year.

The most helpful herb for amenorrhea is **blessed thistle** (*Cnicus benedictus*). Specifically, this herb resolves blood clots and stops uterine bleeding.(Mindell & Colman, 1992). **Blessed thistle** is usually taken in combination with other herbs such as **blue cohosh** (*Caulophyllum thalictroides*), **cramp bark** (*Viburnum opulus*), and **ginger** (*Zingiber officinalis*). The synergistic effect with these other remedies helps regulate the menstrual cycle. Keville (1996) recommended several different herbs to help manage amenorrhea; they are particularly helpful in starting menstruation that has been delayed by illness, stress, or exertion. These herbs are **ginseng** (*Panax quinquefolium, Panax ginseng*), **licorice** (*Glycyrrhiza glabra*), **motherwort** (*Leonurus cardiaca*), and **Siberian ginseng** (*Eleutherococcus senticosus*).

Dysmenorrhea

The severe menstrual cramping that accompanies the menstrual cycle is known as dysmenorrhea. Several herbs are recommended for dysmenorrhea (Starbuck, 1998). **Chaste berry** (*Vitex agnus castus*) is one recommendation. **Dong quai** (*Angelica sinensis*) may be taken during the 2 weeks prior to menstruation (Keville, 1996). If the woman has heavy menstrual bleeding, endometriosis, or uterine fibroids, she should avoid this remedy unless she is under the care of an herbal practitioner (Keville, 1996). In addition, this herb is contraindicated during pregnancy.

Green (1998) and Marti and Hine (1998) recommended several herbs to help reduce menstrual cramping. These include **chamomile flowers** (or camomile) (*Matricaria chamomilla, Matricaria recutita*), **cramp bark** (*Viburnum opulus*), **false unicorn root** (*Chamaelirium luteum, Helonias opulus*), and **raspberry leaves** (*Rubus idaeus*). Chamomile is a member of the daisy family, and anyone who is allergic to other members of the daisy family, including ragweed, should avoid this herb (Mindell & Colman, 1992).

Hoffman (1998) recommended combining tinctures of **black cohosh**, **black haw**, and **skullcap** in equal parts and taking this mixture as needed for menstrual cramps, pain, and heavy bleeding. Black cohosh (*Cimicifuga racemosa*) may cause dizziness and irritate the nerves. If taken in large amounts, this herb can increase blood pressure (Keville, 1996). Black haw (*Viburnum prunifolium*) is well known for its diuretic action and sedative effects along with its actions to reduce menstrual cramping and spasms. Skullcap (*Scutellaria laterifloa*), also known as common skullcap, is a strong tonic that possesses nerve and antispasmodic actions.

For a woman who experiences excess water retention, Hoffman (1998) suggested **dandelion root** (*Taxaracum officinale*), an effective diuretic (Marti & Hine, 1998). Dandelion can cause itching or a skin rash in a sensitive individual (Keville, 1996).

Menorrhagia

Menorrhagia is characterized by excessive, heavy menstrual flow. Three recommended herbal remedies to lessen menstrual bleeding include **nettles** (*Urtica dioica*), **shepherd's purse** (*Capsella bursa-pastoris*), and **yarrow** (*Achillea millefolium*). Shephard's purse has been proven effective in clinical trials in treating both menorrhagia and hemorrhage (Marti & Hine, 1998). This herb should be avoided by women who are breast-feeding (Green, 1998; Herbal Research Publications, 1995; Keville, 1996; Starbuck, 1998). Yarrow (*Achillea millefolium*) controls menstrual bleeding and tones the blood vessels (Green, 1998; Herbal Research Publications, 1995; Keville, 1996).

Other herbs are also sometimes recommended to decrease menstrual bleeding and to strengthen the uterus (Marti & Hine, 1998; Mindell &

Colman, 1992; Starbuck, 1998). These include **agrimony** (*Agrimonia eupatoria*), **birthroot** (*Trillium pendulum*), **blue cohosh** (*Caulophyllum thalictroides*), **chaste berry** (*Vitex agnus castus*), **lady's mantle** (*Alchemilla vulgaris*) (which should be avoided in lactating women), **raspberry leaf** (*Rubus idaeus*), **spotted cranesbill** (*Geranium maculatum*), **vervain** (*Verbena officinalis*), and **witch hazel** (*Hamamelis virginiana*).

Metrorrhagia

Four herbs are recommended to alleviate metrorrhagia. These include **black cohosh** (*Cimicifuga racemosa*), **chaste berry** (*Vitex agnus castus*), **dong quai** (*Angelica sinensis, Angelica polymorpha, Angelica dahurica,* or *Angelica atropurpurea*), and **false unicorn root** (*Chamaelirium luteum* or *Helonias opulus*).

Oligomenorrhea

Four herbs, which have been described previously, are helpful in alleviating oligomenorrhea. These herbs include **black cohosh** (*Cimicifuga racemosa*), **blue cohosh** (*Caulophyllum thalictroides*), **chaste berry** (*Vitex agnus castus*), and **dong quai** (*Angelica sinensis, Angelica polymorpha, Angelica dahurica,* or *Angelica atropurpurea*).

Premenstrual Syndrome

The premenstrual syndrome (PMS) occurs several days prior to the onset of menstruation and terminates a short time after the onset of menstruation. The wide range of symptoms varies among women. Some of the multiple common symptoms experienced by the women include mood swings; anxiety; irritability; tension; headaches; depression; breast soreness; swollen breasts; water retention; abdominal bloating and pain; fatigue; diarrhea or constipation; weight gain; and craving for chocolate, sugary, or salty foods (Northrup, 1998).

The three major herbal remedies for the general overall symptoms of PMS are **black cohosh** (*Cimicifuga racemosa*) (Foster, 1996); **chaste berry** (*Vitex agnus-castus*) (Bilger, 1999; Foster, 1996), which should be taken daily and not just before menstruation; and **dong quai** (*Angelica sinensis*).

Additional herbal remedies to relieve the common overall symptoms experienced with PMS are also recommended (Elias & Masline, 1995; Green, 1998; Keville, 1996; Whittaker, 1999). These include **black walnut** (husk) (*Juglans nigra*); **burdock** (*Arctium lappa*); **dande-**

lion root leaf (*Taxaracum officinale*), which reduces abdominal bloating and swollen breasts (Green, 1998); **evening primrose oil** (*Oenothera biennis*), which reduces irritability, headaches, and breast soreness and tenderness (Green, 1998); **licorice** (*Glycyrrhiza glabra*); **red clover** (*Trifolium pratense*), which contains phytoestrogens, such as genistein and dradzen (Whittaker, 1999); **St. John's wort** (*Hypericum perforatum*), which helps alleviate feelings of depression (Green, 1998), but may increase side effects of photosensitizing drugs, alcohol, and melatonin and may enhance effects of narcotics and selective serotonin reuptake inhibitors (SSRIs).

Wild yam root (*Dioscorea villosa*) is suggested for sore, swollen, tender breasts. To alleviate depression, anxiety, headaches, muscle cramping, nervousness, mood swings, irritability, and depression, the following herbs are recommended: **chamomile, chamomile flowers,** or **camomile** (*Matricaria chamomilla, Matricaria recutita*); **lemon balm** (*Melissa officinalis*); **motherwort** (*Leonurus cardiaca*); **passionflower** (*Passiflora incarnata*); **St. John's wort** (*Hypericum perforatum*); **valerian root** (*Valeriana officinalis*); and **wild yam root** (*Dioscorea villosa*).

For water retention, weight gain, and bloating, several herbs are recommended. **Burdock** (*Arctium lappa*) helps the body to eliminate excess water weight and also acts as nature's best "blood purifier" (Mindell & Colman, 1992). Other herbs used to alleviate these symptoms include **chaste berry** (*Vitex agnus castus*), **dandelion root** (*Taxaracum officinale*), and **pennyroyal** (*Hedeoma pulegioides*).

To ease the food cravings, three herbs are helpful. They include **chamomile, chamomile flowers,** or **camomile** (*Matricaria chamomilla, Matricaria recutita*); **Siberian ginseng** (*Eleutherococcus senticosus*); and **wild yam root** (*Dioscorea villosa*).

Several herbs are helpful in decreasing acne. These include **chaste berry** (*Vitex agnus castus*), **licorice** (*Glycyrrhiza glabra*), **squaw vine** (*Mitchella repens*), and **Sarsaparilla** (*Smilax spp*).

Vaginitis

The organisms that commonly cause vaginitis include *Candida albicans, Trichomonas vaginalis, Gardnerella vaginalis,* and *Chlamydia trachomatis.* At times the woman may develop vaginitis if she is exposed to some irritant that produces either a chemical or allergic reaction. The common symptoms experienced in a woman are moist vaginal discharge, vaginal odor, burning pains, vulval or vaginal itching, irritation, or painful urination after intercourse (Marti & Hine, 1998).

Several different kinds of herbs are useful in alleviating symptoms of vaginitis. These include **black walnut** (*Juglans nigra*), **milk thistle** (*Silybum marianum*), **myrrh** (*Commiphora molmol*), **oak bark** (*Quercus robur*), **pau d'arco** (*Tabecuia impetiginosa*), and **squaw vine** (*Mitchella repens*). **Milk thistle**, also known as silymarin, supports liver functions of the woman with the candidal condition. Damage to the liver is often an underlying factor in chronic candidiasis as well as chronic fatigue (Murray & Pizzorno, 1998). **Myrrh** (*Commiphora molmol*), also known as gum myrrh, karam, or turkey myrrh, is helpful in healing the mucous membranes, although it should not be used by a pregnant woman or a woman with excessive menstrual flow. **Pau d'arco** (*Tabecuia impetiginosa*) helps eliminate fungal and parasitic infections (Mindell & Colman, 1992).

There are many antiseptic herbs that strengthen the immune system to suppress the infection and are useful for douching (if a woman chooses to douche). **Comfrey leaf** (*Symphylum officinale*) has a soothing effect on the membranes. **Echinacea** (*Echinacea angustifolia*) acts against both bacterial and viral infections in addition to strengthening the immune system (Mindell & Colman, 1992). **Garlic** (*Allium salivum*) is known for its antibiotic and antifungal actions, but should be avoided by women who are breast-feeding because it can pass to the breast milk, causing colic in infants (Mindell & Colman, 1992). **Goldenseal** (*Hydrastis canadensis*) is effective against fungal infections and also has an anti-inflammatory action that soothes irritated mucous membranes, but is contraindicated during pregnancy (Mindell & Colman, 1992). **Lavender** (*Lavandula officinalis*) is sometimes used. **Licorice root** (*Glycyrrhiza glabra*) is known for its soothing quality in addition to its effectiveness in specifically treating *Candida albicans,* the fungus responsible for vaginal yeast infections. (Laign, 1998; Mindell & Colman, 1992). Consumption of large amounts of licorice may cause symptoms such as water retention, elevated blood pressure, headaches, lethargy, and perhaps heart failure (Laign, 1998). **Nettles** (*Urtica dioica*) helps to eliminate the vaginal infection. **Plantain** (*Plantago major*) is useful, but the fresh form is recommended. **Slippery elm** (*Ulmus fulva*) is soothing as well as useful in treating yeast infections and trichomoniasias and also has the tendency to draw impurities from the affected areas (Mindell & Coleman, 1992). **Tea tree oil** (*Melaleuca alternifolia*) is another useful herb. **Uva ursi** (*Arctostaphylos uva-ursi*) acts as a disinfectant and astringent. In addition, this remedy dries the discharge caused by an infection.

The berberine-containing plants are also effective in eliminating vaginal infections. The berberine exhibits a broad spectrum of antibiotic action, including activity against bacteria, protozoa, and fungi, particularly *Candida albicans* (Murray & Pizzorno, 1998). The plants that contain berberine include **barberry** (*Berberis vulgaris*), **goldenseal** (*Hydrastis canadensis*), **gold thread** (*Coptis chinensis*), and **Oregon grape** (*Berberis aquifolium*).

Keville (1996) suggested that women drink a tea combining the following herbs for vaginal infections: **burdock root** (*Arcticum lappa*), **chaste berry seeds** (*Vitex agnus castus*) (optional), **cramp bark** (*Viburnum opulus*), **echinacea root** (*Echinacea angustifolia*), and **Oregon grape root** (*Berberis aquifolium*).

Infertility

For infertility that is due to a hormonal imbalance, five common herbs may be helpful. In addition, these herbs may decrease the likelihood of miscarriage (Keville, 1996). **Chaste berry** (*Vitex agnus castus*) acts to normalize and stimulate the pituitary gland functions. This remedy increases the levels of the three key hormones (progesterone, prolactin, and luteinizing hormone) that are related to women's ability to conceive (Keville, 1996). **Damiana** (*Turnera diffusa*) assists in balancing levels of various reproducive hormones. **Dong quai** (*Angelica sinensis, Angelica polymorpha, Angelica dahurica,* or *Angelica atropurpurea*), preferably the one obtained from China, is effective in reestablishing a normal menstrual cycle and strengthening the uterus (Herbal Research Publications, 1995; Keville, 1996). **False unicorn root** (*Chamaelirium luteum*) assists in correcting hormonal imbalances and strengthening the uterus. **Siberian ginseng** (*Eleutherococcus senticosus*), also known as ussurian thorny pepperbush, is a popular general tonic for the body, which enhances stamina and endurance. (Herbal Research Publications, 1995; Keville, 1996). This remedy should be avoided if a person has high blood pressure. Also, any person with human immunodeficiency virus/acquired immune deficiency syndrome (HIV/AIDS) or other autoimmune disorders should not use this herb without professional guidance (Toscano, 1998). Keville (1996) also recommends **motherwort** (*Leonurus cardiaca*) for infertility (Herbal Research Publications, 1995; Keville,1996). The fresh plant of this remedy can cause itching or a skin rash in a sensitive individual (Keville, 1996; Murray & Pizzorno, 1998).

To regulate menstrual flow, **shepherd's purse** (*Capsella bursa-pastoris*) (Green, 1998; Herbal Research Publications, 1995; Keville, 1996) and **yarrow** (*Achillea millefolium*) (Green, 1998; Herbal Research

Publications, 1995; Keville, 1996) are recommended. Yarrow also helps to tone the blood vessels (Green, 1998; Herbal Research Publications, 1995; Keville, 1996).

Pregnancy

Several different herbs are recommended for alleviating many of the common symptoms associated with pregnancy. Morning sickness is often mitigated by **lemon balm** (*Melissa officinalis*), also known as balm, and by **raspberry leaves** (*Rubus idaeus*). Additonally, **burdock** (*Arctium lappa*), **false unicorn root** (*Chamaelirium luteum, Helonias opulus*), **ginger** (*Zingiber officinale*), and **wild yam root** (*Dioscorea villosa*) are recommended. Holmes (1996) noted that ginger is one of the common useful agents in alleviating morning sickness and nausea during pregnancy, but that fresh ginger root, not the dried ginger, must be taken the first thing in the morning and repeated at the first hint of nausea during the day.

Other herbs may help to alleviate nausea. **Ginseng** (*Panax*) is one of these, but it may cause an increase in general discomfort and could potentially cause birth defects. **Licorice** (*Glycyrrhiza glabra*) may worsen the effects of drugs that cause potassium loss, and may lengthen the time of effectiveness of corticosteroids (Hardy, 1998). This herb may lead to sodium and water retention and high blood pressure, and is contraindicated in persons with high blood pressure, congestive heart failure, or kidney or liver problems (Toscano, 1998). **Goldenseal** (*Hydrastis canadensis*), also known by other common names, including eye balm, eye root, ground raspberry, Indian dye, jaundice root, and orange root (Toscano, 1998), may counteract short-acting anticoagulants and may cause uterine contractions (Hardy, 1998).

Herbs for providing nutrients during pregnancy include **oatstraw** (*Avena sativa*) and **nettles** (*Urtica dioica*). Oatstraw contains silica, fiber, and provides trace nutrients, especially calcium that are important for the pregnant woman (Keville, 1996). Nettles provides similar nutrients, especially calcium, that are important during pregnancy, and it enhances the assimilation of these nutrients from other sources (Keville, 1996).

For water retention, **dandelion root** (*Taxaracum officinale*) is useful. This herb, by aiding in prevention of high blood pressure and water retention, helps to prevent eclampsia (Keville,1996).

For pain or uterine cramps that occur during pregnancy, four herbs are suggested: **chaste berry** (*Vitex agnus castus*), **cramp bark** (*Vibur-*

num opulus), **false unicorn root** (*Chamaelirium luteum, Helonias opulus*), and **wild yam root** (*Dioscorea villosa*).

To prevent tension and stretch marks, **lavender** (*Lavandula officinalis*) is recommended (Keville, 1996). This herb is a muscle relaxant and thus eases tension and loosens tight muscles during childbirth.

Childbirth

One herb used to facilitate labor is **raspberry leaves** (*Rubus idaeus*). This herb acts as a uterine tonic that provides relaxant effects, thereby facilitating and possibly shortening length of labor (Keville, 1996). The following herbals, **black cohosh** (*Cimicifuga racemosa*) and **blue cohosh** (*Caulophyllum thalictroides*), are recommended PRIOR TO <u>and</u> FOLLOWING childbirth. Black cohosh is very effective at easing uterine cramping. It is important to note, however, that toxic reactions have been reported if the remedy is taken in large doses. Some people have reported nausea and vomiting with overdoses. This remedy is not recommended during the first trimester of pregnancy. Blue cohosh facilitates childbirth because of its oxytocic effect, contributing to cervical dilation. It is also believed that this herb eases labor pains.

It is suggested that the woman begin to take these two remedies during the last 2 weeks of pregnancy, as it is believed that these herbs prepare the uterus for birth by encouraging the light, early contractions that the woman usually feels a few weeks before labor begins (Braxton Hicks contractions). Also, these two types of cohosh are used to encourage a slow labor once serious contractions begin. Keville (1996) warned that "Although it is suggested in some books that these herbs should be taken throughout pregnancy, this is definitely not a good idea. In other books, women are warned against using them at all because both herbs can affect blood pressure adversely" (p. 234).

After childbirth, several herbs are recommended to assist in decreasing uterine bleeding. **Ginger** (*Zingiber officinale*) is one of these herbs (Mindell & Colman, 1992), although recent reports indicate that heartburn may occur with use of this herb (Consumer Reports, 1999). **Shepherd's purse** (*Capsella bursa-pastoris*) is considered one of the best for regulating uterine bleeding (Green, 1998; Herbal Research Publications, 1995; Keville, 1996). **Yarrow** (*Achillea millefolium*) controls uterine bleeding and tones/strengthens the blood vessels (Green, 1998; Herbal Research Publications, 1995; Keville, 1996), but it may contribute to photosensitivity, whereby sun exposure while taking this herb can lead to a skin reaction.

Calendula (*Calendula officinalis*), **comfrey leaf** (*Symphylum officinale*), **chamomile** (*Anthemis nobilis, Matricaria chamomilla*, or *Matricaria recutita*), and **rosemary** (*Rosmarinus officinalis*) are helpful in easing discomfort after childbirth as well as promoting healing due to their anti-inflammatory action. Adding these herbs to warm water in the form of a sitz bath is recommended.

Breast-feeding

Lactating mothers occasionally experience insufficient or slow milk production. If the milk comes slowly, several herbs are recommended to stimulate lactation and increase milk volume (Mindell & Colman, 1992). One herb is **blessed thistle** (*Cnicus benedictus*), although it is not recommended for the woman with stomach ulcers (Monte, 1997, p. 455). **Caraway** (*Carum carvi*) is another recommended herb. **Chaste berry** (*Vitex angus castus*), commonly referred to as Vitex, acts as a tonic to balance the hormones and stimulate the lactation process. This remedy is not recommended for the woman with heavy menstrual flow or for pregnant women (Mindell & Colman, 1992). **Dill** (*Aniethum graveolens*); **Fennel** (*Foeniculum vulgare*), also known as finocchio or carosella; **goat's rue** (*Galega officinalis*); **milk thistle** (*Cinicus benedictus* or *Silybum marianum*); **nettles** (*Urtica dioica*), also known as stinging nettle; and **vervain** (*Verbena officinalis*) are all herbs that assist in stimulating lactation. Women with excessive menstrual flow or women who are pregnant are not advised to take **chaste berry** or **vervain** (Herbal Research Publications, 1995). Two other helpful herbal seeds are **anise** (*Pimpinella anisum*) and **fenugreek** (*Trigonella foenum-graecum*). **Sage** (*salvia officinalis*) is recommended to assist in slowing the milk flow when the mother wants to wean the baby. The sage extract can cause skin irritation (Kowalchik & Hylton, 1987).

Menopausal Difficulties

Chapter 3, Sexual/Reproductive Health of Women, provides an overview of the various menopausal symptoms. This chapter on herbal remedies presents several recommendations for alleviating many of these symptoms.

There are four well-known herbal remedies for menopausal symptoms. **Black cohosh** (*Cimicifuga racemosa*), used by the Native Americans for many female problems, increases the estrogen levels just enough to minimize and alleviate symptoms of menopause, including hot flashes (frequency and severity), night sweats, heart palpitations, vaginal dryness, and headaches. Also, this remedy helps to increase the libido (Dickstein, 1999; Foster, 1996; Gluck, 1998; Green, 1998; Keville, 1996; Mindell & Colman, 1996). There are no contraindications or drug interactions reported for this herbal remedy when taken for menopausal difficulties; however, a few women have experienced an upset stomach (Foster, 1996). **Chaste berry** (*Vitex agnus-castus*), often referred to as the "menopausal herb," is viewed as a general menopausal tonic that balances the hormones, alleviating symptoms of nervousness and irritability (Foster, 1996). **Dong quai** (*Angelica sinensis, Angelica polymorpha, Angelica dahurica,* or *Angelica atropurpurea*), a common Asian herb, is very effective in alleviating symptoms associated with menopause, particularly fatigue, insomnia, hot flashes, and headaches. Pregnant or lactating women should avoid taking this herbal remedy unless supervised by a qualified medical practitioner (Foster, 1996). Also, this herb can cause photosensitivity (Keville, 1996). **Red clover** (*Trifolium pratense*), considered the most powerful of the plant estrogens (Foster, 1996; Starbuck, 1998), is often recommended as an estrogen source. One of its major benefits in menopause is that it improves the libido (Foster, 1996; Starbuck, 1998).

Other herbs are sometimes recommended for menopausal symptoms. **Flaxseed** (*Linum usitaissmum*) contains omega-3 and omega-6 oils, which assist in decreasing inflammation. Keville (1996) suggests additional herbs for treatment of menopausal symptoms. These herbs are **fenugreek** (*Trigonella foenum-graecum*), **ginseng** (*Panax*), **licorice** (*Glycyrrhiza glabra*), and **stinging nettle** (*Urtica dioica*). Stinging nettle provides nutritional support as it is high in iron and calcium and is considered to be an excellent diuretic for women who retain water (Loecher and O'Donnell, 1997).

Wild yam root (*Dioscorea villosa*) and **motherwort** (*Leonurus cardiaca*) also act to reduce the discomfort and frequency of hot flashes that the woman experiences (Green, 1998). The fresh plant of this motherwort remedy can cause itching or a skin rash in a sensitive person (Keville, 1996; Murray & Pizzorno, 1998).

To alleviate anxiety, nervousness, and irritability, other herbs are recommended. **Hops** (*Humulus lupulus*) helps to increase estrogen levels (Keville, 1996). The fresh plant of hops can cause itching or a skin rash in a sensitive individual (Keville, 1996; Murray & Pizzorno, 1998). **Kava kava** (*Piper methysticum*), known as Kava, is known for its calming properties (Orey, 1998), particularly in reducing anxiety, fatigue, stress-related disorders, and nervousness because of its relaxing effect on the central nervous system. An advantage of this remedy is that it does not lose its effectiveness with time. This herb can cause drowsiness, which is one reason to either discontinue it or reduce the dosage (Sundermann, 1999). **Kava** should not be used with the tranquilizer alprazolam because this combination may result in a coma (Mayo & Mayo, 1999). **Oatstraw** (*Avena sativa*) is considered a tonic for the nervous system, enhancing a restful sleep (Loecher & O'Donnell, 1997). **Ginseng** (*Panax*) also helps to reduce nervousness.

A helpful remedy to increase the estrogen level is **sage** (*Salvia officinalis*). This herb also helps to reduce sweating (Green, 1998). Two herbs are suggested to help alleviate vaginal dryness. These are **evening primrose oil** (*Oenothera biennis*) and **wild yam root** (*Dioscorea villosa*) (Green, 1998).

Hormone Replacement Therapy

Today one of the controversial issues in women's health is whether or not to use hormone replacement therapy (HRT) during the menopausal years. The chapter on pharmacology (Chapter 10) provides an overview of the issues surrounding HRT use. This chapter on herbal remedies presents information on herbal approaches to menopause.

Phytoestrogens are botanicals prepared from plants that contain chemical substances with hormone-type activities or properties described as estrogen-like. These substances protect women against hormone-related illness, including cardiovascular conditions, osteoporosis, colon cancer, and cognitive function. Walker (1998) has reported that current research findings into these phytoestrogens suggest that they can potentially lower the risk of heart disease and osteoporosis by linking up with estrogen receptors on cells in the body.

For HRT, several phytoestrogens are recommended, including **black cohosh** (*Cimicifuga racemosa*), **chaste berry** (*Vitex agnus castus*), and **dong quai** (*Angelica sinensis, Angelica polymorpha, Angelica dahurica,* or *Angelica atropurpurea*). Black cohosh acts to potentially block the entry of undesirable estrogens into sensitive cell membranes. Chaste berry normalizes and stimulates the pituitary gland functions, particularly those of the female sex hormones. It is viewed as a general menopausal tonic that balances the hormones. This remedy also increases the levels of the three key hormones (progesterone, prolactin, and luteinizing hormone) that help women to become pregnant (Gluck, 1998; Keville, 1996). Dong quai, known as the archetypal herbal remedy, is often referred to as the female ginseng. It is most effective for a wide range of women's gynecological conditions. This remedy should not be used during pregnancy, and it is important to note that it may cause photosensitization (Toscano, 1998).

Additional herbs are recommended for HRT, including **false unicorn root** (*Chamaelirium luteum or Helonias opulus*), **fennel** (*Foeniculum vulgare*), **licorice** (*Glycyrrhiza glabra*) (which is not recommended in pregnant women), **unicorn root** (*Aletris farinosa*), and **wild yam root** (*Dioscorea villosa*).

Table 11–2 presents a quick reference for the herbal remedies discussed in this section as they apply to the reproductive system of women.

Table 11–2 Summary of Recommended Herbs for Various Women's Health Conditions

Common Name	Botanical Name
Remedies for Cystitis	
Uva ursi	*Arctostaphylos*
Goldenseal	*Hydrastis canadensis*
Cranberry	*Vaccinium macrocarpon* or *Vaccinium oxycoccos*
Celery	*Apisum graveolens*
Juniper berries	*Juniperus communis*
Licorice	*Glycyrrhiza glabra*
Chronic cystitis	
Gotu kola	*Centella asiatica*
Horsetail	*Equisetum arvense*
Remedies for Cysts and Fibroids	
Fibrocystic Breast Disease	
Evening primrose oil	*Oenothera biennis*
Prickly ash bark	*Xanthoxylum americanum*
To improve lymph drainage	
Burdock root	*Arctium lappa*
Calendula	*Calendula officinalis*
Cleavers	*Galium aparine*
Mullein	*Verbascum thapsus*
Ovarian cysts	
Evening primrose oil	*Oenothera biennis*
Prickly ash bark	*Xanthoxylum americanum*

continues

Table 11–2 continued

Common Name	Botanical Name
Uterine fibroids	
Chaste berry	*Vitex agnus-castus*
Raspberry leaf	*Rubus idaeus*
Wild yam root	*Dioscorea villosa*

Remedies for Endometriosis

Burdock	*Arctium lappa*
Chaste berry	*Vitex agnus castus*
Milk thistle	*Silybum marianum*
For cramping, inflammation, bleeding, and pain	
Cramp bark	*Viburnum opulus*
Wild yam root	*Dioscorea villosa*
For relieving cramping and other related menstrual pain	
Evening primrose oil	*Oenothera biennis*
Ginger	*Zingiber officinale*
For bleeding	
Red raspberry leaf	*Rubus idaeus*
Horsetail	*Equisetum arvense*
For cramping	
Echinacea	*Echinacea angustifolia, Echinacea pallida, Echinacea purpurea*
Milk thistle	*Silybum marianum*
Motherwort	*Leonurus cardiaca*
Nettles	*Urtica dioica*
Passionflower	*Passiflora incarnata*

Remedies for Menstrual Difficulties/Irregularities

For overall menstrual difficulties and irregularities	
Black cohosh	*Cimicifuga racemosa*
Blue cohosh	*Caulophyllum thalictroides*
Chaste berry	*Vitex agnus-castus*
Dong quai	*Angelica sinensis*
Motherwort	*Leonurus cardiaca*
Parsley	*Petroselinum crispum, Petroselinum sativum*
Amenorrhea	
Blessed thistle	*Cnicus benedictus*

continues

Table 11–2 continued

Common Name	Botanical Name
Blue cohosh	*Caulophyllum thalictroides*
Cramp bark	*Viburnum opulus*
Ginger	*Zingiber officinale*
Ginseng	*Panax quinquefolium, Panax ginseng*
Licorice	*Glycyrrhiza glabra*
Motherwort	*Leonurus cardiaca*
Siberian ginseng	*Eleutherococcus senticosus*

Dysmenorrhea

To normalize the menstrual cycle
and alleviate menstrual cramps
and pain

Chaste berry	*Vitex agnus castus*
Dong quai	*Angelica sinensis*

To reduce menstrual cramps

Chamomile flowers (or camomile)	*Matricaria chamomilla, Matricaria recutita)*
Cramp bark	*Viburnum opulus*
False unicorn root	*Chamaelirium luteum, Helonias opulus*
Raspberry leaves	*Rubus idaeus*

For menstrual cramps, pain,
and heavy bleeding

Black cohosh	*Cimicifuga racemosa*
Black haw	*Viburnum prunifolium*
Skullcap	*Scutellaria laterifloa*

For excess water retention

Dandelion root	*Taxaracum officinale*

Menorrhagia

To lessen menstrual bleeding

Nettles	*Urtica dioica*
Shepherd's purse	*Capsella bursa-pastoris*
Yarrow	*Achillea millefolium*

To decrease the menstrual
bleeding and strengthen the uterus

Agrimony	*Agrimonia eupatoria*
Birthroot	*Trillium pendulum*
Blue cohosh	*Caulophyllum thalictroides*
Chaste berry	*Vitex agnus castus*
Lady's mantle	*Alchemilla vulgaris*
Raspberry leaf	*Rubus idaeus*
Spotted cranesbill	*Geranium maculatum*
Vervain	*Verbena officinalis*

continues

Table 11–2 continued

Common Name	Botanical Name
Witch hazel	*Hamamelis virginiana*
Metrorrhagia	
Black cohosh	*Cimicifuga racemosa*
Chaste berry	*Vitex agnus castus*
Dong quai	*Angelica sinensis, Angelica polymorpha, Angelica dahurica,* or *Angelica atropurpurea*
False unicorn root	*Chamaelirium luteum* or *Helonias opulus*
Oligomenorrhea	
Black cohosh	*Cimicifuga racemosa*
Blue cohosh	*Caulophyllum thalictroides*
Chaste berry	*Vitex agnus castus*
Dong quai	*Angelica sinensis, Angelica polymorpha, Angelica dahurica,* or *Angelica atropurpurea*

Recommendations for Premenstrual Syndrome (PMS)

For the general overall symptoms of PMS	
Black cohosh	*Cimicifuga racemosa*
Chaste berry	*Vitex agnus-castus*
Dong quai	*Angelica sinensis*
For common overall symptoms	
Black walnut (husk)	*Juglans nigra*
Burdock	*Arctium lappa*
Dandelion root leaf	*Taxaracum officinale*
Evening primrose oil	*Oenothera biennis*
Licorice	*Glycyrrhiza glabra*
St. John's wort	*Hypericum perforatum*
For sore, swollen, tender breasts	
Wild yam root	*Dioscorea villosa*
To alleviate depression, headaches, muscle cramping and nervousness, mood swings, irritability, and depression	
Valerian root	*Valeriana officinalis*
Passionflower	*Passiflora incarnata*
Wild yam root	*Dioscorea villosa*
Motherwort	*Leonurus cardiaca*
Camomile	*Matricaria chamomilla, Matricaria recutita*

continues

Table 11–2 continued

Common Name	Botanical Name
For water retention, weight gain, bloating, sudden pressure	
Burdock	*Arctium lappa*
Chaste berry	*Vitex agnus castus*
Pennyroyal	*Hedeoma pulegioides*

Recommendations for Vaginitis

Black walnut	*Juglans nigra*
Milk thistle	*Silybum marianum*
Myrrh	*Commiphora molmol*
Oak bark	*Quercus robur*
Pau d'arco	*Tabecuia impetiginosa*
Squaw vine	*Mitchella repens*
Comfrey leaf	*Symphylum officinale*
Echinacea	*Echinacea angustifolia*
Garlic	*Allium salivum*
Goldenseal	*Hydrastis canadensis*
Lavender	*Lavandula officinalis*
Licorice root	*Glycyrrhiza glabra*
Nettles	*Urtica dioica*
Echinacea	*Echinacea angustifolia*
Plantain	*Plantago major*
Slippery elm	*Ulmus fulva*
Tea tree oil	*Melaleuca alternifolia*
Uva ursi	*Arctostaphylos uva-ursi*
The berberine-containing plants	
Goldenseal	*Hydrastis canadensis*
Barberry	*Berberis vulgaris*
Oregon grape	*Berberis aquifolium*
Gold thread	*Coptis chinensis*
Herbal tea drink for vaginal infections	
Cramp bark	*Viburnum opulus*
Burdock root	*Arcticum lappa*
Echinacea root	*Echinacea angustifolia*
Oregon grape root	*Berberis aquifolium*
Chaste berry seeds	*Vitex agnus castus* (optional)

Remedies for Infertility

Chaste berry	*Vitex agnus castus*
Damiana	*Turnera diffusa*

continues

Table 11–2 continued

Common Name	Botanical Name
Dong quai	*Angelica sinensis, Angelica polymorpha, Angelica dahurica, or Angelica atropurpurea*
False unicorn root	*Chamaelirium luteum*
Siberian ginseng	*Eleutherococcus senticosus*
Motherwort	*Leonurus cardiaca*
To regulate menstrual flow	
Shepherd's purse	*Capsella bursa-pastoris*
Yarrow	*Achillea millefolium*

Recommendations during Pregnancy

For morning sickness (and to prevent miscarriage)	
Lemon balm	*Melissa officinalis*
Raspberry leaves	*Rubus idaeus*
For nausea	
Ginseng	*Panax*
Licorice	*Glycyrrhiza glabra*
Goldenseal	*Hydrastis canadensis*
Oatstraw	*Avena sativa*
Nettles	*Urtica dioica*
For water retention	
Dandelion root	*Taxaracum officinale*
For morning sickness and nausea	
Burdock	*Arctium lappa*
False unicorn root	*Chamaelirium luteum, Helonias opulus*
Ginger	*Zingiber officinale*
Wild yam	*Dioscorea villosa*
For pain or uterine cramps	
Chaste berry	*Vitex agnus castus*
Cramp bark	*Viburnum opulus*
False unicorn root	*Chamaelirium luteum, Helonias opulus*
Wild yam root	*Dioscorea villosa*
To prevent tension and stretch marks	
Lavender	*Lavandula officinalis*
To ease food cravings	
Camomile	*Matricaria chamomilla, Matricaria recutita*
Siberian ginseng	*Eleutherococcus senticosus*
Wild yam root	*Dioscorea villosa*
To decrease acne	
Chaste berry	*Vitex agnus castus*

continues

Table 11–2 continued

Common Name	Botanical Name
Licorice	*Glycyrrhiza glabra*
Squaw vine	*Mitchella repens*
Sarsaparilla	*Smilax* spp

Remedies for Childbirth Difficulties

Raspberry leaves	*Rubus idaeus*
Black cohosh	*Cimicifuga racemosa*
Blue cohosh	*Caulophyllum thalictroides*
To slow postpartum bleeding	
Ginger	*Zingiber officinale*
Shepherd's purse	*Capsella bursa-pastoris*
Yarrow	*Achillea millefolium*
Add to daily Sitz baths	
Calendula	*Calendula officinalis*
Comfrey leaf	*Symphylum officinale*
Chamomile	*Anthemis nobilis, Matricaria chamomilla,* or *Matricaria recutita*
Rosemary	*Rosmarinus officinalis*

Remedies for Breast-Feeding Problems

To stimulate milk flow	
Blessed thistle	*Cnicus benedictus*
Caraway	*Carum carvi*
Chaste berry	*Vitex angus castus*
Dill	*Aniethum graveolens*
Fennel	*Foeniculum vulgare*
Goat's rue	*Galega officinalis*
Milk thistle	*Cinicus benedictus* or *Silybum marianum*
Nettles	*Urtica dioica*
Vervain	*Verbena officinalis*
Herbal seeds	
Anise	*Pimpinella anisum*
Dill	*Anethum graveolens*
Fenugreek	
Fennel	*Foeniculum vulgare*
Chaste berry	*Vitex agnus castus*
To slow milk flow	
Sage	*Salvia officinalis*

Remedies for Menopausal Difficulties

For menopausal symptoms	
Black cohosh	*Cimicifuga racemosa*

continues

Table 11–2 continued

Common Name	Botanical Name
Chaste berry	*Vitex agnus-castus*
Dong quai	*Angelica sinensis, Angelica polymorpha, Angelica dahurica,* or *Angelica atropurpurea*
Red clover	*Trifolium pratense*
Flaxseed	*Linum usitaissimum*
Fenugreek	*Trigonella foenumgraecum*
Ginseng	*Panax*
Licorice	*Glycyrrhiza glabra*
Stinging nettle	*Urtica dioica*
To reduce the discomfort and frequency of hot flashes	
Wild yam root	*Dioscorea villosa*
Motherwort	*Leonurus cardiaca*
To alleviate nervousness and irritability	
Hops	*Humulus lupulus*
Kava kava	*Piper methysticum*
Oatstraw	*Avena sativa*
Ginseng	*Panax*
To increase the estrogen level	
Sage	*Salvia officinalis*
To help with vaginal dryness	
Evening primrose oil	*Oenothera biennis*
Wild yam root	*Dioscorea villosa*

Recommendations for Hormone Replacement Therapy

Phytoestrogens	
Black cohosh	*Cimicifuga racemosa*
Chaste berry	*Vitex agnus castus*
Dong quai	*Angelica sinensis, Angelica polymorpha, Angelica dahurica,* or *Angelica atropurpurea*
False unicorn root	*Chamaelirium luteum* or *Helonias opulus*
Fennel	*Foeniculum vulgare*
Licorice	*Glycyrrhiza glabra*
Unicorn root	*Aletris farinosa*
Wild yam root	*Dioscorea villosa*

Source: Data from E. Mindell and C. Colman, *Earl Mindell's Herb Bible,* © 1992, Simon & Schuster.

GENERAL CONDITIONS PREVALENT AMONG WOMEN AND THEIR COMMON HERBAL REMEDIES

This section briefly describes certain common health conditions experienced by women. These include Alzheimer's disease, anxiety and depression, arthritis, chronic fatigue syndrome, digestive problems, edema, fatigue, fibromyalgia, heart problems, high cholesterol, hypertension, insomnia, migraine headaches, osteoporosis, senile dementia (senility), stress, and varicose veins. For each condition, the common remedies, their properties and actions are identified.

Alzheimer's Disease

Alzheimer's disease affects more women than men and researchers have estimated that 4 million Americans have this illness, with the number expected to rise to 6 million by the year 2020. This illness is a degenerative disorder that compromises the brain and includes symptoms such as memory loss, disorientation, dementia, and other debilitating cognitive problems. **Gotu kola** (*Centella asiatica*) and **ginkgo** (*Ginkgo biloba*) are helpful in Alzheimer's disease. Ginkgo enhances circulation and increases oxygen flow, especially to the brain, and it improves memory, concentration, alertness, and general cerebral performance when related to impaired circulation, senile dementia and presenile dementia (Dickstein, 1999; Toscano, 1998). The actions of this remedy have been supported by several European studies (*Consumer Reports,* 1999). Due to ginkgo's actions as an anticoagulant and antiplatelet, women on blood thinners should avoid this remedy. In addition, women with hypersensitivity to poison ivy, cashews, or mangoes should also avoid ginkgo. Potential side effects are gastrointestinal disturbance and headaches (*Consumer Reports,* 1999; Hardy, 1998).

Anxiety and Depression

Anxiety is usually described as an unpleasant feeling of apprehension or tension resulting from an unexpected threat to one's feelings of self-esteem or well-being. The various degrees of anxiety have been grouped as mild, moderate, severe, and panic. This feeling influences our learning, our perceptions, and our performance. As anxiety increases, there is a negative effect on these processes.

Hops (*Humulus lupulus*) alleviates nervousness and irritability due to its calming and relaxing effects. The fresh plant of hops can cause itching or a skin rash in a sensitive individual (Keville, 1996; Murray & Pizzorno, 1998). **Kava kava** (*Piper methysticum*) is effective in easing anxiety, especially in menopause (Sundermann, 1999). Potential side effects that have recently been reported include gastrointestinal disturbance and temporary discoloration of skin, hair, and nails (*Consumer Reports*, 1999).

Passionflower (*Passiflora incarnata*), often referred to as maypop, is a gentle sedative that helps relieve anxiety, insomnia, nervous tension, nervous headaches, muscle spasms and stress-related disorders because of its effect on the sympathetic nervous system. A woman is advised to avoid this herb in high doses during pregnancy (Mindell & Colman, 1992).

Valerian (*Valeriana officinalis*) is known for its natural tranquilizing effect on the central nervous system. This action has been supported by clinical research (Kowalchik & Hylton, 1987; Murray & Pizzorno, 1998). This remedy may be consumed as a tea. If this herb is taken in large doses, it may cause dizziness, stupor, and vomiting.

Depression is characterized by mood changes and loss of interest in pleasurable aspects of life, such as family, friends, work, food, sex, and social community activities. Any of the following symptoms may be experienced: insomnia or excessive sleeping, feelings of hopelessness, fatigue, loss of energy, feelings of helplessness and worthlessness, problems concentrating, weight loss or weight gain, and repeated thoughts of death or suicide. Of note is that the fresh leaf or root of the **gotu kola** (*Centella asiatica*) plant is recommended (Herbal Research Publications, 1995). Also, it is advised that pregnant women avoid **St. John's wort** (*Hypericum perforatum*) (Dickstein, 1999). In addition, it is recommended to avoid taking this herb with antidepressant prescription medications, including monoamine oxidase (MAO) inhibitors and serotonin reuptake inhibitors (Bilger, 1999; Dickstein, 1999). This remedy may cause increased sensitivity to sunlight (Bilger, 1999; *Consumer Reports*, 1999). Other potential side effects reported are dry mouth, bloating, constipation, nausea, and dizziness (*Consumer Reports*, 1999).

Arthritis

Arthritis is a condition that produces inflammation of a joint, often accompanied by pain, swelling, and changes in the physical structure of the joint. Two common types of arthritic conditions are rheumatoid arthritis and the degenerative joint disease known as osteoarthritis. It is noted that **comfrey** (*Symphylum officinale*) has been reported to have a potential side effect of liver damage (*Consumer Reports,* 1999).

Rheumatoid Arthritis

Rheumatoid arthritis is an autoimmune disease resulting in symmetrical joint inflammation. The joints involved are the wrists, hands, ankles, knees, and feet. The major symptoms are morning stiffness lasting several hours, pain in the joints, fatigue, weakness, and malaise. These symptoms experienced over time often produce crippling deformities. It affects three times as many women as men, with the onset occurring between 35 and 50 years of age. (Snyderman, 1996). A few herbal remedies have been helpful in alleviating the symptoms.

Some points to note are that **arnica** (*Arnica montana*) and **cayenne** (*Capsicum annum*) should not be applied on broken skin or open wounds (Khalsa, 1998). If a woman has gastric or duodenal ulcers, **devil's claw** (*Harpagophytum procumbens*) should be avoided because it is a gastrointestinal irritant (Bucco, 1998). Also, it is suggested that pregnant and nursing mothers should avoid this remedy. **Licorice** (*Glycyrrhiza glabra*) is contraindicated for diabetes, liver disorders, severe kidney insufficiency, and hypokalemia. Herbal Research Publications (1995) specifically noted that **wild yam root** (*Dioscorea nillosa*) is rated as an excellent remedy because of its anti-inflammatory action.

Osteoarthritis

This condition occurs 10 times more frequently in women than in men (Bucco, 1998). Postmenopausal women are at greatest risk. The osteoarthritis occurs in the weight-bearing joints—hips, spine, knees, feet, and ankles—and in joints of the fingers. The common experienced symptoms are: swelling, stiffness, tenderness, pain and sometimes deformity. The two most useful herbs for this condition are **boswellia** (*Boswellia serrata*) and **devil's claw** (*Harpagophytum procumbens*). Boswellia is helpful in decreasing the inflammation and managing the pain associated with this condition because the gum resin of the remedy improves circulation to the joints. Also, this remedy may improve the biochemical structure of cartilage (Bucco, 1998). For the most part, this remedy is considered safe. However, on occasion allergic reactions or mild gastrointestinal distress have been reported. Research needs to be conducted to establish whether this remedy is safe for pregnant and nursing mothers (Bucco, 1998). Devil's claw is described under the section on Rheumatoid Arthritis.

Bucco (1998) suggests additional herbal remedies for relief of osteoarthritic symptoms. **Capsaicin** (*Capsicum supp.*) is helpful in relieving pain. One explanation for the pain relief is that this remedy interferes with the body's perception of pain (Bucco, 1998). Research results showed that capsaicin cream applied directly to arthritic joints several times a day provided significant pain relief (Bucco, 1998). Whenever capsaicin cream is used, hands must be thoroughly washed after use and the person must avoid touching the eyes or any mucous membranes. Also, capsaicin cream should never be used on broken skin or skin wounds. Another research study conducted in 1996 in England and reported by Bucco (1998) combined **willow bark** (*Salix alba*), **guaiacum resin** (*Guaiacum officinale*), **black cohosh root** (*Cimicifuga racemosa*), **sarsaparilla** (*Smilax supp.*), and **poplar bark** (*Populus supp.*).

All of these substances are effective in relieving the symptoms. Specifically, the willow bark, an ancient remedy used throughout the ages, sarsaparilla, and poplar bark are useful in reducing the joint pain. Guaiacum resin and black cohosh are helpful for their anti-inflammatory effects (Bucco, 1998). The findings indicated that the study participants experienced a significant decline in pain (Bucco, 1998).

Chronic Fatigue Syndrome

Chronic fatigue syndrome consists of multiple symptoms, including sore throat, tender and sore muscles, multijoint pain, headaches, sleep disturbances, postexertion malaise, impaired memory, lack of concentration, anxiety, depression, irritability, jaundice, loss of appetite, mood swings, muscle spasms, recurrent upper respiratory tract infections, tender and swollen cervical or axillary lymph nodes, and extreme, disabling fatigue (Snyderman, 1996).

These cognitive, physical, and affective symptoms can be reduced with several therapeutic botanical herbs. There are a few important points to note. **Astragalus** (*Astragalus membranaceus*) should be avoided if the woman has a fever. **Burdock root** (*Arctium lappa*), **dandelion leaf** (*Taraxacum officinale*), and **red clover** (*Trifolium pratense*) may be consumed as teas. **Licorice** (*Glycyrrhiza glabra*) should not be used for more than 7 consecutive days. Also, if the woman has high blood pressure, she should avoid this remedy.

Digestive Problems

Digestive problems usually produce any of the symptoms of pain, heartburn, gas, belching, nausea and vomiting. Several herbs are effective in alleviating these symptoms (Bilger, 1999; Elias & Masline, 1995).

Edema

This symptom is characterized by excessive accumulation of water retention in body tissues and cavities. Edema may be associated with premenstrual syndrome, pregnancy, or other conditions such as heart failure or liver and kidney disturbance. **Dandelion root leaf** (*Taraxacum officinale*) is effective for water retention and is a rich source of potassium.

Fatigue

Siberian ginseng (*Eleutherococcus senticosus*) is considered an excellent general tonic that increases one's vitality by increasing resistance to damaging external environmental factors that deplete one's immune system. It is advised that this remedy be taken at least 1 hour before any prescriptive drug (Bilger, 1999).

Fibromyalgia

Fibromyalgia (FM) is increasing among the general public, particularly women. A few precipitating symptoms are overexertion, stress, lack of exercise, and/or humidity changes. LaValle (1999) suggested several herbs for FM. **Astragalus root** (*Astragalus membranaceus*) is useful in oxygenating the peripheral tissues. Also, it appears helpful in stimulating, building, and strengthening the immune system (LaValle, 1999). **Grapeseed extract** (*Vitis vinifera, Vitis coignetiae*) helps to reduce inflammation, and acts as an antioxidant (LaValle, 1999). **Turmeric** (*Curcuma longa*) contains anti-inflammatory properties.

Heart Problems

Hawthorn berries (*Crataegus oxyacantha, Crataegus monogyna, Crataegus laevigata*) are the major remedy for the heart. This remedy has several common names: English hawthorn, oneseed hawthorn, haw, maybush, and whitethorn. This herb enhances cardiovascular health by improving circulation by dilating blood vessels, resulting in greater tone in the heart muscle (Mindell & Colman,1992; Starbuck, 1998). It is helpful in essential hypertension, congestive heart failure, coronary artery disease, and postmyocardial infarction. Often this remedy is promoted as a "heart tonic" (Toscano, 1998). Starbuck (1998) reported that an extract form of this herb reduced heart palpitations in women. This therapeutic agent may enhance action of cardiac glycosides and ease their side effects (Hardy, 1998). Also, high doses may have a sedative effect and can lead to a dangerous drop in blood pressure. It is advised to avoid this remedy with antihypertensive medication (Toscano, 1998). Although most Hawthorn preparations are safe, this herb is also available in a highly concentrated form that should be used only under medical supervision (Mindell & Colman, 1992).

High Cholesterol

Braverman (1999), Marti and Hine (1998), and Mindell and Colman (1992) recommended a few herbs to lower cholesterol. Of particular note is that **flaxseed** (*Linum usitatissimum*) be given in combination with any of the phytoestrogens in order to lower low-density lipoprotein (LDL) cholesterol, lower total serum lipids, promote coronary artery dilation, and increase high-density lipoprotein (HDL) cholesterol. Also, flaxseed binds to drugs in the gut, which may delay absorption of medications taken at the same time (Hardy, 1998). Among the several properties of **garlic** (*Allium sativum*), the vital actions are its blood thinning capacity, and lowering blood pressure as well as blood cholesterol levels (Gottlieb, 1995). While this remedy is considered relatively safe, on occasion it may cause an upset stomach (Bilger, 1999). This remedy is not recommended if a woman is breast-feeding as it may cause flatulence, which, in turn, can cause colic in the baby. Also, this herb enhances the actions of anticoagulant and antiplatelet drugs (Hardy, 1998).

Hypertension

Remedies recommended to reduce blood presssure are those that contain γ-linoleic acid (GLA). These remedies provide a diuretic effect and may also lower cholesterol (Gluck, 1998; Marti & Hine, 1998; Mindell & Colman, 1992).

Insomnia

Several botanicals are strongly recommended to aid in sleep by producing a calming and relaxing effect on the central nervous system. Research findings showed that sleep patterns improved significantly without morning grogginess (*Consumer Reports*, 1999). These remedies should not be used in combination with sedating drugs. (Bilger, 1999). Recently reported side effects are heart palpitations and upset stomach (*Consumer Reports*, 1999).

Migraine Headaches

Migraine headaches are described by a lateralized or generalized throbbing or dull ache associated with nausea, vomiting, blurred vision, and photophobia. These headaches may last several hours or longer (Keville, 1996, p. 36). Of note is that **feverfew** (*Chrysanthemum parthenium*), known also as featherfew or altamisa, is very helpful in vascular-related headaches. British research found that this remedy was effective in reducing the severity as well as the frequency of migraine (Dickstein, 1999; Gottlieb, 1995). A woman who is pregnant should avoid this remedy as it promotes menstruation and stimulates action of the womb (Herbal Research Publications, 1995). Also, if a woman takes **feverfew** by eating the leaves, it is strongly recommended that she take only a few leaves—such as three or four each day. It has been reported that on occasion, a woman develops mouth ulcers (*Consumer Reports,* 1999; Kowalchik & Hylton, 1987). It is also recommended that **ginkgo** (*Ginkgo biloba*) be prepared from the root of this herb (Herbal Research Publications, 1995).

Osteoporosis

Wild yam root (*Dioscorea villosa*) is one herb used in treating osteoporosis.

Senile Dementia

A few herbs are suggested to avoid the severity of symptoms associated with senile dementia. Of particular note is that if a woman has high blood pressure, she should avoid **blue cohosh** (*Caulophyllum thalictroides*).

Stress

Herbs have been used for stress because of their ability to act on the nervous system, by inducing states of relaxation and tranquility; other herbs relax tense muscles, ease stress-related headaches, soothe an upset stomach, or encourage restful sleep (Orey, 1998). Consequently, many of these remedies help with several stress-related symptoms, including fatigue, insomnia, anxiety, and nervousness. Several commonly used herbal relaxants for stress are described.

Several varieties of **ginseng** (*Panax*) are used. Of the three types of ginseng, **Asian ginseng** is the most potent. (Dickstein, 1999). For ages, the **Siberian ginseng** (*Eleutherococcus senticosus*) variations of ginseng have been used to combat stress. Their benefit has been demonstrated in their effects on the adrenal functions, which increase when an individual encounters stress in one's daily life (Orey, 1998). Furthermore, herbalists label ginseng as an "adaptogen" because of its property to be a helpful boost to one's overall health and stamina (Orey, 1998). **American ginseng** (*Panax quinquefolium*) is known to be helpful with fatigue. It is interesting to note that, while side effects are rare with the American ginseng, there have been some reports of insomnia and allergic symptoms while taking the herb. **Asian ginseng—Korean, Chinese** (*Panax ginseng*) helps in states of exhaustion. It is considered more powerful and stimulating than the American ginseng. There are three situations in which to avoid this herb (Orey, 1998): (1) too close to bedtime since it is much more stimulating than the American ginseng; (2) with coffee; and (3) in the presence of high blood pressure. **Siberian ginseng** (*Eleutherococcus senticosus*), also known as eleuthero, helps the body adapt to physical, mental, and emotional stress. It also stimulates the immune system, thereby increasing the body energy and vitality in order to combat fatigue. This ginseng is more powerful than the Asian ginseng. With this herb, the two major precautions are (1) to avoid taking too close to bedtime, since it is much more stimulating than the American ginseng; and (2) to avoid taking in the presence of hypoglycemia, high blood pressure, or heart conditions.

Herbal remedies are relatively safe and effective, but if certain herbs are taken along with prescription medications, the interaction of the herbal remedy with the prescribed drug can be dangerous. Recently the American Medical Association (AMA) conducted several studies on various herbal remedies. The AMA reported that ginseng should not be used with the following: (1) drugs such as warfarin, heparin, aspirin, and other nonsteroidal anti-inflammatory drugs because it can inhibit clotting; and (2) estrogens or corticosteroids because ginseng may increase the side effects of those drugs. Diabetics should not use any ginseng because it can affect the blood glucose levels. Ginseng may cause headache, tremulousness, and manic episodes in patients treated with phenelzine sulfate.

Varicose Veins

Women experience problems with varicose veins approximately three times more often than do men (Bratman, 1998). The predominant symptoms are pain, tiredness, and heaviness in the legs. Research results indicate that **horse chestnut seed** (*Aesculus hippocastanum*) produces significant improvement in leg pain, swelling, and sensation of heaviness (Bratman, 1998). This remedy should be taken orally in a controlled release, enteric-coated form to avoid stomach discomfort. If this remedy is in the form of cream and applied externally to the skin, however, there are no untoward reactions (Khalsa, 1998). This remedy should be avoided if a person is taking anticoagulants or has serious kidney or liver ailments. Safety in pregnancy and nursing has not been established (Bratman, 1998). Occasionally this herb may cause itching (Bilger, 1999). **Gotu kola** (*Centella asiatica*) has been useful in reducing ankle edema and foot swelling (Bratman, 1998). It should be noted, however, that its safety in pregnancy and nursing has not been established.

Additional suggested remedies for varicose veins include **butcher's broom** (*Ruscus aculeatus*) (Bratman, 1998) and **bilberry** (*Vaccinum myrtillus*), also known as whortleberry or huckleberry, and rich in antioxidants (Bratman, 1998; Toscano, 1998). Research findings have shown that this therapeutic agent provided significant symptomatic improvement with varicose veins (Bratman, 1998). **Grapeseed** (*Vitis vinifera, Vitis coignetiae*), also known as muskat, is helpful in improving poor blood circulation (Toscano, 1998).

Table 11–3 presents a quick reference for the herbal remedies discussed in this section as they apply to general conditions prevalent among women.

Table 11–3 Recommended Herbal Remedies for Common Conditions

Common Name	Botanical Name
Recommendations for Alzheimer's Disease	
Gotu Kola	*Centella asiatica*
Ginkgo	*Ginkgo Biloba*
Recommendations for Anxiety	
Hops	*Humulus lupulus*
Kava kava	*Piper methysticum*
Passionflower	*Passiflora incarnata*
Valerian	*Valeriana officinalis*
Recommendations for Depression	
Borage	*Borago officinalis*
Ginseng	*Panax*
Gotu kola	*Centella asiatica*

continues

Table 11–3 continued

Common Name	Botanical Name
Rosemary	*Rosmarinus officinalis*
St. John's wort	*Hypericum perforatum*

Recommendations for Arthritis

General arthritic symptoms
Black cohosh	*Cimicifuga racemosa*
Comfrey	*Symphylum officinale*
Dandelion root	*Taxaracum officinale*
Feverfew	*Chrysanthemum parthenium*
Ginger	*Zingiber officinale*
Goldenrod	*Solidago* spp.
Juniper	*Juniperus communis*
Licorice	*Glycyrrhiza glabra*
Mustard	*Brassica supp.*
Poplar	*Populus supp.*
Wormwood	*Artemisia absinthium*

Osteoarthritis
Boswellia	*Boswellia serrata*
Passionflower	*Passiflora incarnata*
Valerian	*Valeriana officinalis*

Rheumatoid arthritis
Arnica	*Arnica montana*
Cayenne	*Capsicum annum*
Celery seeds	*Apium graveolens*
Cleavers	*Galium aparine*
Turmeric	*Curcuma longa*
Devil's claw	*Harpagophytum procumbens*
Evening primrose oil	*Oenothera biennis*
Ginger	*Zingiber officinale*
Licorice	*Glycyrrhiza glabra*
Meadowsweet	*Filipendula ulmaria or Spiraea ulmaria*
Nettles	*Urtica dioica*
Oatstraw	*Avena sativa*
Prickley ash bark	*Zanthoxylum clava-herculis*
Rosemary	*Rosmarinus officinalis*
Skullcap	*Scutellaria lateriflora*
Vervain	*Verbena officinalis*
Willow bark	*Salix alba*
Wild yam root	*Dioscorea villosa*

continues

Table 11–3 continued

Common Name	Botanical Name

Recommendations for Chronic Fatigue Syndrome

To improve the immune functions

Astragalus	*Astragalus membranaceus*
Burdock root	*Arctium lappa*
Dandelion leaf	*Taraxacum officinale*
Echinacea	*Echinacea angustifolia*
Red clover	*Trifolium pratense*

To improve circulation and brain function

Ginkgo	*Ginkgo biloba*

To improve sleep disturbances

Skullcap	*Scutellaria lateriflora*
Valerian	*Valeriana officinalis*

To support other symptoms

Goldenseal	*Hydrastis canadensis*
Licorice	*Glycyrrhiza glabra*

Recommendations for Digestive Problems

Anise	*Pimpinella anisum*
Camomile	*Matricaria chamomilla, Matricaria recutita*
Meadowsweet	*Filipendula ulmaria* or *Spiraea ulmaria*
Milk thistle	*Silybum marianum*

Recommendations for Edema

Dandelion root leaf	*Taraxacum officinale*

Recommendations for Fatigue

Siberian ginseng	*Eleutherococcus senticosus*

Recommendations for Fibromyalgia

Turmeric	*Curcuma longa*
Grapeseed extract	*Vitis vinifera, Vitis coignetiae*
Astragalus root	*Astragalus membranaceus*

Recommendations for Heart Problems

Hawthorn	*Crataegus oxyacantha, Crataegus monogyna, Crataegus laevigata*

Recommendations for High Cholesterol

Evening primrose oil	*Oenothera biennis*
Fenugreek	*Trigonella foenum-graecum*
Flaxseed	*Linum usitatissimum*
Garlic	*Allium sativum*
Oatstraw	*Avena sativa*

continues

Table 11–3 continued

Common Name	Botanical Name
Linseed oil	*Linum usitatissimum*
Motherwort	*Leonurus cardiaca*
Olive oil	*Olea europaea*
Safflower oil	*Carthamus tinctorius*
Sunflower oil	

Recommendations for Hypertension

Black cohosh	*Cimicifuga racemosa*
Black currant oil	
Borage oil	*Borago officinalis*
Dong quai	*Angelica sinensis*
Evening primrose oil	*Oenothera biennis*
Motherwort	*Leonurus cardiaca*
Herbs containing linoleic acids	
Safflower oil	*Carthamus tinctorius*
Sunflower oil	
Linseed oil	

Recommendations for Insomnia

Chamomile	*Matricaria recutita*
Hops	*Humulus lupulus*
Kava kava	*Piper methysticum*
Lemon balm	*Melissa officinalis*
Passionflower	*Passiflora incarnata*
Skullcap	*Scutellaria lateriflora*
Valerian	*Valeriana officinalis*

Recommendations for Migraine Headaches

Feverfew	*Chrysanthemum parthenium*
Gingko	*Gingko biloba*

Recommendations for Osteoporosis

Wild yam root	*Dioscorea villosa*

Recommendations for Senile Dementia (Senility)

To improve mental function	
Anise	*Pimpinella anisum*
Blue cohosh	*Caulophyllum thalictroides*
To improve cerebral circulation	
Ginkgo	*Ginkgo biloba*

Recommendations for Stress

Varieties of ginseng	*Panax*

continues

Table 11–3 continued

Common Name	Botanical Name
American ginseng	Panax quinquefolium
Asian ginseng	
Korean, Chinese	Panax ginseng
Siberian ginseng	Eleutherococcus senticosus
Gotu kola	Centella asiatica
Kava kava	Piper methysticum
Passionflower	Passiflora incarnata
Skullcap	Scutellaria laterifloa

Recommendations for Varicose Veins

Horse chestnut seed	Aesculus hippocastanum
Gotu kola	Centella asiatica
Additional remedies for varicose veins	
Butcher's broom	Ruscus aculeatus
Bilberry	Vaccinum myrtillus
Grapeseed	Vitis vinifera, Vitis coignetiae

Source: Data from E. Mindell and C. Colman, *Earl Mindell's Herb Bible.* © 1992, Simon & Schuster.

SUMMARY

An overview of herbal remedies has been described. Their importance, safety, and effectiveness were highlighted. In addition, the uses of herbs, their cautions, and the best ways to store herbs were also discussed. Herbal therapy as one approach to helping various women's health conditions and symptoms has become increasingly popular. Several women's conditions have been briefly described with recommended remedies for each condition given. Also, general conditions that are frequently experienced by women were also identified and described with suggested remedies.

REVIEW AND DISCUSSION

See boxes "Patient Education" and "Continuing Questions/Challenges" for discussion topics for this chapter.

Patient Education

Various herbs are useful for various women's conditions:
Cystitis
Fibrocystic breast disease
Ovarian cysts
Uterine fibroids
Endometriosis
Menstrual difficulties
Premenstrual syndrome
Vaginitis
Infertility
Pregnancy
Childbirth
Lactation difficulties
Menopausal difficulties
Hormone replacement

Continuing Questions/Challenges

What issues must be considered in regard to regulation of herbs?
How can health care providers make sure that patients understand that traditional medicines and herbs may interact in ways that can be dangerous?

REFERENCES

Bilger, B. (1999). Herbal lessons from Europe. *Health, 13*(2), 96–99.

Blumenthal, M. (1998). Name that herb? Understanding botanical nomenclature. *Natural Pharmacy, 2*(12), 20–21.

Blumenthal, M. (1999). The roots of herbal medicine. *Natural Pharmacy, 3*(2), 16–19.

Bratman, S. (1998). Alternative view: Varicose veins and venous insufficiency. *Your Health, 37*(6), 21.

Braverman, E. (1999). Nutrition for the heart, Pt. 1: Nutritive approaches for heart health. *Natural Pharmacy, 3*(2), 1, 10.

Brevoort, P. (1998). The booming US botanical market: A new overview. *Herbal Gram, 44*, 33–48.

Bucco, G. (1998). Joint relief: Easing osteoarthritis discomfort. *Herbs for Health, 3*(5), 50–55.

Challem, J., & Berkson, A. (1999). Science literature watch. *Natural Pharmacy, 3*(2), 21.

Consumer Reports. (1999). Herbal rx: The promises and pitfalls. *Consumer Reports, 64*(3), 44–48.

Copstead, L., & Banasik, J. (2000). *Pathophysiology: Biological and behavioral perspectives* (2nd ed.). Philadelphia: W.B. Saunders Co.

Dale, T. (1997). Women, hormones and success. *Explorer, 7*(6), 25.

Dickstein, L. (1999). A guide to natural health. *Psychology Today, 32*(2), 37–52.

Elias, J., & Masline, S. (1995). *Healing herbal remedies.* New York: Dell Publishing.

Emerich, M. (1999). Pharmaceutical giants enter the $400 million herb remedy market. *Natural Pharmacy, 3*(1), 15.

Foster, S. (1996). *Herbs for your health.* Loveland, CA: Interweave Press.

Gardner, C. (1999). Alternative medicine corner: Ease through menopause with homeopathic and herbal medicine. *Pittsburgh Boomers, 1*(1), 14.

Gluck, R. (1998). Natural ways to ease menopause. *Energy Times, 8*(10), 66–72.

Gottlieb, B. (Ed.) (1995). *New choices in natural healing.* Emmaus, PA: Rodale Press.

Green, C. (1998). *Conventional medicine: Alternative medicine.* St. Louis, MO: Mosby.

Greenwalk, J. (1998, November 23). Herbal Healing. *Time* (ed. CAN), 49.

Hardy, M. (1998). Herb-drug interactions: To mix or not to mix? *Herbs for Health, 3*(5), 41.

Herbal Research Publications. (1995). *Naturopathic handbook of herbal formulas: A practical and concise herb users' guide* (4th ed.). Ayer, MA: Author.

Hoffman, D. (1998). *The herbal handbook: A user's guide to medical herbalism.* Rochester, VT: Healing Arts Press.

Holmes, P. (1996). *Jade remedies: A Chinese herbal reference for the west.* Boulder, CO: Snow Lotus Press.

Keville, K. (1996). *Herbs for health and healing.* Emmaus, PA: Rodale Press.

Khalsa, K. (1998). Salvation: Herbal balms for aches and pains. *Herbs for Health, 3*(5), 40–49.

Kowalchik, C., & Hylton, W. (Eds.). (1987). *Rodale's illustrated encyclopedia of herbs.* Emmaus, PA: Rodale Press.

Laign, J. (1998). *1999 Herbal directory.* Boca Raton, FL: Globe International.

LaValle, J. (1999). A contemporary look at fibromyalgia (FM). *Natural Pharmacy, 3*(1), 6–7.

Loecher, B., & O'Donnell, S. (1997). In Faelten. (Ed.). *New choices in natural healing for women: Drug-free remedies from the world of alternative medicine.* Emmaus, PA: Rodale Press.

Marti, J., & Hine, A. (1998). *The alternative health and medical encyclopedia* (2nd ed.). New York: Visible Ink Press.

Mayo, A., & Mayo, J. (1999). 35 Simple ways to manage menopause. *Natural Health, 29*(2), 100.

Mindell, E., & Colman, C. (1992). *Earl Mindell's herb bible.* New York: Simon & Schuster.

Monte, T. (1997). *The Complete Guide to Natural Healing.* New York: Perigee Books.

Murray, M., & Pizzorno, J. (1998). *Encyclopedia of natural medicine* (2nd ed.). Rocklin, CA: Prima Publishing.

Natural Pharmacy. (1998). News wire. *Natural Pharmacy, 2*(12), 4.

Northrup, C. (1998). *Women's bodies, women's wisdom.* New York: Bantam Books.

Orey, C. (1998) Natural ways to feel calm and collected. *Energy Times 8*(10), 33–38.

Pillitteri, A. (1995). *Maternal and child health nursing* (2nd ed.). Philadelphia: J.B. Lippincott.

Snyderman, N. L. (1996). *Dr. Nancy Snyderman's guide to good health for women over forty.* San Diego: Harcourt Brace & Company.

Spencer, J., & Jacobs, J. (Eds.). (1999). *Complementary/alternative medicine: An evidence-based approach.* St Louis: Mosby.

Starbuck, J. (1998). 7 Herbs for women: Herbal wisdom *from* women *for* women. *Better Nutrition, 60*(12), 40–45.

Sundermann, A. (1999). Kava eases menopausal anxiety, studies show. *Herbs for Health, 3*(7), 74.

Toscano, M. (1998, November). Risks and rewards: What you need to know about the 22 bestsellers. *Self,* 163–165.

Walker, L. (1998). New directions in nutrition. *Energy Times 8*(10), 25–30.

Whittaker, D. (1999, March/April). Herbs for balance: PMS relief. *Herbs for Health, 3*(7), 7–10.

Youngkin, E., & Davis, M. (1994). *Women's health.* Norwalk, CT: Appleton, Lange

---

SUGGESTED READINGS

Awang, D. (1998). Legal and regulatory. *Herbal Gram, 44,* 26–27.

Cabrera, C. (1998). Canadian regulatory update. *Herbal Gram, 44,* 42–44.

Chillot, R. (1998). Health news. *Prevention, 50*(11), 34.

Duke, J. (1997). *The green pharmacy.* Emmaus, PA: Rodale Press.

Froemming, P. (1998). *The best guide to alternative medicine.* Los Angeles: Renaissance.

Gladstar, R. (1993). *Herbal healing for women.* New York: Simon & Schuster.

Griggs, B. *Green pharmacy.* Rochester, VT: Healing Arts Press.

Heusel, C. (1998, November). *Self*'s Ultimate guide to herbal medicines. *Self,* 110–167.

Kernion, M. (1998). *Natural with herbs.* Pleasant Grove, UT: Woodland Publishing.

Kessler, D. (1996). *The doctor's complete guide to healing herbs.* New York: Berkeley Books.

Kroeger, H. (1998). *Heal your life with home remedies and herbs.* Carlsbad, CA: Hay House, Inc.

Kroeger, H. (1998). *Healing with herbs a–z.* Carlsbad, CA: Hay House, Inc.

Landis, R. (1997). *Herbal defense: Positioning yourself to triumph over illness and aging.* New York: Warner.

Loecher, B., O'Donnel, S.A., and Editors of *Prevention Magazine*. (1997). *New choices in natural healing for women* (p. 172). Emmaus, PA: Rodale Press, Inc.

Murray, M. (1995). *The healing power of herbs*. Rocklin, CA: Prima Health.

Romm, A. (1998). Understanding phytoestrogens. *Natural Pharmacy, 2*(8), 1, 12.

Shaw, N. (1998). *Herbal medicine: A step-by-step guide*. Boston, MA: Element Books.

Whitaker, J. (1996). *Dr. Whitaker's guide to natural healing*. Rocklin, CA: Prima Publishing Co.

Yarnell, E., & Meserole, L. (1997). Toxic botanicals: Is the poison in the plant or its regulation? *Alternative Complementary Therapy, 4*, 3–19.

CHAPTER 12

Homeopathic Remedies for Women's Wellness

Natalie Pavlovich

Key Points

- Homeopathy stimulates the body's own healing process.
- Homeopathy is based on the theory that illness is a result of a distrubance of the body's vital force, leading to an imbalance in the body's energy (symptoms of a disease represent the body's attempts to heal itself).
- Homeopathic remedies stimulate and increase this vital force and restore balance.
- The person's symptoms are matched with the precise homeopathic remedy.
- There are three major principles of homeopathy (Hahneman's Laws).
  1. The law of similar ("like cures like")
     A substance that can produce symptoms of illness in a well person can, with minute doses, cure similar symptoms in an ill person.
  2. The minimum dose law
     The smallest amount possible is needed to stimulate the body's own natural defense.
  3. The single remedy law
     Only one remedy at a time is administered to a person.
- The healing process (Hering's four laws of cure) occurs in an ordered fashion.
  Healing takes place from the top to the bottom.
  Healing takes place from the inside to the outside.

Healing occurs first in the most important organs and then in the least important organs.

Healing occurs when the symptoms disappear in reverse order of their appearance (emotions usually improve first and then physical symptoms improve).

To better accept the paradox behind homeopathy, it helps to consider other, more conventional medical treatments: If you take allergy desensitization shots, you regularly receive a tiny amount of the very substance that makes you sneeze, wheeze or itch. Eventually, your body will develop a tolerance to that substance and your symptoms will stop.

—Loecher & O'Donnell, 1997, p. 186

Homeopathy, which was originally developed in Europe, is practiced throughout the world. In England, hospitals exist that are devoted exclusively to homeopathy. In France, every apothecary (pharmacy) dispenses homeopathic remedies. Many German physicians practice homeopathy. In the United States at the beginning of the twentieth century, there were many homeopathic hospitals, but these hospitals gradually closed their doors during the century's first four decades. As we approach the twenty-first century, a renewed interest in homeopathy, which is growing at approximately 25% per year, has become apparent in America (White, 1998).

HOMEOPATHIC PRINCIPLES

The root of the word *homeopathy* comes from two Greek words: *homios,* which means *like,* and *pathos,* which means *suffering.* Homeopathy, in modern society, is described as treating "like with like." The science of homeopathy was discovered in the early 1800s by Dr. Samuel Hahnemann (1755–1843), a physician and chemist (Cummings & Ullman, 1997). The basic premise underlying the science of homeopathy is that it stimulates the body's own healing process to cure illnesses naturally. Homeopathy is based on the recognition that illness emerges as a result of a disturbance of the body's vital force, causing an imbalance in the energy within a person. Homeopathic remedies stimulate and increase this vital force and restore balance to it, facilitating the body's innate healing ability. Each homeopathic remedy has several characteristics that influence recommendations for a specific woman. In essence, the homeopathic practitioner aims to match the woman's symptoms with the precise remedy (Fein, 1998).

As a result of Hahnemann's work, three major principles were developed: (1) law of similar, (2) minimum dose, and (3) single remedy. Each of these principles serves a unique role in stimulating the body's healing ability.

The law of similar in Latin is known as *similia similibus curentur*, which, translated literally, means "like cures like." In the law of similar, a substance that can produce symptom(s) of the illness in a well person can, with minute doses, cure similar symptom(s) of the illness (Shealy, 1996). Hahnemann showed that, if a healthy person took a substance from any natural source such as a mineral or plant, the substance produced symptoms. When an ill person took the remedy, it alleviated the similar symptoms that the person experienced with the illness. In this case, the substance was helpful in stimulating the body's vital force in order to alleviate the specific condition or symptoms. The closer the match between the person's symptoms and the remedy symptoms, the more effective the remedy will be.

The minimum dose law is the belief that the smallest dose possible is needed to stimulate the body's own natural defense system within a period of time. Hahneman claimed that when diluting a remedy, its curative properties are enhanced and any side effects are eliminated. This is much more effective in the healing process to alleviate symptoms and cure illnesses. Once the client feels the symptoms are eliminated, indicating that the body's own healing forces are stimulated, the remedy usually is discontinued.

The single remedy law is the notion that only one remedy at a time be administered to the client. A single remedy contains one single homeopathic substance. When given, it produces its own unique set of symptoms. Today, the practitioners who use this approach have become known as classic homeopathic practitioners. Sometimes, in homeopathy, some practitioners use what is known in complementary health as "combinations." This means that two or more homeopathic ingredients are used. Usually these combinations are developed for the treatment of acute symptoms or conditions. The specific formulas contain ingredients that complement one another and cover the total symptom profile of a particular condition. There are health situations for which it is difficult to find a single remedy that will cover all aspects of the person's illness. These combination preparations thus offer a way to handle the entire symptomatic pattern that the client presents.

These three principles of homeopathy reflect the notion that the symptoms of a disease represent the body's attempt to heal itself. By administering minute amounts of a remedy, which produce the same symptoms as the illness, the healing process is reinforced. In other words, homeopathic remedies work with the body, rather than against it. Underpinning these basic philosophical principles is that "a person's constitution is made up of inherited and acquired physical, mental, and emotional characteristics and that these can be matched to a particular remedy that will improve their health no matter what their illness" (Shealy, 1996, p. 83). The application of these principles emphasizes the philosophical foundation of individuality, wherein each person is considered and treated as an individual. The practitioner assesses the person's physical signs and symptoms, emotional aspects, physical responses to daily activities, and of course, personality and body type. All of these aspects together provide a basis for treating the whole person rather than each isolated symptom.

HOMEOPATHY AND THE HEALING PROCESS

Another pioneer in the history of homeopathy was Constantine Hering (1800–1880), who was a student of Dr. Hahnemann. Constantine Hering became known as the "father of homeopathy" in America, as he was the founder of the first schools and hospitals in which homeopathy was taught throughout the United States.

Hering established the *laws of cure,* which are often referred to as "Hering's Laws," based on his observations of how healing occurs. These laws identify the vital aspects of the healing process that occur within the person. These laws are described below.

Healing takes place from the top to the bottom. Any symptom or ailment associated with the head area heals first, before the symptoms in the feet. Another illustration is that the symptoms disappear first from the shoulders, then the elbow, and on down the arm.

Healing takes place from inside to outside. This law refers to the fact that the kidneys, located in the back of the abdominal cavity on each side of the spinal column, heal before the symptoms associated with the toes.

Healing occurs from the most important organs to the least important organs. The symptoms move from the major or vital organs to the less vital or minor ones. Symptoms associated with any conditions of the heart will disappear first before those symptoms associated with the intestines.

*Healing occurs when the symptoms disappear in reverse order of their ap-
pearance, with emotions improving first, then the physical symptoms.* An
example of this law is the instance in which a person developed the flu
or a cold. Meanwhile, that person may have been struggling with
chronic fatigue for several months. Those symptoms related to the flu
or cold will disappear before those chronic fatigue symptoms clear. We
can see that the healing process occurs in the reverse order to the onset
of the symptoms (Hardy & Nonman, 1994).

According to the laws of cure, a person's health seems to get worse
before it improves. When a person shows a reaction during the healing
process, one has to decide if it is a positive reaction. In assessing the
client's responses, Hammond (1995) notes that those more incidental
or peculiar symptoms are the most valuable. Those symptoms tend to
reflect the particular character of the ailment, guiding the choice of
remedy. These most valuable symptoms are known as "rubrics" in homeopathic terminology.

Homeopathy focuses on the entire person, not a particular part. This
holistic approach helps the practitioner to match descriptions of one's
health experience as specifically as possible to a particular homeopathic remedy. The homeopathic practitioner finds in each remedy
the totality of symptoms that reflect the disease in the person. Taylor
described the uniqueness of homeopathic remedies in that the treatment is truly mirrored with the ailment (Taylor 1998). The homeopathic approach emphasizes the uniqueness of each person based on
the belief that no two individuals experience their illnesses in exactly
the same way, even if the ailment is the same. These experiential differences are influenced by one's response to the environment. According to homeopathic theory, everything in our environment has a direct effect on our health status.

HOMEOPATHIC REMEDIES

The homeopathic remedies are made from herbs, plants, and earth
minerals to stimulate the body's vital force. Approximately 80% of the
homeopathic remedies are botanical in origin. A few examples of these
are goldenseal (*Hydrastis canadensis*), mountain arnica (*Arnica
montana*), and deadly nightshade (*Belladonna*). On the other hand,
there are homeopathic remedies prepared from minerals or mineral
ores, such as potassium bichromate (*Kali bichromicum*), and sulfur. Still
other remedies are made from animal sources, such as the honeybee
(*Apis mellifica*), the cuttlefish ink (*Sepia*), or the Spanish fly (*Cantharis*).

Since homeopathy is practiced in many different countries, the homeopathic remedies are identified by their Latin names in order to eliminate the confusion that different languages might cause. Furthermore, the Latin name helps to create a way of standardization of reference for these remedies. Homeopathic practitioners generally refer to the remedies by their abbreviated name. For instance, *Natrum muraticum* is referred to as *Nat. mur.* or *Calcium carbonica* is commonly known as *Calc. carb.*

When a person begins to take a homeopathic remedy, he or she may sometimes experience an initial worsening of the condition. This process is known as a healing crisis or "proving," and is a signal of the body's increased activity toward healing. This healing crisis usually passes quickly. When a healing crisis occurs, the individual is advised to discontinue therapy until the symptoms subside or are minimized. The practitioner will then reintroduce the remedy at a lower dose. A major advantage of the healing crisis is that this phenomenon indicates that the proper remedy has been discovered for the person, that is, the appropriateness of the particular remedy has been "proven."

Preparation and Use of Homeopathic Remedies

Homeopathic remedies are prepared in various forms, including sprays, pellets, tablets, liquids, and a few as suppositories or ointments. The liquid remedy should remain in the mouth for a minimum of 15 seconds before swallowing. When using two or more remedies, it is suggested that the client separate the dosage by 10 minutes. The tablets/pellets should be placed under the tongue and allowed to dissolve slowly without chewing, being held there for a minute or two so that the substance of the remedy may pass through the mucous membranes and into the tiny blood vessels lining the area, bypassing the digestive juices, which can interfere with the action of the remedy. There is no difference in these forms from the standpoint of efficacy; it is a matter of one's preference. Some health care practitioners prefer pellets because they were the first form used by Hahnemann. With children, practitioners prefer the tablets because they are easily crushed for administration, and children are usually less resistant to taking these remedies in that form.

The manufacture and sale of homeopathic remedies are regulated by the Food and Drug Administration (FDA). The FDA provides official recognition of each remedy found in the *Homeopathic Pharmacopoeia of the United States* (HPUS), since the federal agency considers HPUS as the official compendia (reference guide) for homeopathic remedies. In 1988, the FDA approved the Compliance Policy Guide, which provides guidelines for labeling and selling homeopathic remedies.

Clinical "Pearls" Regarding Homeopathic Remedies

The handling, administering, and storing of homeopathic remedies (particularly those in liquid or tablet form) are very important. Five tips for use are the following:

1. The homeopathic remedies or the bottle dropper should be handled as little as possible. This is a source of contamination and may reduce the effectiveness of the product.
2. The mouth should be in its natural condition. That is, these remedies should not be taken at least 15 minutes before or 30 minutes after eating, brushing one's teeth or drinking anything other than water.
3. When using homeopathic remedies, it is best to eliminate the use of certain foods, toiletries, and medications, because they may act as an antidote to the effectiveness of the homeopathic remedy. It is strongly recommended that the client avoid caffeine-containing beverages, alcohol, and tobacco, as well as beverages, candies, medicines, or ointments with mint or menthol ingredients, as these may interfere with the effectiveness of homeopathic therapy. Caffeine is thought to alter the response of the body to the homeopathic remedies. Coffee is a homeopathic remedy in itself, known as *Coffea cruda,* which may alter the body's response to other homeopathic remedies. Examples of camphor products and strong aromatic compounds are strongly perfumed cosmetics, Vicks VapoRub, topical counter irritants, mint foods, aromatic oils, mint toothpastes, and schnapps. It is believed that all of these interfere with the effectiveness of the homeopathic therapy. For anyone taking homeopathic remedies, it is strongly recommended that she refrain from smoking tobacco because nicotine may alter the response of the body to homeopathic remedies.
4. Any homeopathic remedy should be stored at room temperature out of direct sunlight and extremes of temperature. These remedies should also be stored away from any aromatic substances such as perfume, household ammonia, and paint. Homeopathic remedies should be taken only for as long as one needs them.

5. The *Materia Medica* (Kent, 1997) is a resource that describes ho-meopathic remedies. It lists the symptoms, indications, and con-ditions that make the symptoms worse or better.

COMMON HOMEOPATHIC REMEDIES FOR SPECIFIC AILMENTS AND CONDITIONS RELATED TO THE HEALTH OF WOMEN

Ullman (1995, p. 190) reported, ". . . approximately two thirds of homeopathic patients and purchasers of homeopathic products are women." In this section, ailments common to women are identified with a description of the homeopathic remedies appropriate for each ailment or condition. The reference for these descriptions is Kent's *Lectures on Homeopathic Materia Medica* (1997). In the first part of this section, remedies for the symptoms and illnesses common to women are identified. Then, those remedies for general conditions related to women are described briefly.

There are several effective homeopathic remedies used for common problems related to women's health. In homeopathy, the remedy to use is the one whose description most closely resembles the woman's symptoms. In general, if there is no improvement, then a different remedy should be considered. This listing of remedies includes a brief relevant description of symptoms associated with the particular rem-edy. (Among homeopaths, this is referred to as the "symptom-pic-ture.") This symptom brief provides information upon which to choose the remedy, based upon the one remedy that covers most of the main symptoms that the woman experiences. The goal is to select the best fit or the best match between the woman's symptoms and the remedy's characteristics. A few reports of adverse reactions have been reported for some remedies. These are indicated whenever the specific remedy is mentioned. Remedies for the following conditions are listed: cystitis, premenstrual syndrome (PMS), menstrual difficulties/irregu-larities, vaginitis, pregnancy, and menopause.

Cystitis

The remedies for bladder infection are based on three categories: (1) acute or chronic cystitis, (2) acute cystitis, and (3) chronic cystitis.

Acute or Chronic Cystitis

Arsenicum album (white arsenic)—An indication for this remedy is that the woman feels as though her bladder is not emptying properly;

she experiences burning in the bladder; a bloated abdomen; a copious white vaginal discharge; yeast infection; and she feels anxious and restless. These symptoms are often worse in women with diabetes (Kent, 1997; Lockie & Geddes, 1994).

Berberis vulgaris (barberry)—The major indications for this remedy include cutting or shooting pains in the bladder extending down into the pelvic area and thighs during and after urination, and incomplete feeling after urination with the sensation of some urine remaining in the bladder (Jonas & Jacobs, 1996; Kent, 1997).

Cantharis (Spanish fly)—The predominant indications for this remedy include cutting pain in the bladder before, during, and after urination; frequent strong urges to urinate; sensation of severe burning on urination as though it were scalding water; inadequate emptying of the bladder; scanty urine, with urination in painful drops; ache in small of the back that is worse in the afternoon; pain too severe to ignore; merest trickle of urine with blood in it; stricture of the urethra; and constant pain in the urethra that is worse after urination. These symptoms are aggravated by drinking cold water or coffee, before and after urination, and with touch (Jonas & Jacobs, 1996; Kent, 1997; Lockie & Geddes, 1994; Ullman, 1995).

Pulsatilla (windflower)—This remedy is considered in the presence of several symptoms, including constant pain in the urethra during and after urination as well as when lying down, which is worse after urinating; dull aching in the lower abdomen caused by delay in urinating; frequent urination; white, copious, nonirritating vaginal discharge or discharge suggestive of a yeast infection; burning or aching pain in the bladder, which is worse while urinating, upon waking, and after exposure to cold conditions; and chills after urinating. These symptoms are aggravated during the evening, after eating, and in the presence of heat (Kent, 1997; Lockie & Geddes, 1994; Ullman, 1995).

Sarsaparilla—The indications for this remedy are severe painful urination, especially at the end of urination; the presence of blood or pus in the last drops of urine; difficulty passing urine, especially during the day (standing up helps the urine to flow); burning pain; and constant urge to urinate (Ullman, 1995). This remedy is particularly effective for the genitourinary tract.

Sepia (cuttlefish ink)—This remedy is suggested if the following symptoms are experienced: pain in the urethra after urinating; aching, burning or shooting pain in the bladder, which is worse in evening and after urination; leaking of urine with delay in urination; sensation of few drops of urine having been passed; aching, dull pain in the lower abdomen if urination is delayed; copious, white vaginal discharge; and yeast infection. Symptoms are aggravated during pregnancy and during stress. These symptoms are also aggravated with any type of emotional upset, exposure to cold, before menstrual periods, and at dusk (Lockie & Geddes, 1994).

Staphysagria (stavesacre)—The major symptoms for this remedy include hypersensitivity of the genitals, burning during urination, the desire to urinate with a feeling of pressure in the bladder, and psychologically taking offense easily. The symptoms are made worse by indignation, tobacco, humiliation or sadness, and bottled-up anger and are better with warmth, rest, and after breakfast (Jonas & Jacobs, 1996; Kent, 1997). This homeopathic remedy is usually recommended for bladder symptoms that develop after sexual activity, especially with a new partner.

Sulfur (brimstone)—Indications for this remedy are bladder pain associated with cold; chills after urination; constant pain in the urethra, which is worse after urination; urine leakage with delayed urination; urge to urinate at night; frequent urination; bloated abdomen; yeast infection; copious, bland vaginal discharge; worse in diabetics; worse for stress. These symptoms became aggravated under stress, when standing still, washing, heat in all forms, and around 11 AM, as well as in women with diabetes (Kent, 1997; Lockie & Geddes, 1994).

Acute Cystitis

Apis mellifica (honeybee)—The indications for this remedy are frequent urge to urinate; scant, hot, and bloody urine; frequent urination; burning, sharp, stinging pain in the bladder, which is worse after urination; bloated abdomen; a copious, white vaginal discharge; and yeast infection (Ullman, 1995).

Belladonna (deadly nightshade)—The predominant symptoms for which this remedy is used include a burning sensation in the urethra; white vaginal discharge; sensation of lack of proper emptying of the bladder; bladder sensitive to jarring or any other motion; bright red urine and with little clots of blood; feeling of something moving inside the bladder; or restlessness at night with wild dreams. These symptoms are worse with noise, cold air, light, and jolting, as well as during pregnancy and in the presence of feeling anxious (Kent, 1997; Lockie & Geddes, 1994; Ullman, 1995).

Causticum (bisulfate of potash; Hahnemann's tincture)—The indications for this remedy include frequent urge to urinate; involuntary urination when coughing and sneezing; pain after urinating; itching around the opening of the urethra; sense of inadequate emptying of the bladder; copious vaginal discharge; and yeast infection. These symptoms are aggravated by pregnancy, anxiety, and in cold weather (Lockie & Geddes, 1994).

Concium maculatum (bitter apple)—An indication for this remedy is when the bladder feels as if it is not emptying properly; pain in bladder on walking; and a copious, white vaginal discharge. These symptoms are worse under stress or anxiety (Lockie & Geddes, 1994).

Mercurius vivus (quicksilver)—This remedy is recommended if the following symptoms are present: frequent urge to urinate with burning; copious, bland, white vaginal discharge; yeast infection; bloated abdomen; and alternating bouts of chills and sweating. Symptoms worse for stress. The symptoms are aggravated by extreme temperatures, stress, during the night, when not urinating, and with perspiration (Jonas & Jacobs, 1996; Kent,1997).

Chronic Cystitis

Concium maculatum (bitter apple)—The indications for this remedy are that the bladder feels as if it is not emptying properly; pain in bladder on waking; copious white vaginal discharge; worse for stress; feeling anxious.

Premenstrual Syndrome

Belladonna (deadly nightshade)—This remedy is recommended when headache and cramping are present with PMS. Other characteristics that are indicated for this remedy are experiencing acute pain with the menstrual cycle; pains tend to begin and end suddenly. The pain may take the form of cramps or something like labor pains; the woman feels intense weight and pressure in the lower abdomen and pelvis, sometimes as though the pelvic organs are about to fall out (Cummings & Ullman, 1997). This remedy too is indicated when motion, walking, or being jarred worsens it. Pain may be experienced from the region of the uterus and extend to the back; pain may be experienced in the ovaries prior or during the menstrual cycle.

Caulophyllum thalictroides (blue cohosh)—An indication for this remedy is when cramping pains are particularly severe before the menstrual flow begins. Pain in the small of the back or dizziness also may precede menstruation. These symptoms are aggravated by late menstruation, open air, and in the evening (Cummings & Ullman, 1997).

Chamomilla (German chamomile)—The indications for this remedy are marked irritability such as faultfinding or snapping over little things; noticing increase in pain with an increase in anger (emotional changes are the predominant symptom). *Chamomilla* should be given first for these symptoms, but when irritability is present in addition to that remedy's other characteristic symptoms, *Colocynthis* is recommended. The woman may experience sensations of weight, and bearing down also may occur in the pelvis. The menstrual pains are so intense that they may be felt acutely and cause the woman to cry out; especially with this distinguishing symptom, *Chamomilla* is the preferred remedy. These pains are alleviated by warmth.

Cimifuga racemosa (black snake root)—The predominant characteristics for this remedy are sharp pains that dart from side to side in the abdomen, marked lower back pain during the menstrual flow, and menstrual cramps that make the woman double over with pain; motion aggravates the existing pain. These symptoms are aggravated by motion, in the morning, during the menses, and if menstrual periods are missed (Cummings & Ullman, 1997; Kent, 1997).

Colocynthis (bitter cucumber)—The major characteristic for this remedy is that the menstrual cramps are unaccompanied by other symptoms. The woman may experience pain in the ovaries shortly before menses. Symptoms are often relieved with pressure, warmth, or bending forward. The symptoms, especially cramping, are aggravated when the woman becomes angry or if she suppresses angry feelings. Since the symptoms are similar to those that indicate use of *Magnesia phosphorica,* this remedy, too, may be used for these symptoms. The woman for whom *Colcynthis* is recommended is more likely to be irritable or angry than the woman for whom *Magnesia phosphorica* is appropriate (Cummings & Ullman, 1997; Kent, 1997).

Lachesis mutus (bushmaster snake)—A classic characteristic for this remedy is that the symptoms begin or worsen during sleep or immediately upon wakening. Other symptoms that are indicative of this remedy include experience of uterine pains; ovarian pains, especially on the left side; back pain; dizziness; headaches; and diarrhea. The symptoms may extend into the upper abdomen or chest. These symptoms may be severe prior to the beginning of the menstrual flow, and then suddenly decrease once menstruation actually begins. The woman usually feels better with menses, but she often feels worse after sleep and in the presence of heat. Uterine cramps and soreness are likely to be made worse from the pressure of clothing on the abdomen, such as tight belts or elastic bands.

Lycopodium clavatum (club moss)—The indications for this remedy are the following symptoms: irritability, apprehensiveness, bloating, flatulence, heartburn, digestive upset, wrinkled skin, sallow complexion, craving for sugar. Symptoms are better with hot food and drink, cool air, and moving around. The symptoms are worse with tight clothing around waist, after sleep, after eating oysters, and between 4 and 8 PM.

Magnesia phosphorica (phosphate of magnesia)—This remedy is considered with the following symptoms: spasmodic pains, severe cramps, headaches. This remedy is especially recommended if the menstrual cramps are unaccompanied by other symptoms and are relieved with the application of pressure or warmth, or when doubling over or bending forward. This remedy provides relief from the cramping menstrual pains. If the pain is centered in the uterus, it may radiate in all directions, The symptoms are aggravated by touch, movement, cold in any form, and at night (Cummings & Ullman, 1997).

Natrium muriaticum (sodium chloride, table salt)—The predominant symptoms for this remedy are: the women feels sad but cannot weep, craves salty foods, and is thirsty. Symptoms are aggravated by sun, heat, crying, and between 10 and 11 AM (Bellow, 1999).

Nux vomica (poison nut)—The indications include irritability, spasmodic episodes, feeling chilly, and desire for stimulants.

Pulsatilla (windflower)—This remedy helps with alleviating hot flashes and mood changes, including irritability during the menstrual cycle associated with PMS (Natural Pharmacy, Nov. 1998). The woman is usually sensitive, weepy, or depressed and needs and wants gentle comforting. The menstrual pains may be of any type and may be worse before or during the menstrual flow. Additional symptoms that the woman may experience are fainting, nausea and vomiting, diarrhea, back pain, dizziness, and headaches that precede or accompany menstruation. Finally, the woman has no thirst, heat worsens her condition, and open air makes it better (Cummings & Ullman, 1997).

Sepia (cuttlefish ink)—The prevailing characteristic symptoms for this homeopathic remedy are that the woman feels anxious, fearful, sad, and indifferent. The benefit of this remedy is that it helps in reducing the heightened emotional states.

Menstrual Difficulties/Irregularities: Dysmenorrhea

The common homeopathic remedies that are effective in alleviating the symptoms of dysmenorrhea are *Belladonna* (deadly nightshade), which has been previously mentioned; *Chamomilla* (German chamomile), which works well for irritability, moodiness, and unbearable pain, and symptoms that are aggravated by heat, touch, and anger, and at night; *Lachesis mutus* (bushmaster snake), which was previously mentioned; and *Pulsatilla* (windflower), which was previously mentioned.

Additional remedies for dysmenorrhea include **Kali carbonicum** (potassium carbonate), when symptoms are worse in the early morning hours; **Pulsatilla** (windflower), in the presence of scanty, irregular, and painful menstrual flow; restlessness; and alleviation of symptoms in presence of fresh air; **Sepia** (cuttlefish ink), in the presence of painful, irregular menses; heaviness in the abdomen; feeling cold even in a warm room; and when symptoms are alleviated after exercise.

Other herbal remedies that may be considered are listed below.

Cocculus indicus (Indian cockle)—The indications for this remedy are severe cramps, dizziness, weakness, exhaustion, irritability, hypersensitivity to pain, and profuse menses with dark blood. These symptoms are aggravated by tobacco smoke, fresh air, loss of sleep, and the thought or smell of foods.

Coffea cruda (unroasted coffee)—The predominant symptoms are becoming excitable; passing large, dark clots; feeling better with ice water and when lying down. The woman's symptoms are aggravated by warm drinks and by sudden emotions.

Magnesia phosphorica (phosphate of magnesia)—This remedy is considered with the following symptoms: spasmodic pains, severe cramps, headaches, feels better with warmth and bending double. The symptoms are aggravated by touch, movement, cold in any form, and at night.

Sabina (savine)—The major characteristic symptoms for this remedy are pain from the lower back to the lower abdomen (from sacrum to public bone); menses are profuse, heavy, and bright. The symptoms are aggravated by warm air.

Magnesia phosphorica (phosphate of magnesia)—This remedy is for menstrual cramps. It was previously mentioned under Premenstrual Syndrome.

Belladonna (deadly nightshade)—The indications for this remedy are sharp, cutting, or throbbing pain; a feeling of pressure in the pelvis as if the contents would fall out; pains are sudden in onset. These symptoms are worse on the right side (Jonas & Jacobs, 1996; Kent, 1997).

Nux vomica (poison nut)—The major indications for this remedy are that pains can be accompanied by nausea and chills; cramping pains can extend to the lower back with frequent urging to stool; constipation; marked oversensitivity; irritable, touchy; sensitive to light, noise, and odors. The symptoms are worse with exposure to cold; dry winds; after meals and overindulgence in food, drink, and stimulants such as spicy food, coffee, and alcohol; waking 3–4 AM. Symptoms are improved with heat and uninterrupted sleep. *Note:* it is suggested that this remedy is most effective when taken before going to bed.

Pulsatilla (windflower)—Indications for this remedy are nausea, pain in the back; pains are variable in type and can move from place to place at times.

Pregnancy: Morning Sickness

Colchicum (meadow saffron)—The indications for this remedy are nausea that is accompanied by a profound weakness, even to the point of fainting; pain in the stomach; gas; and vomiting of mucus, bile, and food; extreme nausea from the thought, smell, or sight of food, especially fish or eggs; thirst.

Ipecac (ipecac root)—The key symptom for this remedy is that the woman has a constant, persistent nausea with or without vomiting. Additional typical symptoms are that the woman is irritable; undecided as to what she wants; has a relaxed sensation in the stomach as if it is hanging down; has much saliva in the mouth. Symptoms are worse in winter; in dry weather; with a hot, humid wind; and with slightest motion. Symptoms are better with rest and open air.

Kreosotum (beechwood creosote)—As previously described, the nausea is worse in the morning and from the smell or sight of food. The woman feels depressed, wants to be left alone, and is extremely irritable. Symptoms are worse after eating cold foods and are better with warmth.

Phosphorus (phosphorus)—Indications for this remedy are that the woman has difficulty with concentration and uneasiness about being alone; has a strong craving for salt; is extremely thirsty for ice-cold drinks, which are vomited as soon as they become warm in the stomach. Symptoms are worse in the evening, with weather changes, during a thunderstorm, and when lying on the left side; the symptoms are better when eating or sleeping.

Pulsatilla (windflower)—The typical symptoms are very little thirst, even though the mouth is dry; the tongue is coated yellow or white; the woman is moody, weeping easily one minute, then quickly cheered up; has a bad taste in the mouth and a strong aversion to fatty or rich foods, which make the nausea worse.

Sepia (cuttlefish ink)—This remedy is considered with the following symptoms: has a strong desire for vinegar, pickles, and other acids; a yellowish discoloration across the nose and cheeks of some pregnant women, which is indicative of the need for this remedy. The symptoms are worse in the morning and from the smell or sight of food, kneeling, exposure to cold, emotional upset, and at dusk. The symptoms are better with firm pressure, naps, and strenuous exercise.

Vaginitis

Several homeopathic remedies have been helpful in alleviating the symptoms of vaginitis.

Arsenicum album (trioxide of arsenic)—This was previously mentioned under Acute or Chronic Cystitis.

Apis mellifica (honeybee)—This was previously mentioned under Acute Cystitis.

Borax (sodium borate)—The major symptoms are that the discharge is clear and thick, like the white of an egg, or is thick and white, like liquid starch or sometimes even like white paste; the discharge may be irritating to the genitals; there may be a sensation of warmth accompanying the discharge, perhaps as if warm water is flowing over the organs; the discharge may be worse midway between the menstrual cycles; and the woman may have a feeling of a dread, downward motion, digestive problems, and a marked sensitivity to sudden noises. The symptoms become better with cold weather but worse with smoking (Cummings & Ullman,1997). *Note:* These symptoms may not be present with every woman who has vaginitis.

Graphite (black lead-plumbago)—The indications for this remedy are that the woman has a thin, white, and burning discharge; walking may increase the discharge, and the discharge may be worse in the morning. The woman may feel weakness of the back or tension in the abdomen that accompanies the vaginitis (Cummings & Ullman, 1997).

Kreosotum (beechwood creosote)—This was previously mentioned under Pregnancy: Morning Sickness.

Mercurius vivus (quicksilver)—This was previously mentioned under Acute Cystitis.

Nitricum acidum (nitric acid)—The predominant indications for this remedy are that the discharge is greenish, brownish-tan colored or sometimes may appear like transparent, stringy mucus; and the discharge is acid, irritating and contains an offensive odor. As soon as the menstrual cycle begins, the symptoms are aggravated (Cummings & Ullman, 1997).

Pulsatilla (windflower)—This remedy is useful with any type of discharge or if there is the presence of a white discharge with the consistency of cream or milk and particularly if the general symptoms of this remedy are strongly present in the individual. These symptoms are that the women craves affection, has changeable moods; feels worse in a warm room, and has a weepy, clingy mood (Cummings & Ullman, 1997; Jonas & Jacobs, 1996). *Note:* This remedy is safe, and a woman who develops vaginitis during pregnancy can take this remedy without any reservation. Also, this homeopathic remedy has been helpful for pubescent girls with this problem (Cummings & Ullman, 1997; Kent, 1997).

Sepia (cuttlefish ink)—This remedy is indicated when the following characteristics are present: the flow is yellowish or greenish with an accompanying offensive order. The symptoms become worse shortly before the menstrual periods or midway between them. The woman will experience sensations of uncomfortable pressure and weight that are described as "bearing-down pains" in the pelvic organs and lower abdomen. The discharge is likely to be more profuse in the morning and when the woman walks (Cummings & Ullman, 1997; Jonas & Jacobs, 1996). *Note:* This remedy is recommended for a child with vaginitis (Cummings & Ullman, 1997).

Menopause

During menopause women experience several common symptoms that add to their discomfort. A recent survey conducted in London at the Royal London Homeopathic Hospital Women's Clinic indicated that approximately 70% of women felt a definite improvement in menopausal symptoms while using homeopathic remedies. About 25% of the women had some benefit and 5% indicated no change in their symptoms (Bello, 1999).

Cimicifuga racemosa (black snake root)—The indications for this remedy are hot flashes that improve at the onset of the menstrual flow, painful cramps, muscular pain, flushed face, general ill feeling. The symptoms are aggravated by missed menstrual periods, during the menses, and the morning cold.

Graphites (black lead—plumbago)—Major symptoms are hypersensitivity and sensitivity to cold. Symptoms are aggravated by dark; loose clothing (Bello, 1999; Kent, 1997).

Lachesis mutus (bushmaster snake)—This remedy is suggested when the following symptoms are evident: hot flashes, headache, bloating, and irritability; the women becomes talkative, may awaken to waves of bursting headaches, and feels worse from heat, after sleep, and with wearing of tight clothing around the neck or waist.

Natrium muriaticum (sodium chloride—table salt)—The predominant symptoms are that the woman feels sad but cannot weep, craves salty foods, and is thirsty. Symptoms are aggravated by sun, heat, and crying. Symptoms are worse between 10 and 11 AM (Bello, 1999).

Pulsatilla (windflower)—This remedy is considered with the following characteristic symptoms that the woman experiences: hemorrhoids and varicose veins may worsen during this transition; is sensitive to warm or stuffy rooms, desires the open, cold air even more during the hot flashes (Bello, 1999; Kent, 1997).

Sepia (cuttlefish ink)—The major symptoms for this remedy are hot flashes with chill and sweats; she feels worn out, has an aversion to sex, is indifferent to her family, feels fatigue, and feels better after vigorous exercise (Bello, 1999).

Sulfur (brimstone)—The indications are feeling of the need of air; strong desire for sweets; aggravated by heat in all forms; standing still; washing; symptoms worsen around 11 AM.

Cinchona officinalis (cinchona bark)—The indications for this remedy are general fatigue, diarrhea, exhaustion from excessive sweating, distended abdomen. The symptoms are aggravated by the slightest touch.

HERBAL REMEDIES FOR GENERAL CONDITIONS PREVALENT AMONG WOMEN

In this section, symptoms that are commonly experienced by women are listed with recommended homeopathic remedies. The key indications for the specific remedies are described briefly.

Arthritis/Rheumatism

Bryonia alba (wild hops)—The indications for this remedy are joint pain and stiffness that are made worse by any touching, walking, or moving; worse from inhalation, motion, entering a warm room, and about 9 PM.

Calcarea phosphorica (calcium phosphate)—Major characteristic symptoms are cold or a crawling sensation. Symptoms are better in warm, dry, weather and worse when it snows or there are cold drafts.

Dulcamara (bittersweet)—The predominant characteristics for this remedy are puffy joints and extreme sensitivity to damp weather. The symptoms are better after moving around and with heat; they are worse with humidity, cold applications, and rainy weather.

Ferrum phoshoricum (iron phosphate)—This remedy is suggested if the following symptoms prevail: The symptoms improve by slow walking, solitude, and pressure and are worse after physical exertion, exposure to cold air and violent emotion; they are worse between 4 and 6 AM and at night.

Rhododendron or *Chrysanthemum*—The indications for this remedy are severe rheumatic pains, sometimes wandering from joint to joint; stiffness of joints, neck, and back. The symptoms are worse before and during a storm, changes in the weather, especially cold, wet weather; and better with warm wrapping.

Rhus toxicodenron (poison ivy)—The indications for this remedy are rheumatic pains, stiffness, pain in the tendons. The symptoms are made better by moving around and are made worse by resting, cold and damp weather, humidity; symptoms are worse in the evening and during menstruation.

Cramps and Spasms

Cocculus indicus (Indian cockle)—The major indications for this remedy are painful menstruation and feeling weak.

Colocynthis (bitter cucumber)—The key indication is abdominal pain, causing one to bend over double.

Magnesia phosphorica (phosphate of magnesia)—This is remedy is indicated for the following symptoms: feels better from warmth, experiences pressure, and finds herself bending double.

Fatigue

Arsenicum album (white arsenic)—The indications for this remedy are fear, worry, restlessness, anxiety, burning pains relieved by heat, intense weakness, feeling chilly, desires fresh air. Symptoms are worse with the cold.

Echinacea angustifolia (purple coneflower)—The classic symptoms are a weak and tired feeling accompanied by aching limbs. The symptoms are improved with rest and worse with cold air, eating , and injury. Hardy and Nonman, (1994) classified fatigue as acute and chronic.

Acute Fatigue

Arnica montana (mountain daisy)—This remedy is often referred to as *Arnica*. Muscular fatigue occurs after much exertion and after a rapid growth spurt.

Calcera phosphorica (calcium phosphate)—The major indications for this remedy are loss of a large amount of body fluids (diarrhea, heavy menstrual periods, heavy sweating, vomiting).

Iodum—The key symptoms of acute fatigue are fatigue and thinness despite healthy appetite.

Rhus toxicodendron (poison ivy)—This remedy is considered for stiffness after participation in sports.

Chronic Fatigue

Cinchona officinalis (cinchona bark)—The indications for this remedy are exhaustion from excessive sweating, diarrhea, debility from exhausting discharges and from loss of vital fluids, especially accompanied by overexcitement or nervousness. The symptoms are improved at night or in wet weather and are worse with the slightest touch.

Gelsemium sempervirens (yellow jasmine)—This remedy is often referred to as *Gelsemium*. The major indications for this remedy are muscular weakness, drowsiness, slow pulse, general depression, apprehension, dread of important events, migraine headaches. The symptoms improve with urination and sweating and are worse with heat, hot weather, and bad news.

Iodum—The key indications for this remedy are great debility, when the slightest effort induces perspiration.

Kali phosphoricum (potassium phosphate)—This nerve remedy is indicated when weak and tired; for mental and physical depression, mental anxiety, extreme lassitude and depression, brain fatigue; when slightest labor seems a heavy task; for exhaustion after diarrhea (Hardy & Nonman, 1994).

Pulsatilla (windflower)—The major indication is fatigue due to convalescing from an infectious disease.

Sepia (cuttlefish ink)—This remedy is suggested for fatigue after childbirth.

Flatulence/Belching

Carbo vegetabilis (vegetable charcoal)—The indications for this remedy are digestive problems, stomach gas, and greatly distended abdomen; the person feels better after expelling flatulence and being fanned, and worse with heat, humid atmosphere, and alcohol consumption.

Cinchona officinalis (cinchona bark)—Major symptoms for this remedy are belching for which bitter fluid gives no relief, and a bloated feeling; the person feels better by motion.

Headaches

Belladonna (deadly nightshade)—This remedy is considered for the following symptoms: sudden onset; throbbing pain; very sensitive to light, noise, and motion.

Gelsemium sempervirens (yellow jasmine)—The major indications for this remedy are headaches that feel as if a tight band is around the person's head; the individual feels drowsy.

Kali bichromicum (potassium bichromate)—The indications for this remedy are sinus headaches with pressure; colds; sore throat; a mucous discharge that is thick, yellow. Symptoms are better in hot weather, while eating, and in open air; they are worse when drinking beer, in cold damp weather, when undressing, and between 2 and 3 AM.

Lachesis mutus (bushmaster snake)—An outstanding symptom for this remedy is a left-sided headache that seems worse with heat, after sleep, or while wearing tight clothing.

Natrum muriaticum (sodium chloride—table salt)—This remedy is considered if there is a throbbing migraine headache that may be one-sided or worsened by heat or the sun.

Nux vomica (poison nut)—The key indication for this remedy is headache that occurs after overindulgence in food or drink.

Thuja occidentalis (arborvitae—tree of life)—This remedy is recommended if the woman experiences headaches during which the head feels as if pierced by a nail. The symptoms are worse when drinking tea, eating onions, when there is humidity, and between 3 AM and 3 PM.

Insomnia/Sleeplessness

Coffea cruda (unroasted coffee)—The indications for this remedy are agitation, nervousness and restlessness.

Ignatia amara (St. Ignatius bean)—The major symptoms for this remedy are anxiety, stress due to an emotional upset, grief, or shock; the person feels hopeless.

Kali phosphoricum (potassium phosphate)—This remedy is used with the following symptoms: stress or nervousness due to excitement, worry, or overwork.

Osteoporosis

Calcarea phosphorica (calcium phosphate)—This was discussed under Arthritis/Rheumatism and Acute Fatigue.

Sinusitis

Kali bichromicum (potassium birchromate)—(This homeopathic substance is considered the main remedy for sinus conditions.) The person feels pressure in the nasal passages; experiences pain over the eyes; and describes a stringy, sticky, tough mucus.

Mercurius vivus (mercury)—This remedy is indicated if the woman has a bad taste in the mouth or produces greenish or yellow mucus.

Thuja occidentalis (arborvitae—tree of life)—This remedy is for the woman who experiences sinusitis.

Stress

Ignatia amara (St. Ignatius bean)—This remedy is often referred to as *Ignatia*. The indications for this remedy are nervousness, irritability, headaches, general weakness, and sighing. It helps the woman to relax emotional tension causing stress. It is effective especially during times of great grief or loss. The symptoms are better when the woman is exposed to heat or is having a pleasant time, and the symptoms are worse when there are strong smells such as coffee or tobacco and when she is experiencing unpleasant emotions.

SUMMARY

Homeopathy is a popular natural approach aimed at promoting general health by reinforcing the body's own natural healing capacity. Homeopathy relies upon the energy of an individual's vital force, and treating the whole person is essential. When the closest match between the client's symptoms and the remedy characteristics is chosen correctly, symptoms have a greater chance of being alleviated. Symptoms may become worse before they get better, which can be part of the healing process. The homeopathic remedies that are helpful to women experiencing particular symptoms and conditions specific to women were briefly discussed as well as those general health concerns prevalent among women as well as men (see Table 11–1).

REVIEW AND DISCUSSION

See boxes "Patient Education" and "Continuing Questions/Challenges" for discussion topics for this chapter.

Table 12–1 Summary of Homeopathic Remedies

Ailment or Condition	Remedy
Acute and chronic cystitis	*Arsenicum Album* (While Arsenic)
	Berberis vulgaris (barberry)
	Cantharis (Spanish fly)
	Pulsatilla (windflower)
	Sarsaparilla
	Sepia (culttlefish ink)
	Staphysagria (stavesacre)
	Sulfur (brimstone)
Acute cystitis	*Apis mellifica* (honeybee)
	Belladonna (deadly nightshade)
	Causticum (bisulfate of potash— Hahnemann's tincture)
	Concium caculatum (bitter apple)
	Mercurius vivus (quicksilver)
Chronic cystitis	*Concium caculatum* (bitter apple)
Menopause	
Hot flashes that improve at the onset of menstrual flow	*Cimicifuga racemosa* (black snake root)
	Graphites (black lead—plumbago)
	Lachesis mutus (bushmaster snake)
	Natrium muriaticum (sodium chloride— table salt)
	Pulsatilla (windflower)
	Sepia (cuttlefish ink)
Need of air	*Sulfur* (brimstone)
General fatigue	*Cinchona officinalis* (cinchona bark)
Menstrual difficulties/irregularities	
Dysmenorrhea	*Belladonna* (deadly nightshade)
	Chamomilla (German chamomile)
	Lachesis mutus (bushmaster snake)
	Pulsatilla (windflower)
	Kali carbonicum (potassium carbonate)
	Sepia (cuttlefish ink)
	Cocculus indicus (Indian cockle)
	Coffea cruda (Unroasted coffee)
	Magnesia phosphorica (phosphate of magnesium)
	Sabina (savine)
Menstrual cramps	*Magnesia phosphorica* (phosphate of magnesium)

continues

Table 12–1 continued

Ailment or Condition	Remedy
	Belladonna (deadly nightshade)
	Nux vomica (poison nut)
	Pulsatilla (windflower)
Pregnancy: morning sickness	*Colchicum* (meadow saffron)
	Ipecac (ipecac root)
	Kreosotum (beechwood creosote)
	Pulsatilla (windflower)
	Sepia (cuttlefish ink)
Premenstrual syndrome	*Belladonna* (deadly nightshade)
	Caulophyllum thalictroides (blue cohosh)
	Chamomilla (German chamomile)
	Cimifuga racemosa (black snake root)
	Colocynthis (bitter cucumber)
	Lachesis mutus (bushmaster snake)
	Lycopodium clavatum (club moss)
	Magnesia phosphorica (phosphate of magnesium)
	Natrum muriaticum (sodium chloride—table salt)
	Nux vomica (poison nut)
	Pulsatilla (windflower)
	Sepia (cuttlefish ink)
Vaginitis	*Arsenium album* (trioxide of arsenic)
	Apis mellifica (honeybee)
	Borax (sodium borate)
	Graphite (black lead—plumbago)
	Kreosotum (beechwood creosote)
	Mercurius vivus (quicksilver)
	Nitricum acidum (nitric acid)
	Pulsatilla (windflower)
	Sepia (cuttlefish ink)
Arthritis/rheumatism	*Bryonia alba* (wild hops)
	Calcarea phosphorica (calcium phosphate)
	Dulcamara (bittersweet)
	Ferrum phosphoricum (iron phosphate)
	Rhododendron or *Chrysanthemum*
	Rhus toxicodenron (poison ivy)

continues

Table 12–1 continued

Ailment or Condition	Remedy
Cramps/spasms	*Cocculus indicus* (Indian cockle)
	Colocynthis (bitter cucumber)
	Magnesia phosphorica (phosphate of magnesium)
Fatigue	*Arsenicum album* (white arsenic)
	Echinacea angustifolia (purple cone-flower)
Acute fatigue	*Arnica montana* (mountain daisy)
	Calcera phosphorica (calcium phosphate)
	Iodum
	Rhus toxicodendron (poison ivy)
Chronic fatigue	*Cinchona officinalis* (cinchona bark)
	Gelsemium sempervirens (yellow jasmine)
	Iodum
	Kali phosphoricum (potassium phosphate)
	Pulsatilla (windflower)
	Sepia (cuttlefish ink)
Flatulence/belching	*Carbo vegetabilis* (vegetable charcoal)
	Cinchona officinalis (cinchona bark)
Headaches	*Belladonna* (deadly nightshade)
	Gelsemium sempervirens (yellow jasmine)
	Kali bichromicum (potassium bichromate)
	Lachesis mutus (bushmaster snake)
	Natrum muriaticum (sodium chloride—table salt)
	Nux vomica (poison nut)
	Thuja occidentalis (arborvitae—tree of life)
Insomnia/sleeplessness	*Coffea cruda* (unroasted coffee)
	Ignatia amara (St. Ignatius bean)
	Kali phosphoricum (potassium phosphate)
Osteoporosis	*Calcarea phosphate* (calcium phosphate)
Sinusitis	*Kali bichromicum* (potassium bichromate)
	Mercurius vivus (mercury)
	Thuja occidentalis (arborvitae—tree of life)
Stress	*Ignatia amara* (St. Ignatius bean)

Patient Education

- Homeopathic remedies or the bottle dropper should be handled as little as possible
- The mouth should be in its natural condition when homeopathic remedies administered
- When using homeopathic remedies, may be recommended to discontinue use of certain foods, toiletries, medication
- Store homeopathic remedies at room temperature, out of direct sunlight
- Homeopathic remedies may be effective for a variety of conditions affecting women.

Continuing Questions/Challenges

What issues are important in relation to regulation of homeopathic remedies?

What are the implications for patient education related to self-administration of homeopathic remedies?

What resources are available for additional information on homeopathic remedies?

What are some recommendations for the woman if her condition persists or if the illness/symptoms reoccur?

If the woman seeks professional help from a qualified homeopath, what factors are essential in selection of this professional health care practitioner?

REFERENCES

Bello, L. (1999). Women's health: Menopause—a natural transition. *Homeopathy Today, 19*(3), 22–23.

Cummings, S., & Ullman, D. (1997). *Everybody's guide to homeopathic medicines* (3rd ed.). New York: Tarcher/Putnam.

Fein, J. (1998, March–April). Consumer guide: Three alternative therapies. *Natural Health,* 120–132.

Hammond, C. (1995). *The complete family guide to homeopathy.* New York: Penguin Studio.

Hardy, M., & Nonman, D. (1994). *The alchemist's handbook to homeopathy.* Allergan, Michigan: Delta K Trust.

Jonas, W., & Jacobs, J. (1996). *Healing with homeopathy: The doctors' guide.* New York: Warner Books.

Kent, J. (1997). *Lectures on homeopathic materia medica.* New Delhi, India: B. Jain Publishers.

Lockie, A., & Geddes, N. (1994). *The women's guide to homeopathy.* New York: St. Martin's Press.

Loecher, B., & O'Donnell, S. (1997). In Faelten (Ed.) *New choices in natural healing for women: Drug-free remedies from the world of alternative medicine.* Emmaus, PA: Rodale Press.

Natural Pharmacy, 2(11) (1998, Nov.)

Shealy, C. (Ed.). (1996). *The complete family guide to alternative medicine.* Rockport, MA: Element Books.

Taylor, W. (1998). Appreciating Wholeness: Implications of the Totality of Symptoms. *Newsletter for the Ohio State Homeopathic Medical Society.*

Ullman, D. (1995). *Consumer's guide to homeopathy.* New York: Tarcher/Putnam.

White, L. (1998). Homeopathy: From placebo effect to clear science? *Natural Pharmacy, 2*(8), 14.

SUGGESTED READINGS

Castro, M. (1990). *The complete homeopathy handbook.* New York: St. Martin's Press.

Gottlieb, B. (Ed.). (1995). *New choices in natural healing.* Emmaus: Rodale Press.

Horvilleur, A. (1986). *The family guide to homeopathy.* VA: Health and Homeopathy Publishing, Inc.

Koehler, G. (1989). *The handbook of homeopathy: Its principles and practice.* Rochester, VT: Healing Arts Press.

Kruzel, T. (1992). *The homeopathic emergency guide.* Berkeley, CA: North Atlantic Books.

Lockie, A. (1993). *The family guide to homeopathy.* New York: Fireside.

Murray, M., & Pizzorno, J. (1998). *Encyclopedia of natural medicine* (2nd ed.). Rocklin, CA: Prima.

Page, L. (1998). *Healthy healing* (10th ed.). Carmel Valley, CA: Healthy Healing Publications.

Weiner, M. (1989). *The complete book of homeopathy.* New York: MJF Books.

CHAPTER 13

Acupuncture/ Acupressure

Christine D. Meyer

Key Points

- Acupuncture and acupressure are based on the belief that wellness is maintained when Qi is in balance.
  - Qi is divided into yin and yang.
  - Acupuncture points are manipulated to achieve balance between yin and yang.
- Acupoints are manipulated in two ways:
  - Acupressure (stimulation by finger pressure)
  - Acupuncture (stimulation by insertion of needle)
- There are 12 meridians (pathways) in the body through which Qi flows.
  - Each meridian is connected to a specific organ or body system.
  - Stimulation of acupoints affects the specific meridian to which they are attached.
  - Stimulation releases endogenous endorphins.
- There are various certification boards for acupuncture practitioners:
  - Accreditation Commission for Acupuncture and Oriental Medicine
  - Council of Colleges of Acupuncture and Oriental Medicine
  - National Commission for Certification of Acupuncturists
- Typical acupuncture session
  - Minimum of 3 to maximum of 12 needles used per session
  - Length of needles range from 1.25 cm to 15 cm
  - Gauge of needles range from 26 to 36

— Needles usually in place between 5 and 20 minutes, but may be in for seconds and up to an hour
— Normally 12 sessions is considered a "full trial"
— Length of time between visits is gradually extended as treatment continues
— Symptoms may get worse before they get better.

Because the benefits of acupuncture are often immediate and measurable, the practice has steadily gained the respect of medical practitioners in the United States.

—Judelson & Dell, 1998, p. 265

ACUPUNCTURE: ITS HISTORY

Acupuncture is one component of traditional Chinese medicine (TCM). TCM, which dates back between 2,500 and 3,000 years (Bareta, 1998; Beal, 1992a; Beinfield & Korngold, 1995; Helms, 1998; Hsu & Diehl, 1998; Pomeranz, 1996; Ulett, Han, & Han, 1998b), consists of three intervention modalities: herbal medicine, Qi Gong, and acupuncture (Rubik, 1995). The National Institutes of Health (NIH) Consensus (1998) estimated that more than one million Americans use acupuncture each year. Another study (Eisenberg et al., 1998) stated that approximately 1% of the population used acupuncture in the past 12 months. Further, the Landmark Study (1998) found that 42% of Americans were either very likely or somewhat likely to use acupuncture, and that 67% had a similar regard toward acupressure. Interest in acupuncture in the United States was ignited in 1971 when President Richard Nixon visited China and an accompanying reporter, James Reston, required an emergency appendectomy (Ulett, 1996). When he experienced severe gas pains after the surgery, the Chinese physicians used acupuncture to help relieve the pain. Reston was so enthralled with the results that, when he returned to the United States, he wrote an article about his experience in the July 26, 1971, issue of the *New York Times* (Reston, 1971a; Reston, 1971b). As a result, the general public in the West became more aware of the benefits of acupuncture (Beal, 1992a; Beinfield & Korngold, 1995; Helms, 1998; NIH Consensus Conference, 1998).

Eight years later, in 1979, the Beijing Neurosurgical Institute in China invited David Eisenberg, M.D., from Harvard University to study and to observe major surgeries in which Chinese physicians were using only acupuncture for the relief of pain (Burton Goldberg Group, 1997). One of the most impressive operations was the removal of a brain tumor that was adjacent to the pituitary gland. The patient was awake and alert throughout the procedure and walked out of the operating room when surgery was completed. According to the Beijing Institute, acupuncture is more effective for pain relief in areas of the upper body or above the waistline. For this reason acupuncture is often the anesthesia of choice for thyroidectomies, tonsillectomies, and other surgeries involving the head and neck (Beal, 1992a). Like other interventions, acupuncture analgesia has its limitations and is generally not considered for abdominal, gynecological, cardiac, or pulmonary operations (Burton Goldberg Group, 1997). The use of exogenous analgesics is greatly reduced when they are used in conjunction with acupuncture (Bareta, 1998).

In November 1997, the NIH created a 12-member panel to evaluate the scientific documentation on various aspects of acupuncture, which was presented by experts in acupuncture (Marwick, 1997). After all the presentations were completed within 3 days, the panel created a consensus statement for each topic. Studies supported acupuncture's effectiveness for managing numerous health-related problems. These problems include nausea and vomiting related to pregnancy, surgery, and chemotherapy; the pain due to migraine headaches, surgical wounds, dental surgery, dysmenorrhea, and back pain; addiction to alcohol, drugs, and tobacco; Carpal tunnel syndrome; stroke rehabilitation; labor induction, and the conversion of a breech to a vertex presentation (Beal, 1992b; Bullock, Culliton, & Oleander, 1989; Cardini & Weixin, 1998; Dundee & McMillan, 1991; Hsu & Diehl, 1998; Landmark Report, 1998; Marwick, 1997; NIH Consensus Conference, 1998; Schulte, 1996). Future research funded by the NIH includes further studies of acupuncture on knee osteoarthritis, back pain, dental pain and depression (Hsu & Diehl, 1998). Other studies demonstrated that acupuncture is also effective for asthma, tennis elbow, Raynaud's syndrome, post-herpetic neuralgia, and nonallergic rhinitis (Appiah, Hiller, Caspary, Alexander, & Creutzig, 1997; Davies, Lewith, Goddard, & Howarth, 1998; Hsu & Diehl, 1998; NIH Consensus Conference, 1998).

Acupuncture is based on the belief that wellness is maintained when a vital life energy, called Qi or Chi (pronounced chee), which is present in all living organisms, remains balanced and flows easily along 12 major meridians or energy pathways in the body. Each meridian runs along the body surface and through the internal organs, and is named for the organ through which it travels. Each meridian is connected to specific organs or systems. Illness or disease is the result if Qi becomes depleted, blocked, or congested in an area (Beal, 1992a; Beinfield & Korngold, 1995). According to Beal (1992a), there are two basic types of treatment for out-of-kilter Qi: (1) tonification, if Qi is depleted, and (2) sedation, if Qi is congested.

Qi is divided into two complementary and interdependent forces, yin and yang. Yin is defined as a feminine force and is considered to possess a negative charge. In contrast, yang is believed to possess masculine characteristics with a positive charge (Beal, 1992a). Acupuncture points, sometimes called *tsubos,* are found in small indentations in the skin along the meridians, and are manipulated in order to achieve an energy balance between the yin and the yang (Beinfield & Korngold, 1995; Jimenez, 1992; Pomeranz, 1996). Ulett, Han, and Han (1998a) believe that there are 365 specific acupuncture points, abbreviated as acupoints, along the meridians, but other experts are convinced there are well over 1,000 points (Burton Goldberg Group, 1997; Rubik, 1995). Acupoints tend to be more tender than the surrounding tissue (Oleson & Flocco, 1993). The goal of acupuncture is to stimulate the acupoints to enhance the flow of Qi.

Acupoints can be stimulated by a variety of methods. Among these methods is stimulation either by finger pressure (acupressure) or by the insertion of very fine, sterile, disposable, solid, stainless steel needles (acupuncture). Applying pressure with the thumbs or needles to specific points serves to stimulate the movement of Qi. Once the needles are inserted, the acupuncturist may augment the strength of the stimulation of the acupuncture point by twirling the needles, by applying a low-voltage electrical current to them via a battery (electroacupuncture), or by using lasers, infrared light, or suction-cupping devices such as bamboo cups. The United States Food and Drug Administration (FDA) classifies laser acupuncture investigational and so its use requires a signed informed consent to that effect (NIH, 1997) There is also evidence that injections of water into acupoints can substitute for needles. An analgesic effect can also be achieved by stimulating the acupoints with a transcutaneous electrical nerve stimulation (TENS) device (Ulett, Han, & Han, 1998a). Heating the acupoint (moxibustion) is yet another method of stimulating an acupoint. Moxibustion entails burning small cones of an herb, such as artemis vulgaris (mugwort), over the chosen acupoint, or igniting it atop an object like a slice of ginger placed on the skin (Beal, 1992a; Burton

Goldberg Group, 1997; Cadwell, 1998; NIH Consensus Conference, 1998; Ulett et al, 1998b). Table 13–1 lists common conditions that can be treated by acupuncture.

Closely related to acupuncture and acupressure is reflexology. Reflexology is based on the idea that certain body parts such as the foot, hand and ear are "reflex microsystems" that contain circumscribed zones or acupoints that correspond to every part of the body (Burton Goldberg Group, 1997; Oleson & Flocco, 1993; Pomeranz, 1996; Rubik, 1995). Acupoints on the ear are said to be distributed as though the body is in a fetal position "with its head at the earlobe, and lower limbs at the antihelix" (Beal, 1992a, p. 258). In 1989 auriculotherapy was formally acknowledged by the World Health Organization (WHO) as an acceptable healing intervention (Burton Goldberg Group, 1997).

HOW DOES ACUPUNCTURE/ACUPRESSURE WORK?

The predominant theory to explain the dynamics of acupuncture is that the stimulation of an acupoint promotes the release of endogenous endorphins: meta-enkephalins, beta-endorphins, and dynorphins (NIH, 1997; Pomeranz, 1996). Endorphins are amino acid peptides that are chemically similar to opiate or morphine and therefore bind to opiate receptor sites in the central nervous system (CNS) and block the pain pathways. Endorphins have been found to occur naturally in the brain (pituitary, midbrain, and hypothalamus) and in the spinal cord (Beal, 1992a; Pomeranz, 1996; Rubik, 1995; Ulett, 1996). Ulett et al. (1998a) confirmed that neurotransmitters such as serotonin and endorphins are primary factors in acupuncture analgesia. They performed acupuncture analgesia in a rabbit. When a portion of the rabbit's cerebrospinal fluid (CSF) was transferred into the third ventricle of a naïve rabbit, the second rabbit experienced the analgesic effect (Ulett, Han, & Han, 1998a).

Ulett, Han, and Han (1998a) discovered that the health care practitioner could stimulate the release of select neuropeptides by changing the frequency and intensity of electroacupuncture. In other words, different frequencies of electrical stimulation released specific neuropeptides. For instance, low-frequency (2 to 4 Hz), high-intensity electroacupuncture tends to increase the level of beta-endorphin and enkephalin in the CSF, with a slow onset and a generalized effect that is cumulative. On the other hand, high frequency (70 to 100 Hz), low intensity increases the release of dynorphin in the spinal cord (NIH, 1997), with a quick onset and a more localized effect that is not cumu-

Table 13–1 Conditions Recommended for Acupuncture by WHO

Condition	Specific Manifestations
Respiratory diseases	• Acute sinusitis • Acute rhinitis • Common cold • Acute tonsillitis
Bronchopulmonary diseases	• Acute bronchitis • Bronchial asthma
Eye disorders	• Acute conjunctivitis • Cataract (without complications) • Myopia • Central retinitis
Disorders of the mouth cavity	• Toothache • Pain after tooth extraction • Gingivitis • Pharyngitis
Orthopedic disorders	• Periarthritis humeroscapularis • Tennis elbow • Sciatica • Low back pain • Rheumatoid arthritis
Gastrointestinal disorders	• Spasm of the esophagus and cardia • Hiccups • Gastroptosis • Acute and chronic gastritis • Gastric hyperacidity • Chronic duodenal ulcer • Acute and chronic colitis • Acute bacterial dysentery • Constipation • Diarrhea • Paralytic ileus
Neurologic disorders	• Headache • Migraine • Trigeminal neuralgia • Facial paralysis • Paralysis after apoplectic fit • Peripheral neuropathy • Paralysis caused by poliomyelitis • Meniere's syndrome • Neurogenic bladder dysfunction • Nocturnal enuresis • Intercostal neuralgia

Courtesy of American Academy of Medical Acupuncture, Los Angeles, California.

lative (Helms, in press). Some researchers have suggested that if the practitioner alternates the administration of electroacupuncture at 2 Hz for 3 seconds followed by 100 Hz for 3 seconds, all three types of the opioid peptides can be released. The synergistic action among the three endorphins would induce a powerful analgesic outcome (NIH, 1997).

Rubik (1995), Schulte (1996), and Ulett, Han, and Han (1998a) reported that acupuncture also increases the level of glucocorticoids. It is surmised that the release of the glucocorticoids helps to relieve inflammatory conditions such as asthma and arthritis (Ulett, Han, & Han, 1998). Pomeranz (1996), a well-known expert on acupuncture, asserted that there is plenty of evidence to support the acupuncture-endorphin hypothesis. He explained that acupuncture, like the endogenous release of endorphins, is cumulative (Pomeranz, 1996). Each successive treatment becomes more effective or stronger because "endorphins have memory" (Pomeranz, 1996). The first session may have little or no noticeable effect, but the fifth or sixth treatment may be the one that begins to make a difference. Pomeranz emphasized that acupuncture takes time and will not work quickly, like medications often will. Because healing is subtle, it is so important for a patient to have several treatments before deciding that acupuncture is not helpful.

In addition to the release of endorphins, other mechanisms such as the relaxation response, the halo effect, and the Hawthorne effect may contribute to acupuncture's effectiveness in pain management (Jiminez, 1992; Plawecki & Plawecki, 1998). Stimulation of the acupoints may help to induce the gate control mechanism, a phenomenon in which stimulation of large, myelinated fibers through touch, pressure, heat, cold, and movement transmits high-speed impulses that overload and close the "substantia gelatinosa" (pain gate) in the dorsal horn of the spinal cord.

Another theory for the mechanics of acupuncture is the interaction of electromagnetic fields and the life force of Qi. (Rubik, 1995). Becker (1982, as cited in Rubik, 1995) proposed that the needling of an acupuncture point might reestablish a wave pattern or a shift in the electromagnetic field, promoting healing.

Scientists who discredit acupuncture contend that the relief of pain is due to the placebo effect. There are, however, several studies refuting this assertion. Pomeranz (1996) demonstrated that naloxone, an opiate receptor antagonist, is able to block the analgesic effects of acupuncture. It is also important to note that in order to have a placebo effect the recipient would need to be aware of the treatment. Yet, acupuncture tends to be effective and endorphin levels increase when acupuncture is performed on young babies and animals (Plawecki & Plawecki, 1998, Pomeranz, 1996). Pomeranz supported the notion that acupuncture does not behave like a placebo. For instance, acupuncture in clinically controlled studies is effective for 70% to 80% of patients with pain versus the 30% associated with a placebo. He also contended that acupuncture becomes more effective with each successive treatment. In contrast, the strength and effect of a placebo diminishes with each exposure (Helms, 1998; Pomeranz, 1996).

Acupuncture points along the meridians are uniquely different from other types of tissue. Liu et al. (1975, as cited in Rubik, 1995) stated that a map of the acupuncture points could be superimposed on the areas where the motor neurons enter the skeletal muscle and where there is a greater density of motor nerve terminals at the surface. Watari (1987, as cited in Rubik, 1995) provided further support of this concept. He maintained that acupuncture sites not only possess a greater concentration of neuroreceptors, that is, 1.4 times more nerve fibers, but also contain 4 times more blood vessels that merged to create a "glomerular structure" (Rubik, 1995). Acupuncture sites also demonstrate a higher capacity for electrical conductivity (Jimenez, 1992; Schulte, 1996; Ulett et al., 1998a). It should be noted that needles are not used in the areas of the navel, nipples, and penis (Burton Goldberg Group, 1997).

The effectiveness of acupuncture depends on many variables. First, it is important to note that all acupoints are not the same. The Chinese have identified distinct acupoints for various results such as the relief of pain or nausea. For example, to relieve pain, a needle or pressure would have to be used on an acupoint that contained a specific nerve in a specific muscle that is capable of releasing endorphins. This acupoint, which may work quite well for pain relief, may not necessarily relieve nausea.

Second, the acupuncturist needs to insert the needle to a certain depth and twirl it in order to produce a phenomenon called d'ai chi , defined as an aching, tingling, or numbness sensation that radiates out from the insertion point when the nerve is stimulated properly (Helms, 1998; Hoo, 1997; Pomeranz, 1996; Ulett et al., 1998b). Similarly, when acupressure is used, it is recommended that the therapist inquire about these sensations to ensure that pressure is applied to the correct site (Hoo, 1997). Pomeranz implied that the d'ai chi phenomenon indicates adequate stimulation of the acupoint (Pomeranz, 1996).

A third factor in the relief of pain is that acupuncture does not work immediately, but is a cumulative process. Initial pain relief with acupuncture may take up to 30 minutes due to the gradual release of the endorphins, but each successive treatment becomes more potent. Because of this summation characteristic, acupuncturists will normally recommend several acupuncture sessions before deciding upon its effectiveness (Pomeranz, 1996).

TYPICAL TREATMENT SESSION

More than half of acupuncture in the United States is done on an outpatient basis (Nasir, 1998). A typical treatment session begins with a history and a physical and a lengthy discussion of the patient's life (job, stressors, multiple roles). This initial session also includes an assessment of the tongue (color and texture), the 12 radial pulses, the external ear, and a review of past medical records, x-rays, and laboratory tests (Burton Goldberg Group, 1997; Helms, 1998; Pomeranz, 1996). The number of needles that may be used varies, although 3 is the minimum and 10 to 12 is the maximum (Burton Goldberg Group, 1997). The length and the gauge of the needles vary with the intended treatment, ranging from 1.25 to 15 cm in length and from 26 to 36 gauge (Ceniceros & Brown, 1998). The needles are generally in place between 5 and 20 minutes, but may be retained from only seconds to a maximum of an hour (Ceniceros & Brown, 1998). The frequency of visits to the acupuncturist depends on the severity and acuity of the problem, but 12 visits is considered a "full trial." The length of time between visits is gradually extended, determined by the length of time that the patient can maintain the desired response. For example, if the patient maintains the desired outcome for 1 week, then the next visit may be scheduled 2 weeks later. Chronic problems may require monthly or bi-monthly visits (Helms, 1998). Finally, patients need to understand that any change in the signs or symptoms of the problem during treatment, even an exacerbation, is considered a "favorable response." For example, the intensity of pain may initially intensify before it improves (Cadwell, 1998; NIH, 1997).

Since acupuncture is believed to stimulate the endogenous release of endorphins, continued acupuncture over several hours' duration may induce a tolerance to the acupuncture with a simultaneous decrease in the acupuncture-induced analgesia. In his presentation to the NIH Consensus Development Conference on Acupuncture (1997), Han compared the "acupuncture tolerance" phenomenon to the development of morphine tolerance associated with the heavy use of opioids. He explained that prolonged electrostimulation of the acupuncture points increases the production of cholecystokinin (CCK), which competes with the endorphins for the same receptor sites in the CNS. In experiments with rats, the administration of CKK can prevent or reverse acupuncture tolerance (Han, Ding & Fan, 1986).

ADVERSE INCIDENTS RELATED TO ACUPUNCTURE, ACUPRESSURE

As with other treatment interventions, there are adverse reactions to acupuncture. While adverse reactions are infrequent, the literature indicates the occurrence of some common non–life-threatening reactions. Such reactions include fainting (due to the vasovagal reflex), contact dermatitis, hematoma, chondritis associated with acupuncture of the ear, local infections, increased pain, and tissue trauma secondary to improper needling (Bareta, 1998; NIH, 1997; Yamashita, Tsukayama, Tanno, & Nishijo, 1998). Less common, but more serious major adverse reactions can also occur. These reactions include pneumothorax, pneumoperitoneum, hemothorax, cardiac tamponade, penetration of the kidney bladder or spinal medulla, hepatitis B, human immunodeficiency virus (HIV), septicemia, osteomyelitis, endocarditis, migration of broken needles to critical areas, and spinal lesions (Kent, Brondum, Keenlyside, LaFazia, & Scott, 1988; Lee, & McLwian, 1985; NIH Consensus, 1998; Norheim, 1996; Norheim & Fonnebo, 1995; Yamashita et al., 1998). Interestingly, medical doctors educated in Western medical schools who performed acupuncture, did not have a lower number of pneumothorax complications when compared with acupuncturists (Norheim & Fonnebo, 1995).

In 1972, the FDA originally classified acupuncture needles as a class III or "research and investigation only" devices because, at that time, there was insufficient information on the efficacy of acupuncture (NIH, 1997). In 1996, however, the FDA reclassified them as a class II, legitimate medical instruments to be regulated like syringes (Bareta, 1998; Cadwell, 1998; NIH, 1997; Plawecki & Plawecki, 1998). This classification mandates that acupuncture needles be packaged as sterile, single-use instruments, and sold only to authorized practitioners (NIH, 1997). This change has greatly reduced the threat of infection secondary to contaminated or reused needles.

Some researchers imply that medically trained professionals should only do acupuncture and that acupuncturists who are "nonmedically qualified" are more likely to cause or experience negative consequences associated with acupuncture than medically trained acupuncturists (Ernst & White, 1997). After citing several untoward incidents that were linked to acupuncture, Ernst and White (1997) proposed a strict curriculum and registration process to minimize these complications. Representatives from schools of acupuncture defended their education and credentialing programs, stating that these measures have been in place for some time. They believe that the quality of the practitioner's schooling in acupuncture is the important predictor of outcomes (Hicks, Hicks, Mole & Smith, 1997). Yamashita et al. (1998) conducted a 5-year study in a Japanese clinic with 76 acupuncturists. Based on 55,291 acupuncture treatments, a total of 64 adverse events were reported. In order of descending frequency, these untoward effects included: forgotten needles ($n = 16$), transient hypotension-induced dizziness and perspiration ($n = 16$), ecchymosis ($n = 11$), thermal injuries associated with thermotherapies such as moxibustion ($n = 7$), malaise ($n = 5$), minor bleeding ($n = 3$), aggravation of presenting problem ($n = 3$), local itching/redness ($n = 3$), pain in the treatment area ($n = 2$), and a fall out of bed ($n = 1$). There was not a single case of pneumothorax, septicemia, or hemorrhaging. Yamashita et al. propose that the more serious untoward reactions to acupuncture reported in the literature are directly related either to the practitioners' lack of knowledge of anatomy and physiology or to asepsis or negligence. This study accentuates the importance of high-quality education, certification, and licensure of professionally trained acupuncturists.

LICENSURE, EDUCATION, AND CERTIFICATION OF ACUPUNCTURE PRACTITIONERS

There are currently about 10,000 acupuncture practitioners in the United States. Thirty percent of them are medical doctors (MDs) or doctors of osteopathy (DOs), with the remaining being nonphysician practitioners (Bareta, 1998; NIH, 1997). Today, there are at least 70 schools of acupuncture with formal education ranging from instruction in an accredited program to a 4-year college degree for both nonphysician and physician providers (NIH, 1997). Schools may be certified by the Accreditation Commission for Acupuncture and Oriental Medicine (ACAOM) and/or the Council of Colleges of Acupuncture and Oriental Medicine (Bareta, 1998). Some states have strict laws regulating acupuncture instruction and practice, while others have minimal requirements (Acupuncture Laws by State, 1999). Similarly, the number of hours of classroom instruction, observation, and practicum for students in acupuncture varies tremendously from state to state, as well as whether the student is an MD, a DO, a chiropractor, a podiatrist, or a nonphysician (Helms, in press; Ulett, 1996).

For physicians, the practice of acupuncture is considered within the scope of practice of medicine in 35 states. This means that these physicians are not required to obtain additional education in order to perform acupuncture (Helms, in press). However, the remaining 15 states mandate that physicians who intend to employ acupuncture submit evidence of attendance in a structured curriculum of 200 to 300 hours (Bareta, 1998; Helms, 1998; Helms, in press). The American Academy of Medical Acupuncture (AAMA) (1999) is an organization that was created exclusively for MDs and DOs who are well educated in acupuncture. It requires a minimal 220 hours of formal education and 2 years of clinical practice. The AAMA also offers a competency examination, which is the first component of a two-step board certification examination.

Acupuncture performed by nonphysicians is strictly regulated in 33 states, but 12 other states are considering similar measures (Helms, 1998.). The certification exam prerequisites and process are different in each state and are controlled by either the National Certification Commission for Acupuncture and Oriental Medicine (NCAA) or by each state certification board, or by both (Bareta, 1998). Another organization is the National Commission for Certification of Acupuncturists (NCCA). The NCCA was established in 1984 to administer a written- and performance-based examination. Candidates who pass this exam are permitted to use the title "Diplomate in Acupuncture," abbreviated as Dipl.Ac (NCCA) (Cadwell, 1998). California and Nevada are the only two states that do not honor the certification examination by the NCCA (Helms, In press).

It is highly recommended that patients who seek acupuncture treatments investigate the regulations of the state in which they live. A listing of these organizations and their addresses is provided in Exhibit 13–1. Two places to locate and examine acupuncture laws by state on the Internet are (1) http://acupuncture.com/StateLaws/StateLaws.htm and (2) http://www.aaom.org/resource/legsource.html.

ACUPUNCTURE STUDIES

The literature indicates that there are many variations in the administration of acupuncture, which makes it difficult to evaluate acupuncture treatments across multiple studies. Needles or pressure may be used, needles may be twirled or connected to a low-voltage battery for

Exhibit 13–1 Listing of Organizations Related to Acupuncture

Accreditation Commission for Acupuncture and Oriental Medicine (ACAOM)
Previously known as: National Accreditation Commission for Schools and Colleges of Acupuncture and Oriental Medicine. (NACSCAOM)
8403 Colesville Rd., Suite 370
Silver Spring, MD 20910

American Academy of Medical Acupuncture and Medical Acupuncture Research Foundation (AAMA/MARF)
5820 Wilshire Blvd, Suite 500
Los Angeles, CA 90036
Telephone: (323) 937-5514
Web: http://www.medicalacupuncture.org

American Association of Oriental Medicine (AAOM)
Previously known as American Association of Acupuncture and Oriental Medicine (AAAOM)
433 Front St.
Catasaugua, PA 18032
Telephone: (610) 266-1433 or (610) 433-2448
FAX:(610) 264-2768
Web: http://www.aaom.org/aboutaaom.html

American College of Acupuncture & Oriental Medicine (ACAOM)
9100 Park West Drive
Houston, TX 77063
Telephone: (713) 780-9777
FAX: (713) 781-5781
Email: webmaster@acaom.edu

Council of Colleges of Acupuncture and Colleges (CCAOM)
Previously known as National Council of Acupuncture Schools and Colleges (NCASC)
1010 Wayne Avenue, Suite 1270
Silver Spring, MD 20910
(301) 608-9175

National Academy of Acupuncture and Oriental Medicine (NAAOM)
Box 62
Tarrytown, NY 10591
Telephone: (914) 332-4576
Email: 75776.1734@compuserve.com   *continues*

Exhibit 13–1 continued

> **National Accreditation Commission for Schools and Colleges of**
> **Acupuncture and Oriental Medicine (ACAOM)**
> Previously known as NACSCAOM
> 8403 Colesville Rd., Suite 370
> Silver Spring, MD 20910
>
> **National Acupuncture and Oriental Medicine Alliance**
> 14637 Starr Road S.E.
> Olalla, WA 98359
> Telephone: (253) 851-6896
>
> **National Acupuncture Detoxification Association (NADA)**
> 3115 Broadway, Suite 51
> New York, New York 10027
> Telephone: (212) 993-3100
>
> **National Commission for Certification of Acupuncturists (NCCA)**
> 1424 16th St. NW, Suite 601   P.O. Box 97075
> Washington, DC 20036   Washington, D.C. 20090-7075
> (202) 232-1404
>
> **Society for Acupuncture Research**
> 6900 Wisconsin Avenue, Suite 700
> Bethesda, MD 20815
> Fax: (301) 961-5340
> Email: hannahb@erols.com

electroacupuncture, or heat may be applied via moxibustion. The size and number of needles used, the depth of needling, the entry points, length of time, and intensity of stimulation used are yet more variables that can modify the desired outcomes of the treatment. Notations on whether d'ai chi was achieved are often missing. Few studies on acupuncture include this kind of detailed information, and this lack of uniformity makes it difficult to compare and evaluate the efficacy of the treatment. With this in mind, White and Ernst (1998), with the assistance of six experts in acupuncture, recommended a checklist of 13 factors that they believed should be well defined in future studies on acupuncture. These 13 variables are (1) position of the patient, (2) number of needles, (3) needle size and manufacturer, (4) rationale and justification for the selection of acupoints, (5) acupoints used, (6) laterality, (7) depth, (8) stimulation, (9) presence of d'ai chi, (10) length of time, (11) repetitive treatments, (12) other concurrent treatments, and (13) outcomes (White & Ernst, 1998).

Establishing a control group for acupuncture studies is also very difficult due to the very nature of acupressure or acupuncture. Critics state that any improvement in the problem being studied is easily attributed to the placebo effect (Aikens, 1998). In addiction, when sham acupoints are used in a control group, participants in a study are able frequently to identify the correct point in self-help books (Aikens, 1998). A final note is that several studies have revealed that even the incorrect placement of pressure or needles may produce the desired therapeutic response.

MOST COMMON USES FOR ACUPUNCTURE

The NIH Consensus Panel on acupuncture has determined that there are convincing data that acupuncture is quite effective for postoperative and chemotherapy nausea and vomiting, postoperative pain, and pregnancy-induced nausea (NIH, 1997). This 12-member panel also concluded that acupuncture is probably helpful in other conditions such as addictions, headache, stroke rehabilitation, tennis elbow, fibromyalgia, myofacial pain, osteoarthritis, carpal tunnel syndrome, spasticity associated with cerebral palsy, Bell's palsy, and asthma (NIH, 1997). It also found that the two largest groups of acupuncture users in the United States are those persons seeking treatment for addictions and chronic conditions, particularly pain such as musculoskeletal problems, headaches, and low back pain (Nasir, 1998; NIH, 1997).

Like other medical interventions, acupuncture is not effective for every disease or disorder. For instance, White, Resch, and Ernst (1998) found, in their experimental study, that acupuncture did not decrease the signs and symptoms of smoking cessation any more than in the control group. In the cases of spinal cord injuries and cerebrovascular accidents (CVA), the effectiveness of acupuncture is decreased while the number of required sessions is increased. In addition, acupuncture is not highly effective as the sole therapy in severe and chronic inflammatory conditions such as asthma, ulcerative colitis, and rheumatoid arthritis (Helms, in press).

USE OF ACUPUNCTURE IN WOMEN'S' HEALTH-RELATED ISSUES

Studies conducted in Israel, Belgium, and other European countries on the personal use of complementary and alternative medicine (CAM) therapy indicate that women in general tend to employ integrative treatments more frequently than men, but that they used CAM interventions in conjunction with contemporary medical practices (Beal, 1998). Similar findings were obtained in an Australian study in which over 3,000 adults in Australia were questioned on their use of CAM treatments. It revealed that perimenopausal women in particular tended to employ integrative modalities at a higher rate than men (MacLennan, Wilson, & Taylor, 1996). Pain was identified as the most common reason for using CAM, but women used acupuncture for a number of different health disorders such as dysmenorrhea; lactation problems; nausea and vomiting associated with pregnancy; chemotherapy, and surgery; breech presentation; Raynaud's syndrome; and migraines (Aikens, 1998; Beal, 1998).

Nausea and Vomiting

Using acupuncture to control nausea and/or vomiting associated with pregnancy, chemotherapy, and postoperatively has been studied by several researchers (Aikens, 1998; Dundee, & McMillan, 1991). A review of the literature on the effects of acupuncture, acupressure, electroacupuncture, and TENS of the pericardium 6 point (P6), also referred to as the Neiguan point, revealed a positive effect in most cases (Vickers, 1996). The P6 point is located on the anterior surface of the forearm, approximately "2 'cun' proximal from the wrist crease and P5 3 'cun' proximal from the wrist crease between the tendons of m. palaris longus and m. flexor radialis" (Hoo, 1997, p. 1395). Hoo (1997) explained that pressure to either point would probably produce an antiemetic effect, but pressure between the two points would be totally ineffective. The exact length of a Chinese inch, a "cun" is different for every person. It is defined by measuring the "width of the interphalangeal joint of the patient's thumb or the width of the two radial ends of the flexor creases of a flexed middle finger" (Hoo, 1997, p. 1395).

The most common way to stimulate the P6 acupoint is to apply an elasticized wristband with a blunt button that exerts continuous pressure to the P6 acupoint. The most cited brands in the literature are

AcuBands (AcuBand, Lifestyle Enterprises, Inc., PO Box 355, Little Silver, New Jersey, or Marine products, which can be located at http://www.marineproducts.com.au/default.asp). These wristbands are adjustable and are closed with Velcro, or SeaBands (SeaBand, SeaBand UK Ltd., Leicestershire, United Kingdom), a closed elasticized band. SeaBands are available from Kinakin International Holdings, Inc., #439, 177 Telegraph Bellingham, Washington 98226, or LandFall Navigation (e-mail: infor@landfallnav.com). Another type of acupressure wrist band is the MorningGarde from Marine Logic, Inc., 450 Australian Avenue, Suite 603, West Palm Beach, Florida 33401.

A study of 60 women between 7 and 12 weeks of gestation on the effectiveness of Neiguan point acupressure revealed that the women in the treatment group experienced more than a 60% reduction in morning sickness frequency when compared to the control group ($P < 0.05$) (De Aloysio & Penacchioni, 1992). Additionally, there were no statistically significant differences if the acupressure was unilateral or bilateral.

Another clinical trial of 27 women between 5 and 22 weeks of gestation who used the SeaBands found that the SeaBands decreased the nausea and vomiting by 50% (Stainton & Neff, 1994). The authors also listed specific directions in the use of acupressure bands that were not found anywhere else. These directions include (1) correct positioning of the band, (2) placing acupressure bands bilaterally, (3) applying band on right wrist first, and then left (according to yin-yang principles), and (4) applying additional pressure to the button with episodes of increased nausea and/or vomiting (Stainton & Neff, 1994).

Belluomini, Litt, Lee, and Katz (1994) obtained similar results in the use of acupressure wristbands for pregnancy-associated nausea and vomiting. Their findings revealed that acupressure at the P6 acupoint significantly decreased the nausea ($P = 0.0021$), but had no effect on the frequency of vomiting. The study by Hyde (1987) supported the above findings in that the use of acupressure wristbands significantly reduced nausea in pregnancy ($P < 0.025$).

In contrast to the studies listed above, a clinical trial to investigate the efficacy of pressure on the P6 anatomical site in the management of pregnancy-induced nausea and vomiting found no relief with the use of P6 acupressure (O'Brien, Relyea, & Taerum, 1996). Hoo (1997) responded to this study in a letter to the editor in the *American Journal of Obstetrics and Gynecology*, questioning whether the patients in that study applied the acupressure wristband to the correct acupoint.

Barsoum, Perry, and Fraser (1990) randomized 162 surgical patients to three groups. The groups consisted of (1) an acupressure group using an elasticized band with a button that exerts continuous pressure into the P6 acupoint, (2) a control group with buttonless bands, and (3) a group that received prochlorperazine, an antiemetic with each administered opiate. The degree of nausea was determined using a linear analogue scale, and was found to be significantly ($P = 0.002$) decreased in the acupressure band group on the first 2 days postoperatively when compared with the sham and antiemetic groups (Barsoum et al., 1990). A similar investigation was done by Stein et al. (1997) on 75 patients on the effects of acupressure versus intravenous metoclopramide on nausea and vomiting during spinal anesthesia for cesarean section. Group I received the authentic acupressure band and 2 mL of saline, group II received sham wrist bands and 10 mg of metoclopramide IV, and group III received the sham wrist bands and 2 mL of saline. There was no difference in the incidence of nausea between patients who received only acupressure and patients who received only metoclopramide ($P > 0.05$). Acupressure, however, was not as effective as metoclopramide in controlling episodes of vomiting. ($P = 0.23$). A study done by Fan et al. (1997) further supports these findings. Thus, studies are conflicting regarding the effectiveness of accupressure in helping to alleviate nausea and vomiting.

Labor

There are numerous clinical trials that examine the influence of acupuncture and electroacupuncture on labor induction, inhibition, duration, and pain. Tsuei and Lai (1974) did a study to determine the effects of acupuncture with and without electrical stimulation on the induction of labor. They found that, "in every case, uterine contractions occurred as soon as the patient experienced the needle sensation from the sites of needle insertion but that the success rate was 83%" (Tsuei & Lai, 1974, p. 340). They also reported that none of the mothers received any pain medications during the first stage of labor, which they attribute to the analgesic qualities of acupuncture. In 1977, Tsuei, Lai, and Sharma expanded this study to look at the effects of acupuncture on induction of labor in full- and postterm pregnancies, intrauterine fetal demise, and midterm abortion ($n = 48$), as well as the arrest of premature labor ($n = 12$). Seventy-eight percent of the labor inductions were successful but all attempts at terminating pregnancy at midterm ($n = 7$) were unsuccessful. The success rate for stopping premature labor was 91% (Tsuei et al., 1977).

The use of acupuncture to shorten the duration of labor is controversial. Zeisler, Tempfer, Mayerhofer, Barrada, and Husslein (1998) found that the women who received acupuncture prenatally had a labor that was approximately 61% shorter ($P < 0.0001$), and received significantly less oxytocin during the first stage of labor than the women in the control group ($P = 0.01$). Contrary to these findings, Lyrenas, Lutsch, Hetta, and Lindberg (1987) concluded that acupuncture, in fact, lengthens pregnancy and the time of labor.

Another intervention closely related to electroacupuncture is TENS. The difference is that the electrical charge is administered through electrodes that are placed directly on the skin, instead of needles that have been inserted into precise anatomical locations. It is believed that TENS helps to decrease pain perception by the patient through two mechanisms. The first mechanism is that electrical stimulation blocks the conduction of the painful stimulus to the brain by bombarding the "pain gate" with messages from fibers (Melzack & Wall, 1965). The second mechanism is that local stimulation of the area promotes the release of endorphins. Kemp (1996) noted that TENS would be a helpful tool for women in labor because it provides a degree of control by the patient with minimal additional attention by the medical staff. However, she added that there is a concern that it may cause premature labor if TENS is used before the 37th week of gestation (Kemp, 1996).

Several researchers have tested the benefits of using TENS versus needles in labor For instance, Harrison, Woods, Shore, Mathews, and Unwin (1986) conducted a randomized, placebo-controlled clinical trial to study the effects of TENS on 100 primigravidae and 50 women in their third labor experience. Two pairs of electrodes were applied to the lumbosacral area corresponding to the dermatomes of the posterior rami from T10 to L1 and from S2 to S4. There were no significant differences between the TENS and the TENS placebo groups for pain relief reported by the mothers and the midwives' assessment of pain relief. Also, there were no significant differences for women who completed labor without additional analgesia. The researchers do report, however, that there were highly significant differences in the comments that were solicited from the mothers and the attending midwives 1 hour and 24 hours postbirth. The first-time mothers in the TENS groups offered more favorable statements whether or not they had additional analgesia. In contrast, most of the participants in the TENS placebo group who received additional analgesia reported more unfavorable statements than those who did not receive supplementary analgesia. It is a common practice in this hospital for mothers to administer Entonox (nitrous oxide and oxygen), a particular kind of analgesia, to themselves. The authors noted that if the use of Entonox is omitted from the analysis, the percentage of primigravidae not declining additional analgesia increased to 41% and 24% in the TENS and placebo groups, respectively, and for the para 2 group to 81% and 65%, respectively.

A similar study was done by Dunn, Rogers, and Halford (1989) on postdue pregnant women, but the skin electrodes were applied to acupuncture sites traditionally associated with uterine stimulation, the "spleen 6" on the inner aspect of the lower leg, and the "liver 3," on the foot. Mothers in the experimental group experienced significantly more and stronger contractions than the mothers in the placebo group ($P < 0.01$). The authors hypothesized that stimulation of the peripheral acupoints activates the hypothalamic-anterior pituitary system and the subsequent release of oxytocin (Dunn et al., 1989).

Carroll, Tramer, McQuay, Nye, and Moore (1997) conducted a systematic review of the literature on the effectiveness for labor pain, and found that TENS provided weak analgesic properties in the management of labor pain. These findings may be explained in part by the differences in the location of the electrodes and the intensity and frequency of the electrical stimulation that was administered.

Another way to stimulate the acupoints on the body is by the injection of a solution into the acupoint. Ader, Hansson, and Wallin (1990) conducted an interesting study in which intracutaneous solutions of 0.1 mL of sterile water were injected into four different areas of the lumbosacral area to manage intense lower back pain during the first stage of labor. Women in the treatment group reported significantly less pain 10 minutes after the injection than the placebo group who received 0.01 mL of sterile saline injections ($P < 0.001$). These differences in pain levels continued to be significantly different at 45 minutes ($P < 0.02$) and at 90 minutes ($P < 0.05$) following the treatment. However, their need for meperidine and Entonox was not different.

A related study to the effects of acupuncture on labor done by Tempfer et al. (1998) examined the effects of acupuncture on the length of labor and changes in serum levels of interleukin-8, prostaglandin $F_{2\alpha}$, and beta-endorphin. They concluded that prenatal acupuncture significantly reduces the duration of labor but has no effect on intereukin-8, prostaglandin $F_{2\alpha}$, and beta-endorphin.

Premenstrual Syndrome/Primary Dysmenorrhea

Many studies report that premenstrual syndrome (PMS) and primary dysmenorrhea (PD) affect a large percentage of women. Various studies indicate that prevalence rates of PMS range widely from 30% to

80%, but that 85% of the respondents experience one or more of the signs and symptoms associated with PMS (Nader, 1991; Oleson & Flocco, 1993). A study by Singh, Berman, Simpson, and Annechild (1998), which involved a national telephone survey of 1,052 women, concluded that 58% of women suffered with PMS. PD affects 50% of all teenagers (Kaplan et al., 1997) and is the most common factor in missed days of school or work (Andersch & Milsom, 1982).

The most frequent problems associated with PMS or PD include headaches, moodiness, weight gain, bloating, and increased appetite (Singh et al., 1998). Forty-five percent of women who complain of PMS state that they would like more assistance in coping with it (Campbell, Peterkin, O'Grady, & Sanson-Fisher, 1997). Oleson and Flocco (1993) randomized 35 women to an ear, hand, and foot reflexology group or to a sham reflexology group. Results showed that patients who received reflexology experienced at least a 46% reduction of the somatic and psychological signs and symptoms associated with PMS as compared with the placebo group ($P < 0.01$). In addition, these effects tended to linger for 2 months after the reflexology. Study participants in the reflexology group also reported a deep relaxation state.

Helms (1987) has provided evidence in a randomized controlled trial that acupuncture is quite effective for PD. He reported that 90.9% of the respondents in the real acupuncture group improved versus 36.4% in the placebo acupuncture group, 18.2% in a control group (no acupuncture or medical intervention), and 10% in a visitation control group. Furthermore, there was a 41% decrease in pain medication usd by the women in the real acupuncture group after the acupuncture intervention, and no difference in intake of analgesic medication seen in the other groups (Helms, 1997).

As was mentioned earlier, acupuncture can be administered via pressure (reflexology or acupressure), needling, and electrical stimulation of the acupoints (acupuncture). TENS has been used successfully for different types and sources of pain. Kaplan et al. (1997) evaluated a new TENS device (Freelady, Life Care, Tiberias, Israel), for primary dysmenorrhea. This acupuncture-like TENS provided "marked" pain reduction for 56.9%, and "moderate" alleviation for 30.4%. These findings were substantiated by the fact that the same percentage of patients reported stopping or decreasing their analgesic use. Lewers, Clelland, Jackson, Varner, and Bergman (1989) conducted a similar study using a TENS unit to alleviate primary dysmenorrhea. The experimental group reported at least a 50% reduction in pain immediately after the treatment. This study also suggested that auriculotherapy may be helpful in reducing dysmenorrhea.

Addictions

Using acupuncture in the treatment of addictions was first explored in 1972, when patients who had a known history of addictions to opium and heroin reported a marked decrease in their cravings after experiencing electroacupuncture preoperatively (NIH, 1997). Subsequent studies indicated that 90% were drug free over a two week period, and another study suggested a 51% success rate at a 1-year follow-up (NIH, 1997). Most of the addiction treatment centers in the United States now use the "five-point auricular" model advocated by the National Addiction Detoxification Association (Bullock et al., 1989; NIH, 1997). Significantly more patients in the treatment group in Bullock's study completed the trial of acupuncture treatments than the control group. They also reported reduced cravings for alcohol, fewer drinking incidents, and lower incidence of admissions to detoxification units (Bullock et al, 1989).

Another study in the management of cocaine addiction used three auricular acupoints generally known to be effective for addictions, and control sites a few millimeters removed from the treatment site. The use of cocaine dropped considerably for patients in the control and the treatment groups. However, there were significant differences on their ratings of cravings (Avants, Margolin, Chang, Kosten, & Birch, 1995). Patients in the treatment group reported significantly less cravings than those in the control group.

It is believed that placing needles in the area of the concha stimulates the vagus nerve and reduces cravings for the abused substance (Ulett et al., 1998b). Other studies support the idea of acupuncture for addictions. Ulett et al. (1998b) cited a study in which Han used a TENS unit to stimulate acupoints on the body using alternating high (100 Hz) and low (2 Hz) frequencies, which clearly showed a reduction in withdrawal symptoms.

Pain

In general, acupuncture has a long history in the treatment of acute and chronic pain. Ulett et al. (1998b) reported four studies that indicate that acupuncture has a 70% success rate for the reduction of low back pain, arthritis, headaches, and other painful conditions.

Headache Pain

Acupuncture has been known to be effective for short-term relief of migraine headaches. A 3 year prospective study suggested that over half of the participants reported at least a 50% reduction in symptoms associated with migraine headaches and reduced their use of analgesics from a mean of 19.5 before treatment to 9.2 after treatment (Baischer, 1995). The acupressure point that is traditionally used for headaches is called the "large intestine 4." It is located by pinching the fleshy part of the web between the thumb and index finger with the thumb and index finger of the opposite hand (Milton, 1998). Massaging the tips of the toes on both feet, which corresponds to the top of the head, is another recommended location (Milton, 1998).

Dental Pain

Acupuncture in the management of dental pain has been used for centuries in China. A systematic review of the literature produced 16 controlled studies on the effectiveness of acupuncture on dental pain (Ernst & Phittler, 1998). Ernst and Phittler (1998) concluded that acupuncture can serve as dental analgesia to lessen dental pain but that certain information was lacking. They recommended that future studies include the mechanics of the procedure and compare its effectiveness to prevailing methods of controlling dental pain.

Phantom Pain

Lixing Lao reported to the NIH Panel (Bareta, 1998) that acupuncture was as effective as medication, but that acupuncture used with medication gave more pain relief than either one alone. Lu (1998) published a case report on the use of acupuncture in the treatment of phantom limb pain on a 34-year-old female athlete whose right leg was amputated following a boating accident. Postoperatively she experienced excruciating and incapacitating "contraction pain" that occurred "in waves" throughout the stump. She described the pain by saying, "My right big toe and heel [are] trapped inside the stump." She then requested information on CAM. In place of using traditional acupuncture, several acupoints were stimulated with percutaneous electrical nerve stimulation (PENS) with increasing electrical strength (2.5 Hz to 30 Hz) twice a week for a month.

After 2 weeks, the patient reported an 80% improvement, and after a month of PENS, she was able to resume full-time employment with the assistance of crutches (Lu, 1998).

Back Pain

Back pain is one of the most common health problems and the most frequent reason for using CAM (Eisenberg et al., 1993). Ernst and White (1998) conducted a meta–analysis of clinical studies of acupuncture and back pain. They concluded that acupuncture was more effective than control interventions, but they were unable to state whether acupuncture was more effective than a placebo (Ernst & White, 1998).

Postoperative Pain

A study was done in England to determine the efficacy of electroacupuncture on postoperative pain, nausea, and drowsiness among 20 healthy women who had had abdominal surgery (Christensen, Noreng, Andersen, & Nielsen, 1989). Electroacupuncture was used right after closure of the surgical wound but while the patient was still anesthetized. The group that received electroacupuncture used 50% less of the patient-controlled analgesia via infusion pump as compared with the group who did not receive the electroacupuncture ($P = 0.01$) (Christensen et al., 1989). However, another study by Christensen et al. (1993) on the effects of electroacupuncture on postoperative pain on fifty women undergoing a hysterectomy indicated that there were no significant differences between the treatment and control groups. The authors suspected that the effects of the electroacupuncture may have worn off prior to the assessment of postoperative pain. They referred to previous studies that suggest that electroacupuncture effects last approximately 2 hours post-operatively (Christensen, et al., 1993). Other studies have indicated that the frequency and intensity of the current can modulate the effectiveness of the electroacupuncture (Ulett, 1996).

Renal Colic

Acupuncture has also been effective in the management of renal colic. Lee et al. (1992) reported that acupuncture was equally effective but had a more rapid onset than Avafortan, and had no reported side effects.

OTHER USES FOR ACUPUNCTURE

Acupuncture has been successfully used for many other conditions. For instance, the incidence of laryngospasm following tracheal extubation in children was significantly less in those receiving acupuncture when compared with a control group ($P < 0.05$) (Lee et al., 1998). Raynaud's syndrome is responsive too, indicated by patients receiving acupuncture demonstrating a marked decrease of attacks by 63% ($P = 0.03$) and a drop in the mean duration of capillary flow stop ($P = 0.02$) with acupuncture (Appiah et al., 1997). Chen and Yu (1998) reviewed the literature on acupuncture treatment for urticaria, showing that there are six different kinds of acupuncture approaches that are effective for urticaria. For instance, they refer to the combined technique of ordinary acupuncture and auricular acupuncture. Another method is the injection of thiamine hydrochloride (Vitamin B_1) into the acupoints. Severe itching in patients with uremic pruritis was dramatically reduced with electroacupuncture. The reduction in the itching allowed these patients to obtain more sleep time, which, in turn, increased their quality of life (Duo, 1987).

Insomnia and Urinary Problems in Women

Acupuncture is used for additional problems as well. For instance, in a review article on the use of acupuncture in the management of insomnia, Lin (1995) cited a 90% success rate. In a study by Sprott, Franke, Kluge, and Hein (1998), acupuncture decreased pain levels and positive tender points by 50% ($P < 0.001$) and 31% ($P < 0.01$), respectively, in patients with fibromyalagia. Additional findings revealed that serum substance P and serotonin levels increased by 54% ($P < 0.01$) and 28% ($P = 0.01$), respectively. Acupuncture also seems to be effective for urinary frequency, urgency, and dysuria in women (Chang, 1988; Culligan & Sand, 1998). One study by Aune, Alraek, LiHua, and Baerheim (1998) suggested that acupuncture is even useful for the prevention of recurrent lower urinary tract infections in adult women.

Menopausal Symptoms

Acupuncture has also been used in the treatment of menopausal symptoms such as hot flashes, night sweats, and urogenital dryness. Cohen, Carey, and Rousseau (1988) compared acupuncture administered to no more than 10 established menopause-related acupoints to a control group that received acupuncture to acupoints not appropriate for these symptoms. Hot flashes in the treatment group were decreased by 30% but remained unchanged in the control group (Cohen, Carey, & Rousseau, 1998).

Version of Breech Presentations in Labor

Using acupuncture with and without moxibustion to convert breech babies to a vertex position has been practiced in China for years, but has not been widely offered as an option in the United States. Nonetheless, a recent clinical trial of 260 women in their 33rd week of gestation suggested that a significant increase in fetal activity and a cephalic presentation was observed in those women who received acupuncture with moxibustion for 1 to 2 weeks (Cardini & Weixin, 1998). Beal (1992a) referred to similar studies in which the conversion to vertex rate for the treatment groups ranged between 75% and 80%, with 39% for the control group. The sites most frequently chosen for the version of breech babies are the BL67 or the end point of the bladder meridian, and the SP6, spleen meridian. BL67 is found bordering the outer, proximal corner of the nail of the little toe (Beal, 1992b). The SP6 is on the inferior side of the ankle, four fingerbreadths above the top of the internal malleolus (Beal, 1992b).

Female Infertility

There is some research to support the use of acupuncture in female infertility. Stener-Victorin, Waldenstrom, Andersson, and Wikland (1996) conducted a study to access the effects of electroacupuncture on blood flow impedance in the uterine arteries in women with infertility problems. After eight electroacupuncture treatments over 4 weeks, the pulsatility index in the uterine arteries was significantly reduced ($P < 0.0001$). The authors explained that this effect is probably due to the inhibition of sympathetic activity. The presentation by Yu (1998) on the induction of ovulation with acupuncture to the NIH Consensus Development Conference on Acupuncture indicated that the rate of successful induction of ovulation varies greatly, depending on the medical history of the woman. Yu stated that the success rate for acupuncture-induced ovulation is 86.7 % in pubertal dysfunctional uterine bleeding, 60% in pubertal oligomenorrhea, and 36.87% in polycystic ovarian syndrome (Yu, 1998).

SUMMARY

Acupressure and acupuncture are components of an ancient Chinese art and treatment modality that is not well understood within the Western paradigm. However, in the past several years the World Health Organization and the National Institutes of Health officially recognized acupressure and acupuncture as effective interventions for a wide variety of health problems. These problems include the management of nausea and vomiting, surgical wounds, back pain, headache, addictions, labor induction, Raynaud's syndrome, depression, breech presentations, and others.

Acupuncture can be performed by using needles, burning herbs (moxibustion), TENS units and by injecting solutions into the acupoints. It is believed that the healing effects of acupressure and acupuncture are due to the release of endogenous endorphins and glucocorticoids and blocking of the pain gate. Adverse effects are possible but generally are benign and uncommon. The licensure, education requirements, and certification requirements for acupuncture are different in each state. Persons who are interested in receiving acupuncture are encouraged to investigate the credentials and qualifications of the individual practitioner.

Web sites that provide additional information on acupuncture are:

- http://www.americanwholehealth.com/library/acupuncture/tcm.htm
- http://www.nlm.nih.gov/pubs/cbm/acupuncture.html.

REVIEW AND DISCUSSION

See boxes "Patient Education" and "Continuing Questions/Challenges" for discussion topics for this chapter.

Patient Education

- Acupuncture is appropriate for a variety of conditions:
  —Postoperative and chemotherapy nausea and vomiting
  —Postoperative pain
  —Pregnancy-induced nausea
- Acupuncture may be helpful for a variety of conditions:
  —Addictions
  —Headaches

—Stroke rehabilitation
—Tennis elbow
—Fibromyalgia
—Myofacial pain
—Osteoarthritis
—Carpal tunnel syndrome
—Spasticity associated with cerebral palsy
—Bell's palsy
—Asthma
—Induction of labor
—Premenstrual syndrome and primary dysmenorrhea
• Most treatments are done on an outpatient basis.
• Symptoms often worsen before they get better.

Continuing Questions/Challenges

Are some people more amenable and responsive to acupuncture
treatment than others? If so, what explains this phenomenon?
How can acupuncture work in conjunction with other treatments?

REFERENCES

Acupuncture Laws by State. (1999). (on-line). Available: http://acupuncture.com/StateLaws/StateLaws.htm

Ader, L., Hansson, B., & Wallin, G. (1990). Parturition pain treated by intracutaneous injections of sterile water. *Pain, 41,* 133–138.

Aikens, M.P. (1998). Alternative therapies for nausea and vomiting of pregnancy. *Obstetrics and Gynecology, 91*(1), 149–155.

American Academy of Medical Acupuncture. (1999). Medical acupuncture research foundation. (on-line). Available: http://acupuncture.com/StateLaws/StateLaws.htm

Andersch, B., & Milsom, I. (1982). An epidemiologic study of young women with dysmenorrhea. *American Journal of Obstetrics and Gynecology, 144,* 655–660.

Appiah, R., Hiller, S., Caspary, L, Alexander, K., & Creutzig, A. (1997). Treatment of primary Raynaud's syndrome with traditional Chinese acupuncture. *Journal of Internal Medicine, 241*(2), 119–124.

Aune, A., Alraek, T., LiHua, H., & Baerheim, A. (1998). Acupuncture in the prophylaxis of recurrent lower urinary tract infection in adult women (abstract). *Scandinavian Journal of Primary Health Care, 1,* 37–39.

Avants, S.K., Margolin, A., Chang, P., Kosten, T.R., & Birch, S. (1995). Acupuncture for the treatment of cocaine addiction: investigation of a needle puncture control. *Journal of Substance Abuse Treatment, 12*(3), 195–205.

Baischer, M.D. (1995). Acupuncture in migraine: Long term outcome and predicting factors (abstract). *Headache, 35*(8), 472–474. From *Alternative Therapies in Health and Medicine,* 1999, *5*(1), 90

Bareta, J. C. (1998). Evidence presented to consensus panel on acupuncture's efficacy. *Alternative Therapies in Health and Medicine, 4*(1), 22–30, 102.

Barsoum, G., Perry, E.P., & Fraser, I.A. (1990). Postoperative nausea is relieved by acupressure. *Journal of the Royal Society of Medicine, 83*(2), 86–89.

Beal, M.W. (1992a). Acupuncture and related treatment modalities. Pt. I: Theoretical background. *Journal of Nurse-Midwifery, 37*(4), 254–259.

Beal, M.W. (1992b). Acupuncture and related treatment modalities. Pt. II: Applications to antepartal and intrapartal care. *Journal of Nurse-Midwifery, 37*(4), 260–268.

Beal, M.W. (1998). Women's use of complementary and alternative therapies in reproductive health care. *Journal of Nurse-Midwifery, 43*(3), 224–234.

Beinfield, H., & Korngold, E. (1995). Chinese traditional medicine: An introductory overview. *Alternative Therapies in Health and Medicine, 1*(1), 44–52.

Belluomini, J., Litt, R.C., Lee, K.A., & Katz, M. (1994). Acupressure for nausea and vomiting of pregnancy: A randomized, blinded study. *Obstetrics and Gynaecology, 84*(2), 245–248.

Bullock, M.L., Culliton, P.D., & Oleander, R.T. (1989). Controlled trial of acupuncture for severe recidivistic alcoholism. *Lancet, 1*(8652), 1435–1439.

Burton Goldberg Group. (1997). Acupuncture. In *Alternative medicine: The definitive guide.* Tiburon, CA: Future Medicine Publishing, Inc.

Cadwell, V. (1998). A primer on acupuncture. *Journal of Emergency Nursing, 24*(6), 514–517.

Campbell, E.M., Peterkin, D., O'Grady, K., & Sanson-Fisher, R. (1997). Premenstrual symptoms in general practice patients. Prevalence and treatment. *Journal of Reproductive Medicine, 42*(10), 637–646.

Cardini, F., & Weixin, H. (1998). Moxibustion for correction of breech presentation: A randomized controlled trial. *JAMA, 280*(18), 1580–1584.

Carroll, D., Tramer, M., McQuay, H., Nye, B., & Moore, A. (1997). Transcutaneous electrical nerve stimulation in labour pain: A systematic review. *British Journal of Obstetrics and Gynaecology, 104*(2), 169–175.

Ceniceros, S., & Brown, G.R. (1998). Acupuncture: A review of its history, theories, and indications. *Southern Medical Journal, 91*(12), 1121–1125.

Chang, P.L. (1988). Urodynamic studies in acupuncture for women with frequency, urgency and dysuria. *Journal of Urology, 140*(3), 563–566.

Chen, C.J., & Yu, H.S. (1998). Acupuncture treatment of urticaria. *Archives of Dermatology, 134,* 1397–1399.

Christensen, P.A., Noreng, M., Andersen, P.E., & Nielsen, J.W. (1989). Electroacupuncture and postoperative pain. *British Journal of Anesthesia, 62*(3), 258–262.

Christensen, P.A., Rotne, M, Vedelsdal, R.H., Jensen, K., Jacobsen, K., & Husted, C. (1993). Electroacupuncture in anaesthesia for hysterectomy. *British Journal of Anesthesia, 71*(6), 835–838.

Cohen, S.M., Carey, B., & Rousseau, M.E. (1998). Menopausal symptom management with acupuncture (Abstract). *Menopause, 5,* 257.

Culligan, P.J., & Sand, P.K. (1998). Involuntary urine loss in women: Help for a hidden problem. *Patient Care, 32*(2), 141–162.

Davies, A., Lewith, G., Goddard, J., Howarth, P. (1998). The effect of acupuncture on nonallergic rhinitis: A controlled pilot study. *Alternative Therapies in Health and Medicine, 4*(1), 70–74.

De Aloysio, D., & Penacchioni, P. (1992). Morning sickness control in early pregnancy by Neiguan point acupressure. *Obstetrics and Gynecology, 80*(5), 852–854.

Dundee, J.W., & McMillan, C. (1991). Positive evidence for P6 acupuncture antiemesis. *Postgraduate Medicine Journal, 67*(787), 417–422.

Dunn, P.A., Rogers, D., & Halford, K. (1989). Transcutaneous electrical nerve stimulation at acupuncture points in the induction of uterine contractions. *Obstetrics and Gynecology, 73*(2), 286–290.

Duo, L.J. (1987). Electrical needle therapy of uremic pruritus. *Nephron, 47*(3), 179–183.

Eisenberg, D.M., Davis, R.B., Ettner, S.L., Appel, S., Wilkey, S., Rompay, M.V., & Kessler, R.C. (1998). Trends in alternative medicine use in the United States, 1990–1997. *Journal of the American Medical Association, 280*(18), 1569–1575.

Eisenberg, D.M., Kessler, R.C., Foster, C., Norlock, F.E., Calkins, D., & Delbanco, T.L. (1993). Unconventional medicine in the United States. *New England Journal of Medicine, 328*(4), 246–252.

Ernst, E., & Phittler, M. (1998). The effectiveness of acupuncture in treating acute dental pain: A systematic review (abstract). *British Dental Journal, 184,* 443–447. From *Alternative Therapies in Health and Medicine, 5*(1), 90.

Ernst, E, & White, A. (1997). Acupuncture: Safety first (letter to the editor). *British Medical Journal, 314,* 1362.

Ernst, E., & White, A. (1998). Acupuncture for back pain. *Archives of Internal Medicine, 158,* 2235–2241.

Fan, C.F., Tanhui, E., Joshi, S., Trivedi, S., Hong, Y., & Shevde, K. (1997). Acupressure treatment for prevention of postoperative nausea and vomiting. *Anesthesia Analog, 84*(4), 821–825.

Han, J.S., Ding, X.Z., & Fan, S.G. (1986). CCK-8: Antagonism on electroacupuncture analgesia and a possible role in electoacupuncture tolerance. *Pain, 27,* 101–115.

Harrison, R.F., Woods, T., Shore, M., Mathews, G., & Unwin, A. (1986). Pain relief in labour using transcutaneous electrical nerve stimulation (TENS): A TENS/TENS placebo controlled study in two parity groups. *British Journal of Obstetrics and Gynaecology, 93*(7), 739–746.

Helms, J.M. (1987). Acupuncture for the management of primary dysmenorrhea. *Obstetrics and Gynecology, 69*(1), 51–56.

Helms, J. M. (1998). An overview of medical acupuncture. *Alternative Therapies in Health and Medicine, 4*(3), 35–45.

Helms, J. M. (In press). An overview of medical acupuncture. In W.B. Jonas & J.S. Levin (Eds.). *Essentials of complementary and alternative medicine* (on-line). Available: http://www.medicalacupuncture.org/helmsarticle.htm

Hicks, J., Hicks, A., Mole, P., & Smith, C. (1997). Core curriculum is important. *British Medical Journal, 315,* 429–430.

Hoo, J.J. (1997). Acupressure for hyperemesis gravidarum. *American Journal of Obstetrics and Gynecology, 176*(6), 1395–1397.

Hsu, D.T., & Diehl, D.L. (1998). Acupuncture: The West gets the point. *Lancet, 352s*(Suppl. 5), SIV1.

Hyde, E. (1989). Acupressure therapy for morning sickness. A controlled clinical trial [Abstract]. *Journal of Nurse Midwifery, 34*(4), 171–178.

Jimenez, S.L.M. (1992). Teaching acupressure for pregnancy and birth. *Journal of Perinatal Education, 1*(1), 58–60.

Judelson, D.R., & Dell, D.L. (1998). *The complete women's wellness book.* New York: Golden Books.

Kaplan, B., Rabinerson, D., Lurie, S., Peled, Y., Royburt, M., & Neri, A. (1997). Clinical evaluation of a new model of a transcutaneous electrical nerve stimulation device for the management of primary dysmenorrhea. *Gynecologic and Obstetric Investigation, 44*(4), 255–259.

Kemp, T. (1996). The use of transcutaneous electrical nerve stimulation on acupuncture points in labour. *Midwives, 109*(1307), 318–320.

Kent, G.P., Brondum, J., Keenlyside, R.A., LaFazia, L.M., & Scott, H.D. (1988). Large outbreak of acupuncture-associated hepatitis B (abstract). *American Journal of Epidemiology, 127*(3), 1591–1598.

Landmark Healthcare & Interactive Solutions. (1998). *Landmark report on public perceptions of alternative care.* Sacramento, CA: Landmark Healthcare.

Lee, C.K., Chien, T.J., Hsu, J.C., Yang, C.Y., Hsiao, J.M., Huang, Y.R., & Chang, C.L. (1998). The effect of acupuncture on the incidence of postextubation laryngospasm in children. *Anaesthesia, 53*(9), 917–920.

Lee, Y.H., Lee, W.C., Chen, M.T., Huang, J.K., Chung, C., & Chang, L.S. (1992). Acupuncture in the treatment of renal colic. *Journal of Urology, 147,* 16–18.

Lee, R.J.E., & McLwian, J.C. (1985). Subacute bacterial endocarditis following ear acupuncture. *International Journal of Cardiology, 7,* 62–63.

Lewers, D., Clelland, J.A., Jackson, J.R., Varner, R.E., & Bergman, J. (1989). Transcutaneous electrical nerve stimulation in the relief of primary dysmenorrhea. *Physical Therapy, 69*(1), 3–9.

Lin, Y. (1995). Acupuncture treatment for insomnia and acupuncture analgesia. *Psychiatry and Clinical Neurosciences, 49*(2), 119–120.

Lu, T.V. (1998). Acupuncture treatment for phantom limb pain. *Alternative Therapies in Health and Medicine,4*(5), 124.

Lyrenas, S., Lutsch, H., Hetta, J., & Lindberg, B. (1987). Acupuncture before delivery: Effect on labor. *Gynecologic and Obstetric Investigation, 24*(4), 217–224.

Lyrenas, S., Lutsch, H., Hetta, J., & Nyberg, F. (1990). Acupuncture before delivery: Effect on pain perception and the need for analgesics. *Gynecologic and Obstetric Investigation, 29*(2), 118–124.

MacLennan, A.H., Wilson, D.H., & Taylor, A.W. (1996). Prevalence and cost of alternative medicine in Australia. *Lancet, 347,* 569–573.

Marwick, C. (1997). Acceptance of some acupuncture applications. *Journal of the American Medical Association, 278,* 1725–1727.

Melzack, R., & Wall, P.D. (1965). Pain mechanisms: A new theory. *Science, 150,* 971–979.

Milton, D. (1998). Using alternative and complementary therapies in the emergency setting. *Journal of Emergency Nursing, 24*(6), 500–508.

Nader, S. (1991). Premenstrual syndrome: Tailoring treatment to symptoms. *Postgraduate Medicine, 90,* 173–178.

Nasir, L. (1998). Acupuncture in a university hospital: Implications for an inpatient consulting service. *Archives of Family Medicine, 7*(6), 593–596.

NIH Consensus Development Conference on Acupuncture. (1997, November 3–5). [online]. Available: http://odp.od.nih.gov/consensus/cons/107/107_abstract.pdf

NIH Consensus Development Panel on Acupuncture. (1998). Acupuncture. *Journal of the American Medical Association, 280*(17), 1518–1524.

Norheim, A.J. (1996). Adverse effects of acupuncture: A study of the literature for the years 1981–1994 (abstract). *Journal of Alternative and Complementary Medicine, 2*(2), 291–297.

Norheim, A.J., & Fonnebo, V. (1995). Adverse effects of acupuncture [letter to the editor]. *Lancet, 345*(8964), 1576.

O'Brien, B., Relyea, M.J., & Taerum, T. (1996). Efficacy of P6 acupressure in the treatment of nausea and vomiting during pregnancy. *American Journal of Obstetrics and Gynecology, 174*(2), 708–715.

Oleson, T., & Flocco, W. (1993). Randomized controlled study of premenstrual symptoms treated with ear, hand, and foot reflexology. *Obstetrics and Gynecology, 82*(6), 906–911.

Plawecki, H.M., & Plawecki, J.A. (1998). Acupuncture the same difference. *Journal of Gerontology Nursing, 24*(7), 45–46.

Pomeranz, B. (1996). Acupuncture and the raison d'etre for alternative medicine. *Alternative Therapies in Health and Medicine, 2*(6), 85–91.

Reston, J. (1971a, July 26). Now about my operation in Peking. *New York Times,* pp. A1, A6.

Reston, J. (1971b, August 22). A view from Shanghai. *New York Times,* pp. E 13.

Rubik, B. (1995). Can Western science provide a foundation for acupuncture? *Alternative Therapies in Health and Medicine, 1*(4), 41–47.

Schulte, E. (1996). Acupuncture: Where East meets West. *RN, 10,* 55–57.

Singh, B.B., Berman, B.M., Simpson, R.L., & Annechild, A. (1998). Incidence of premenstrual syndrome and remedy usage: A national probability sample study. *Alternative Therapies in Health and Medicine, 4*(3), 75–79.

Sprott, H., Franke, S., Kluge, H., & Hein, G. (1998). Pain treatment of fibromyalgia by acupuncture (abstract). *Rheumatology International, 18*(1), 35–36.

Stainton, M.C., & Neff, E.J. (1994). The efficacy of seabands for the control of nausea and vomiting in pregnancy. *Health Care for Women International, 15*(6), 563–575.

Stein, D.J., Birnbach, D.J., Danzer, B.I., Kuroda, M.M., Grunebaum, A., & Thys, D.M. (1997). Acupressure versus intravenous metoclopramide to prevent nausea and vomiting during spinal anesthesia for cesarean section. *Anesthesia Analog, 84*(2), 342–345.

Stener-Victorin, E., Waldenstrom, U., Andersson, S.A., & Wikland, M. (1996). Reduction of blood flow impedance in the uterine arteries of infertile women with electro-acupuncture (abstract). *Human Reproduction, 11*(6), 1314–1317.

Tempfer, C., Zeisler, H., Heinzl, H., Hefler, L., Husslein, P., & Kainz, C. (1998). Influence of acupuncture on maternal serum levels of interleukin-8, prostaglandin F2alpha, and beta-endorphin: A matched pair study. *Obstetrics and Gynecology 92*(2), 245–248.

Tsuei, J.J., & Lai, Y.F. (1974). Induction of labor by acupuncture and electrical stimulation. *Obstetrics and Gynecology, 43*(3), 337–342.

Tsuei, J.J., Lai, Y.F., & Sharma, S.D. (1977). The influence of acupuncture stimulation during pregnancy: The induction and inhibition of labor. *Obstetrics and Gynecology, 50*(4), 479–478.

Ulett, G.A. (1996). Conditioned healing with electroacupuncture. *Alternative Therapies in Health and Medicine, 2*(5), 56–60.

Ulett, G. A., Han, S, & Han J. (1998a). Electroacupuncture: Mechanisms and clinical application. *Biological Psychiatry, 44*, 129–138.

Ulett, G. A., Han, S, & Han J. (1998b). Traditional and evidence-based acupuncture: History, mechanisms, and present status. *Southern Medical Journal, 91*(12), 1115–1120.

Vickers, A. (1996). Can acupuncture have specific effects on health? A systematic review of acupuncture antiemesis trials. *Journal of the Royal Society of Medicine, 89*, 303–311.

White, A.R., & Ernst, E. (1998). A trial method for assessing the adequacy of acupuncture treatments. *Alternative Therapies in Health and Medicine, 4*(6), 66–71.

White, A.R., Resch, K., & Ernst, E. (1998). Randomized trial of acupuncture for nicotine withdrawal symptoms. *Archives of Internal Medicine, 158*, 2251–2255.

Yamashita H., Tsukayama, H., Tanno, Y., & Nishijo, K. (1998). Adverse events related to acupuncture (letter to the editor). *Journal of the American Medical Association, 280*(18), 1563–1564.

Yu, J. (1998). Induction of ovulation with acupuncture. *NIH Consensus Development Conference on Acupuncture* (1997, November 3–5). (on-line). Available: http://odp.od.nih.gov/consensus/cons/107/107_abstract.pdf

Zeisler, H., Tempfer, C., Mayerhofer, K., Barrada, M., & Husslein, P. (1998). Influence of acupuncture on duration of labor. *Gynecologic and Obstetric Investigation, 46*(1), 22–25.

CHAPTER 14

Biofeedback

Christine D. Meyer

Key Points

- Some physiological changes are related to stress.
- These changes can be controlled by controlling the stress response.
- Biofeedback teaches people how to control these responses.
- The patient will be taught to become very sensitive to bodily cues and to control responses.
- These bodily cues are related to specific physiological activities.
- A variety of instruments may be used during a biofeedback session:
  —Electromyelogram (EMG)
  —Electrogastrography (EGG)
  —Electroencephalogram (EEG)
  —Electrocardiogram (EKG)
  —Galvanic Skin Response machine (GSR)
  —Thermal sensor
  —Strain gauges
  —Moisture sensors
  —Pressure sensors

We are accustomed to employing conscious feedback, the type used when we learn to play darts or to drive a car. Through training and technology (biofeedback), we can also gain access to many previously unconscious sources of feedback, such as heart rate, peripheral skin temperature, blood pressure, and muscle tension.

—Dossey, Keegan, Guzzetta, & Kolkmeier, 1995, p. 579

In the 1960s, most students in the health sciences were taught that certain body processes, such as heart rate, blood pressure, brain wave patterns, muscle function, and digestion were not under a person's voluntary control, but were solely governed by the autonomic nervous system (Burton Goldberg Group, 1997). Since then, we have learned that we can influence these functions through biofeedback and other self-regulatory interventions, such as guided imagery and progressive relaxation. The earliest known biofeedback machine was developed by O. Hobart Mowrer in 1938 to help children stop bed-wetting. He designed a device that sounded an alarm when moisture was detected (Burton Goldberg Group, 1997). But it was not until 1969 when the term *biofeedback* first appeared in the literature (Association for Applied Psychophysiology and Biofeedback, 1998).

Biofeedback may or may not be classified as a type of complementary or alternative medicine (CAM). However if one were to rank order CAM interventions based on current medical education curricula, clinical experience, and practice, biofeedback would be positioned at the "less alternative" end of the continuum (Eisenberg et al., 1998). Supporting this stance is a study by Boucher and Lenz (1998) in which biofeedback was found to be the best understood of the listed CAM therapies, and that 94.5% of physicians reported that they possessed a fundamental or more advanced understanding of biofeedback.

While the use of CAM is rapidly becoming more acceptable, the use of biofeedback has not increased since 1990. Eisenberg's study (1998) revealed that 1% of all visits to practitioners of alternative therapies were for biofeedback, and that this rate remained unchanged between 1990 to 1997 (Eisenberg, 1998). The Landmark Report on Public Perceptions of Alternative Care (1998), which interviewed 1,500 Americans in 1997, found that while only 2% of the respondents employed biofeedback within the past year, 56% reported that they would be very likely or somewhat likely to try biofeedback. Similar findings were found in a study by Burg, Hatch and Neims (1998) in which 62% of 1,012 Florida residents reported that they had used one or more of 11 CAM modalities, but only 2% had ever used biofeedback. A survey of

764 faculty members in a major Health Science Center in Florida indicates that less than 10% of the faculty used biofeedback at some time (Burg, Kosch, et al., 1998). Ten percent of the respondents in a study of Emergency Department staff stated they had used biofeedback, and 8.5% reported recommendation of biofeedback in their practice (Taylor, Lin, Snyder, & Eggleston, 1998).

BIOFEEDBACK DEFINED

Biofeedback was defined by the U.S. Department of Health and Human Services (1994b). Their document described biofeedback as a process in which a person learns how to and is able to reliably influence physiologic responses. These physiological responses include those that are not ordinarily under voluntary control or those that ordinarily are easily regulated but for which regulation has broken down because of trauma or disease.

Biofeedback is a procedure whereby individuals are taught to become very sensitive to subtle bodily cues that correspond to specific physiological activities within their bodies. The most common types of instruments used in biofeedback are the electromylogram (EMG), the electroencephalogram (EEG), the electrocardiogram (EKG), a thermal sensor, and a galvanic skin response (GSR) machine (Jennings et al., 1999; Burton Goldberg Group, 1997; National Institutes of Health, 1995). For example, an EMG would be an appropriate tool to help a patient with tension headaches to learn to decrease voluntarily the muscle tension in the neck and upper back. The beep may grow either louder or faster as muscular tension increases, and become softer or slower as tension decreases. With practice, the patient learns how to lower the tone or slow the beeps, and also begins to associate "what it feels like" when muscular tension is low (Alexander & Steefel, 1995). Eventually, the patient is able to "control" tension headaches by consciously relaxing the neck muscles. EMGs may also be employed for back, neck and temporomandibular pain, and urinary problems. They may be used to reduce the level of depression in alcoholics and to improve treatment retention for cocaine users (Kearney, 1997).

An EEG, a device to monitor electrical brain wave activity, may be used in the treatment of insomnia or anxiety. Temperature or thermal sensors are typically used to assist patients to learn to elevate skin temperature. Through the feedback from the sensor, the patient learns to control blood flow to selected areas and thus raise or lower the skin temperature at will. Temperature sensors are typically used for patients with Raynaud's syndrome and hypertension.

Less common biofeedback instruments include an electrogastrography (EGG), strain gauges to evaluate penile dysfunctions, and moisture sensors to monitor bladder incontinence. In 1999, Jennings et al., reported on a new diagnostic tool, called a Thermal Vascular Test, used to determine Raynaud's syndrome. This instrument measures digital blood pressure responses to a combined cooling and occlusion condition.

ADVANTAGES AND DISADVANTAGES OF BIOFEEDBACK

Certain advantages and disadvantages of biofeedback have been identified. Advantages to biofeedback include the following: there are no known adverse effects; it is low cost; it provides a degree of control for the patient; and it can be used as adjuvant therapy with other interventions. Probably the most significant barrier to its use is a lack of understanding by Western medical professionals, whose education was based predominantly on the biomedical model. Thus they were not exposed to nontraditional or non–Western approaches to health care. However, a recent survey revealed that 53 medical schools out of 124 members of the Association of American Medical Colleges now offer courses or "brown-bag" lecture series on complementary and alternative medicine (Moore, 1998). In fact, one school, the University of Pennsylvania, lists CAM as a required component in the curriculum.

Other obstacles range from a lack of reimbursement by health insurance companies and lack of well-established outcome measures on what is regarded as success (Chilton, 1996). Furthermore, biofeedback requires special training and the purchase of biofeedback equipment for the practitioner, and an ability to follow directions and a high level of motivation and commitment by the patient (U.S. Department of Health and Human Services, 1994b).

GENERAL USES FOR BIOFEEDBACK

Biofeedback is frequently incorporated into the plan of care for specific disorders. Various studies indicated that biofeedback is beneficial for stress-related disorders such as tension and migraine headaches, chronic neck and back pain, and temporomandibular joint (TMJ) pain (Burton Goldberg Group, 1997; Chilton, 1996; Fynes, et al., 1999). It is also useful for vascular-related problems such as hypertension and

Raynaud's syndrome; gastrointestinal disorders such as irritable bowel syndrome; insomnia; urinary incontinence; bowel incontinence and retention; mild to moderate acute pain and postoperative incisional pain; asthma; twitching of the eyelids; cardiac problems; and panic and anxiety disorders (Alexander & Steefel, 1995; Bleijenberg & Kuijpers, 1994; Burton Goldberg Group, 1997; U.S. Department of Health and Human Services, 1992a). The Association for Applied Psychophysiology and Biofeedback (1998) states that biofeedback techniques can be used for other health conditions such as premenstrual syndrome (PMS), bed-wetting, epilepsy paralysis, spinal cord injury and attention deficit hyperactive disorder (ADD/ADHD).

Biofeedback is not a panacea for any condition or medical disorder. For instance, biofeedback is not helpful for serious anatomical problems such as fractured bones and herniated disks (Burton Goldberg Group, 1997). Additionally, the panel on the Agency for Health Care Policy and Research (1994a) does not recommend biofeedback in the treatment of acute low back pain. Jablon, Naliboff, Gilmore, and Rosenthal (1997) conducted an interesting study to evaluate the effects of progressive relaxation and EMG biofeedback on glucose tolerance and fructosamine levels in non-insulin-using Type II diabetic patients. Their findings indicated that biofeedback-assisted relaxation training did not improve diabetic control.

A study to evaluate the effectiveness of EMG and skin-temperature biofeedback with relaxation training to decrease chemotherapy-induced nausea and vomiting revealed that relaxation training was effective in reducing nausea and anxiety during chemotherapy, but the EMG and skin-temperature biofeedback alone produced no effect on the nausea and anxiety during chemotherapy (Burish & Jenkins, 1992).

USE OF BIOFEEDBACK IN SPECIFIC MEDICAL CONDITIONS

Headaches

Headache disorders are the second leading complaint of chronic pain in the United States, but tend to afflict a higher percentage of women in a lower socioeconomic group (Barrett, 1996). Epidemiological studies have shown that 29% of women and 14% of men have headaches every few days, or headaches which cause a great deal of stress. They have also been directly linked to a loss of more than 150 million work days and are the seventh most common reason for visits to ambulatory care centers (Barrett, 1996).

In the early 1960s Elmer Green, PhD, and Alyce Green of the Menninger Clinic inadvertently discovered that biofeedback could be used to treat headaches (Burton Goldberg Group, 1997). They noticed that at the moment a woman experienced an abrupt 10-degree increase in the temperature of her hand, she reported that her headache had just suddenly disappeared too. By using this information they created a temperature-sensing biofeedback instrument and then educated patients to curtail their migraines merely by using a relaxation technique to raise the temperature of their hands (Burton Goldberg Group, 1997). The National Institutes of Health Technology Assessment Conference (1995) issued a statement that there is moderate evidence to believe that EMG biofeedback in conjunction with other therapies such as relaxation is effective for tension and migraine headaches.

Studies by Wauquier, McGrady, Aloe, Klausner, and Collins (1995) and McGrady, Wauquier, McNeil, and Gerard (1994) provide further support that biofeedback is effective in the management of headaches.

Nonpharmacological interventions in the management of headaches are especially appealing for pregnant women. Marcus, Scharff, and Turk (1995) report that a combined therapy approach consisting of relaxation, thermal biofeedback, and physical therapy reduced headaches by 72%, and that this improvement was still evident after 12 months for 50% of the participants (Scharff, Marcus, & Turk, 1995).

Cardiovascular Disorders

Biofeedback is quite effective in the management of hypertension, especially if it is combined with other changes in one's lifestyle. In fact, one study determined that home training with a direct blood pressure biofeedback was effective in reducing the blood pressure in unmedicated, mild hypertensives (Marcus, Scharff, Mercer & Turk, 1998). Nakao et al. (1997) conducted a study to determine the effectiveness of blood pressure biofeedback on hypertension by autoshaping. Respondents were assigned to either a treatment group that experienced biofeedback once a week for 4 weeks or a placebo group that monitored their own blood pressure during the study, but received biofeedback at a later time. Results indicate that the participants in the treatment group were able to lower their blood pressure significantly by $17 \pm 18/8 \pm 7$ ($P < 0.01$) mm Hg and were able to minimize an elevation of blood pressure brought on by mental stress by 8 ± 9 ($P < 0.05$)/4 ± 8 mm Hg. The blood pressure measurements of participants in the control group remained the same during the study, but were significantly decreased by 20 ± 15/9 ± 7 ($p < .01$), and .11 + 10 ($p < .05$) 5 ± 9 when they received the biofeedback.

Since biofeedback is so effective in increasing skin temperature, it is often used in the treatment of Raynaud's disease. It is estimated that Raynaud's disease affects women 5 times more often than men (Sedlacek & Taub, 1996). Sedlacek and Taub (1996) cite several studies in which biofeedback decreased the average number of ischemic attacks anywhere between 67% and 93%. Moser, Dracup, Woo, and Stevenson (1997) report on studies done by Freedman showing that biofeedback significantly decreased the frequency of vasospastic episodes by up to 92% and that these beneficial effects continued for 2 years.

A recent study was done to determine whether a single biofeedback treatment could change the pathophysiological effects of advanced heart failure (Moser et al., 1997). It found that patients in the treatment group experienced the following changes: an increase in finger and toe temperature ($P < 0.001$), a decrease in systemic vascular resistance ($P < 0.005$) in 76% of the patients, an increase in cardiac output ($P > 0.001$) in 80% of the patients, and a decrease in respiratory rate ($P < 0.001$) in 84% of the patients.

Insomnia

There are basically three kinds of insomnia: (1) difficulty in falling asleep, (2) trouble remaining asleep, and (3) early awakening. Any of these types can be caused by very different factors. Possible causes of insomnia are muscle tension, racing thoughts, pain, or depression. Melvyn Werbach, MD, Assistant Clinical Professor of UCLA School of Medicine and Director of the Biofeedback Medical Clinic in Tarzana, California, states that "biofeedback is appropriate when insomnia is due to overstimulation of the autonomic nervous system" (Burton Goldberg Group, 1997, p. 75). Dr. Werbach explains that the underlying cause of the insomnia is a factor in deciding the best biofeedback approach. For instance, for patients who report that they are able to relax their body physiologically but are having trouble falling asleep because they can't seem to stop thinking about things, biofeedback using EEG would probably be the first-line choice. However, for patients who experience extreme muscular tension and moist skin, biofeedback using the EMG and GSR would be appropriate (Burton Goldberg Group, 1997).

Urinary Incontinence

Urinary incontinence is defined by the urinary incontinence panel for the Agency for Health Care Policy and Research as, "involuntary loss of urine which is sufficient to be a problem" (U.S. Department of Health and Human Services, 1992b). The three major types of urinary incontinence and incidence are stress incontinence (50–70%), urge incontinence (20–40%), and overflow incontinence (5–10%). It is a common problem among men and women, affecting approximately 10 million Americans (U.S. Department of Health and Human Services, 1992b). For persons between 15–64 years of age, it is estimated that 10 to 25% of women and 1.5–5% of men experience urinary incontinence (Thomas, Plymat, Blannin, & Meade, 1980). Burns et al. (1993) reports that 30% of noninstitutionalized postmenopausal women experience stress urinary incontinence. Another study by Ferguson et al. (1990) determined that 22% of a group of women who were 45 years old reported stress incontinence. It is estimated that urinary incontinence in noninstitutionalized persons older than 60 years of age ranges from 15 to 30% (Diokno, Brock, Brown, & Herzog, 1986). The prevalence of urinary incontinence for individuals who live in a nursing facility is 50% or higher (National Center for Health Statistics, 1979).

The types of biofeedback instruments that are typically used in the treatment of urinary incontinence are an EMG and manometric devices. These devices are used to evaluate muscular activity of the pelvic and abdominal muscles, post-void residual volume defined as the quantity of urine remaining in the bladder immediately after voiding, and pressure readings of the detruser muscle in the bladder wall responsible for contracting and expelling the urine from the bladder. When biofeedback is employed in the treatment of urinary incontinence, the Clinical Practice Guideline for Urinary Incontinence in Adults recommends that it should be used in combination with behavioral therapies such as bladder training, prompted voidings, voiding diary, Kegel exercises, and electrical stimulation of the pelvic muscles and viscera (1992b). Glavind, Laursen, and Jaquet (1998) provided biofeedback directions on how to perform pelvic floor exercises correctly to women with stress incontinence. At 3 months, 39% were symptom-free and 42% reported improvement. Two years later, 27% remained symptom-free and 47% verbalized improvement. A questionnaire revealed that 78% possessed an accurate understanding of the exact location of the pelvic floor muscles.

Further support of the effectiveness of bladder training exercises with biofeedback is provided by McDowell et al. (1999). Another study on 197 women between the ages of 55 and 92 years showed that biofeedback was significantly more effective with a mean 80% reduction in urinary incontinence than with oxytatynin chloride with a mean 68.5% reduction (Burgio et al., 1998). In a study using 135 community-dwelling women, Burns et al. (1993) compared the effects of biofeedback alone, Kegel exercises alone, and a control group. They found that urinary incontinence significantly decreased in both treatment groups and persisted for at least 6 months. However, the biofeedback group demonstrated a significant increase in their EMG's measurements. Another study by Stein, Discippio, Davia, and Taub (1995) found that biofeedback helped 36% of the women with stress incontinence and 43% of women with urgency incontinence. They also discovered that daytime frequency (P=0.038) and nocturia (P=0.044) was significantly reduced. However, these authors stated that not many patients chose biofeedback as a first line of treatment and doubted that biofeedback will ever be a standard treatment choice.

An overall review of studies which was done by the Panel on Urinary Incontinence reveals that there is a 54 to 94% improvement in incontinence when biofeedback is used with other behavioral interventions (USDHHS, 1992b). These studies also suggest that biofeedback coupled with other behavioral interventions can be beneficial in decreasing symptoms associated with neurologic problems. However, individuals who experience incontinence through extraurethral devices are not candidates for biofeedback. The U.S. Department of Health and Human Services, Agency of Health Care Policy and Research on Urinary Incontinence advises that a behavioral intervention like biofeedback be used initially before a surgical or other invasive procedure. Unfortunately, even though the Clinical Practice Guideline for Urinary Incontinence in Adults reports that bladder training via biofeedback significantly reduces urinary incontinence, biofeedback is seldom integrated in the initial plan of care (USDHHS, 1992b).

Defecation Disorders

Defecation disorders may include a wide range of disorders such as anal incontinence for flatus, anal incontinence for feces, and constipation with obstructive defecation. Females are eight times more likely to experience anal incontinence than males. A major cause of fecal and gas incontinence in women is obstetrical trauma to the anal sphincter. The incidence rate for fecal incontinence for women following their first vaginal delivery varies widely from 5% to 22%, whereas the incidence rate for women who are 50 years old or older is approximately 15% (Fynes et al., 1999; Meyer, Schreyer, De Grandi, & Hohl-feld, 1998; Roberts, et al., 1999).

The goals and the type of most biofeedback techniques in the treatment of defecation disorders depend on the specific problem. For example, the goals of biofeedback for patients with incontinence are to strengthen anal sphincter tone and increase the patient's sensory perception, whereas the goal for patients with obstruction constipation is to relax the anal sphincter (Rao, 1998). Studies indicate that biofeedback is effective in increasing anorectal manometry (resting and squeezing pressures), and thus improves overall rectal and anal control to decrease anal incontinence (Fynes et al., 1999; Rao, 1998).

Miscellaneous Conditions

Even though most of the literature supports the use of biofeedback in the treatment of headaches, insomnia, and urinary and bowel disorders, there are isolated studies that indicate that biofeedback-assisted procedures may be helpful for other conditions. For instance, a study by Podoshin, Ben-David, Fradis, Gerstel, and Felner (1991) suggested that biofeedback is more effective than acupuncture and Cinnarizine in patients who have idiopathic subjective tinnitis. Another study found that electromyographic feedback in patients who experienced an ischemic stroke with subsequent hemiplegia and foot drop increased their muscle strength and ability to walk (Intiso, Santilli, Grasso, Rossi, & Caruso, 1994). Another interesting study was done by Leahy, Clayman, Mason, Lloyd, and Epstein (1998) in which a new computerized biofeedback game was developed to teach patients with Irritable Bowel Syndrome to achieve a relaxation state in order to decrease the number of symptomatic episodes.

Tyson (1996) has recommended the use of biofeedback-controlled systematic desensitization to decrease the stress of child care providers precipitated by infant crying. Based on the assumption that the adult's perception of infant crying will define if the event will evoke a physical and psychological stress mediated response, Tyson and Sobschak (1994) investigated if biofeedback-assisted stress management training while listening to an infant crying could reduce their perceived arousal, anxiety, physiological responses, and evaluation of the crying. They named this procedure "biodesensitization." Compared to the results of the adults in the control group, biofeedback assisted stress management training significantly decreased the electroencephalogram cortical arousal, perceived arousal, and anxiety levels. Tyson continues to investigate this new intervention as a preemptive technique to possibly prevent child abuse as a response to physiological hyperre-activity.

Individuals who are interested in using biofeedback can obtain a list of educated practitioners from the Association for Applied Psycho-physiology and Biofeedback, 10200 W. 44th Avenue, Suite 304, Wheat Ridge, CO, 80033-2840, Phone: 1-800-477-8892/303-422-8436, Fax: 303-422-8894, E-mail: AAPB@resourcenter.com, Internet: http:/// www.aapb.org

SUMMARY

Biofeedback is an effective tool in the treatment of many health problems. It provides to the patient a way to learn to adapt or regulate body functions that were once believed not to be under one's control. It has been found to be especially useful for headaches, insomnia, spe-cific cardiovascular disorders, and urinary incontinence. However, biofeedback seems to be more effective when used in conjunction with other behavioral interventions.

REVIEW AND DISCUSSION

See boxes "Patient Education" and "Continuing Questions/Chal-lenges" for discussion topics for this chapter.

Patient Education

Biofeedback may be helpful for the following conditions:
- Stress-related disorders (tension and migraine headaches, chronic neck/back pain, temporomandibular joint pain, irritable bowel syndrome, and stress as response to infant crying)
- Vascular-related problems (hypertension, Raynaud's syndrome)
- Insomnia
- Urinary incontinence
- Defecation disorders
- Mild to moderate acute pain and postoperative incisional pain
- Asthma
- Twitching of the eyelids
- Cardiac problems
- Panic and anxiety disorders
- Congestive heart failures
- Foot drop

Continuing Questions/Challenges

Does biofeedback work better in some patients than other patients? If
so, what explains this phenomenon?
Can biofeedback work in conjunction with other treatment modalities?
What risks exist with biofeedback?
Name five conditions for which biofeedback is not very helpful.

REFERENCES

Alexander, C.J., & Steefel, L. (1995). Biofeedback: listen to the body. *RN, 58*(8), 51–52.

Association for Applied Psychophysiology and Biofeedback. (1998). What is biofeedback? (on-line). http://www.aapb.org.

Barrett, E. (1996). Primary care for women: Assessment and management of headache. *Journal of Nurse-Midwifery, 41*(2), 117–124.

Bleijenberg, G., & Kuijpers, H.C. (1994). Biofeedback treatment of constipation: A comparison of two methods (Abstract). *The American Journal of Gastroenterology, 89*(7), 1021–1026.

Boucher, T.A., & Lenz, S.K. (1998). An organizational study of physicians' attitudes about and practice of complementary and alternative medicine. *Alternative Therapies in Health and Medicine, 4*(6), 59–65.

Burg, M.A., Hatch, R.L., & Neims, A.H. (1998). Lifetime use of alternative therapy: A study of Florida residents. Personal use of alternative medicine therapies by health science center faculty. *Southern Medical Journal 91*(12), 1126–1131.

Burg, M.A., Kosch, S.G., Neims, A.H., & Stoller, E.P. (1998). Personal use of alternative medicine therapies by health science center faculty. *Journal of the American Medical Association, 280*(18), 1563.

Burgio, K.K., Locher, J.L., Goode, P.S., Hardin, J.M., McDowell, B.J., Dombroski, M., & Candib, D. (1998). Behavioral vs drug treatment for urge urinary incontinence in older women: A randomized controlled trial. *Journal of the American Medical Association, 280*(23), 1995–2000.

Burish, T.G., & Jenkins, R.A. (1992). Effectiveness of biofeedback and relaxation training in reducing the side effects of cancer chemotherapy. *Health Psychology, 11*(1), 17–23.

Burns, P.A., Pranikoff, K., Nochajski, T.H., Hadley, E.C., Levy, K.J., & Ory, M.G. (1993). A comparison of effectiveness of biofeedback and pelvic muscle exercise treatment of stress incontinence in older community-dwelling women. *Journal of Gerontology, 48,* 167–174.

Burton Goldberg Group. (1997). Biofeedback training. In *Alternative medicine: The definitive guide*. Tiburon, CA: Future Medicine Publishing, Inc.

Chilton, M. (1996). Panel recommends integrating behavioral and relaxation approaches into medical treatment of chronic pain, insomnia. *Alternative Therapies in Health and Medicine, 2*(1), 18–20, 22, 24, 26, 28.

Diokno, I.A., Brock, B.M., Brown, M.B., & Herzog, A.R. (1986). Prevalence of urinary incontinence and other urological symptoms in the noninstitutionalized elderly. *Journal of Urology, 136,* 1022–1025.

Dossey, B.M., Keegan, L., Guzzetta, C.E., & Kolkmeier, L.G. (1995). *Holistic nursing: A handbook for practice* (2nd ed.). Gaithersburg, MD: Aspen Publishers, Inc.

Eisenberg, D.M., Davis, R.B., Ettner, S.L., Appel, S., Wilkey, S., Rompay, M.V., & Kessler, R.C. (1998). Trends in alternative medicine use in the United States, 1990–1997. *JAMA, 280*(18), 1569–1575.

Ferguson, K.L., McKey, P.L., Bishop, K.R., Kloen, P., Verheul, J.B., & Dougherty, M.C. (1990). Stress urinary incontinence. Effect of pelvic muscles exercises. *Obstetrics and Gynecology, 75*(4), 671–675.

Fynes, M., Donnelly, V., Behan, M., O'Connell, P.R., & O'Herlihy, C. (1999). Effect of second vaginal delivery on anorectal physiology and faecal continence: A prospective study. *Lancet, 354* (9183), 883–986.

Fynes, M.M., Marchall, K., Cassidy, M., Behan, M., Walsh, D., O'Connell, P.R., & O'Herliny, C. (1999). A prospective, randomized study comparing the effect of augmented biofeedback with sensory biofeedback alone on fecal incontinence after obstetric trauma (Abstract). *Diseases of the Colon and Rectum, 42*(6), 753–761.

Glavind, K., Laursen, B., & Jaquet, A. (1998).Efficacy of biofeedback in the treatment of urinary stress incontinence (abstract). *International Urogynecology Journal and Pelvic Floor Dysfunction, 9*(3), 151–153.

Intiso, D., Santilli, V., Grasso, M.G., Rossi, R., & Caruso, I. (1994). Rehabilitation of walking with electromyographic biofeedback in foot-drop after stroke [Abstract]. *Stroke, 25*(6), 1189–1192.

Jablon, S.L., Naliboff, B.D., Gilmore, S.L., & Rosenthal, M.J. (1997). Effects of relaxation training on glucose tolerance and diabetic control in type II diabetes [Abstract]. *Applied Psychophysiology and Biofeedback, 22*(3), 155–169.

Jennings, J.R., Maricq, H.R., Canner, J., Thompson, B., Freedman, R.R., Wise, R., & Kaufmann, P.G. (1999). A thermal vascular test for distinguishing between patients with Raynaud's phenomenon and health controls. *Health Psychology, 18*(4), 421–426.

Kearney, M.H. (1997). Drug treatment for women: Traditional models and new directions. *Journal of Obstetric, Gynecologic and Neonatal Nursing, 26,* 459–468.

Landmark Healthcare & Interactive Solutions. (1998). Landmark report on public perceptions of alternative care. Sacramento: Landmark Healthcare.

Leahy, A., Clayman, C., Mason, I., Lloyd, G., & Epstein, O. (1998). Computerized biofeedback games: A new method for teaching stress management and its use in irritable bowel syndrome. *Journal of the Royal College of Physicians, 32*(6), 552–556.

Marcus, D.A., Scharff, L., Mercer, S., & Turk, D.C. (1998). Nonpharmacological treatment for migraine: Incremental utility of physical therapy with relaxation and thermal biofeedback. *Cephalalgia, 5,* 262–272.

Marcus, D.A., Scharff, L., & Turk, D.C. (1995). Nonpharmacological management of headaches during pregnancy. *Psychosomatic Medicine, 57,* 527–535.

McDowell, B.J., Engberg, S., Sereika, S., Donaovan, N., Jubeck, M.E., & Engberg, R. (1999). Effectiveness of behavioral therapy to treat incontinence in homebound older adults. *Journal of the American Geriatrics Society, 47*(3), 309–318.

McGrady, A., Wauquier, A., McNeil, A., & Gerard, G. (1994). Effect of biofeedback-assisted relaxation on migraine headache and changes in cerebral blood flow velocity in the middle cerebral artery [Abstract]. *Headache, 34*(7), 424–428.

Meyer, S., Schreyer, A., DeGrandi, P., & Hohlfeld, P. (1998). The effects of birth on urinary continence mechanisms and other pelvic-floor characteristics. *Obstetrics and Gynecology, 92*(4), 613–618.

Moore, N.G. (1998). A review of alternative medicine courses taught at US medical schools. *Alternative Therapies in Health and Medicine, 4*(3), 90–101.

Moser, D.K., Dracup, K., Woo, M.A., & Stevenson, L.W. (1997). Voluntary control of vascular tone by using skin-temperature biofeedback-relaxation in patients with advanced heart failure. *Alternative Therapies in Health and Medicine, 4*(1), 51–59.

Nakao, M., Nomura, S., Shimosawa, T., Yoshiuchi, K., Kumano, H., Kuboki, T., Suematsu, H., & Fujita, T. (1997). Clinical effects of blood pressure biofeedback treatment on hypertension by auto-shaping. *Psychosomatic Medicine 59*, 331–338.

National Center for Health Statistics. (1979). The national nursing home survey: 1977 summary for the United States by Van Nostrand J.F., et al. (DHEW Publication No. 79-1794). Vital and Health Statistics. Series 13, No. 43. Washington, DC: Health Resources Administration, U.S. Government Printing Office.

National Institutes of Health Technology Assessment Conference statement. (1995). Integration of behavioral and relaxation approaches into the treatment of chronic pain and insomnia. (on-line) http://nlm.nih.gov/nih/ta/www/017txt.html

Podoshin, L., Ben-David, Y., Fradis, M., Gerstel, R., & Felner, H. (1991). Idiopathic subjective tinnitis treated by biofeedback, acupuncture and drug therapy [Abstract]. *Ear, Nose and Throat Journal, 70*(5), 284–289.

Rao, S.S. (1998). The technical aspects of biofeedback therapy for defecation disorders. *Gastroenterologist, 6*(2), 96–103.

Roberts, R.O., Jacobsen, S.J., Reilly, W.T., Pemberton, J.H., Lieber, N.M., & Talley, N.J. (1999). Prevalence of combined fecal and urinary incontinence: A community-based study. *Journal of the American Geriatrics Society, 47*(7), 309–318.

Scharff, L., Marcus, D.A., & Turk, D.C. (1996). Maintenance of effects in the nonmedical treatment of headaches during pregnancy. *Headache, 36*(5), 285–290.

Sedlacek, K., & Taub, E. (1996). Biofeedback treatment of Raynaud's disease. *Professional Psychology: Research and Practice, 27*, 548–553.

Stein, M., Discippio, W., Davia, M., & Taub, H. (1995). Biofeedback for the treatment of stress and urge incontinence. *Journal of Urology, 153*(Pt a), 641–643.

Taylor, A.G., Lin, Y., Snyder, A., & Eggleston, K. (1998). ED staff members' personal use of complementary therapies and their recommendations to ED patients: A southeastern US regional survey. *Journal of Emergency Nursing, 24*(6), 495–499.

Thomas, T.M., Plymat, K.R., Blannin, J., & Meade, T.W. (1980). Prevalence of urinary incontinence. *British Medical Journal, 281*, 1243–1245.

Tyson, P.D. (1996). Biodesensitization: Biofeedback-controlled systematic desensitization of the stress response to infant crying [Abstract]. *Biofeedback and Self Regulation, 21*(3), 273–290.

Tyson, P.D., & Sobschak, K.B. (1994). Perceptual responses to infant crying after EEG biofeedback assisted stress management training: Implications for physical child abuse [Abstract]. *Child Abuse and Neglect, 18*(11), 933–943.

U.S. Department of Health and Human Services. (1992a). *Acute pain management: Operative or medical procedures and trauma: Clinical practice guideline.* (AHCPR Publication No. 92-0032). Rockville, MD: Agency for Health Care Policy and Research, Public Health Service.

U.S. Department of Health and Human Services. (1992b). *Urinary incontinence in adults: Clinical practice guidelines.* (AHCPR Publication No. 92-0038). Rockville, MD: Agency for Health Care Policy and Research, Public Health Service.

U.S. Department of Health and Human Services. (1994a). *Acute low back problems in adults: Clinical practice guidelines.* (AHCPR Publication No. 95-0642). Rockville, MD: Agency for Health Care Policy and Research, Public Health Service.

U.S. Department of Health and Human Services. (1994b). *Management of cancer pain* (AHCPR Publication No. 94-0592). Rockville, MD: Agency for Health Care Policy and Research, Public Health Service.

Wauquier, A., McGrady, A., Aloe, L., Klausner, T., & Collins, B. (1995). Changes in cerebral blood flow velocity associated with biofeedback-assisted relaxation treatment of migraine headaches are specific for the middle cerebral artery [Abstract]. *Headache, 35*(6), 358–362.

CHAPTER 15

Spiritual Approaches

Michele Maloy

Key Points

Concepts of spirituality and religiosity are different, but overlapping.
Spirituality is involved with developing meaning.
Spirituality occurs across the life span.
Spirituality is a facet of optimal health and well-being.

There are many ways we can stay in touch with ourselves . . . for some of us, being connected with a spiritual community helps.

—Boston Women's Health Collective, 1998, p. 582

This chapter presents a discussion of the concept of spirituality with a particular focus on women, with emphasis on some specific cultural groups of women. Spirituality as contributing to women's health and well-being is emphasized. Some specific ways of integrating spirituality into one's life are suggested, including storytelling and poetry.

SPIRITUALITY, RELIGIOSITY, AND MEANING

A discussion of spirituality requires differentiating between what is termed religious, or religiosity, and what is termed spiritual, or spirituality. One does not negate the other, nor does one necessarily imply the presence of the other. One is not inherently better than the other one. Religion, or religiosity, describes the nature of the divine (God) and prescribes ways of relating to this God, which involve commonly held beliefs, symbols, and rituals such as prayer, meditation, and eating patterns (Miller, 1995). Spirituality refers to a "dynamic balance that allows and creates healing of body-mind-spirit" (Dossey & Guzzetta, 1995, p. 6) and, according to Dossey and Guzzetta (1995), may sometimes involve organized religion.

Today's contemporary religions are societal institutions that have evolved over thousands of years. While religion often provides comfort and a sense of purpose to many men and women, some believe that the religions of Western civilization can be particularly detrimental to women. King (1989), in discussing women's roles and status in religious institutions, stated that cross-cultural studies note that the more undifferentiated religion and society are, the greater is the participation of women in religion. In contrast to our modern religions, women have held higher powers in archaic, ancient, and tribal religions, or in nonhierarchical groups, such as Quakers. Female visionaries with prophetic powers, called *sibyls*, existed in ancient Rome, and were considered the oracles of God.

Barker (1989) emphasized that women have historically viewed most spiritual development in the context of male religious formation. Such religions are androgenic, meaning that the creator is male and the tenets of the religious code have men as the dominant figures. These organized religions may be found lacking for women. For some women, spiritual development begins with developing their own meanings for religious rituals; although not without pain and feelings of alienation. Through this development, the woman moves toward peace, wholeness, and a sense of power.

Apart from religious rituals, another way of viewing spirituality is to emphasize its relationship with the development of meaning. The notion that spirituality is related to searching for and finding meaning is highlighted in the following examples.

Viktor Frankl, a Viennese psychiatrist, survived the German concentration camps of the Second World War. As a result of his experiences and observations, he determined that the single most important motivation in an individual's life is spiritual. Frankl (1984) believed that spiritual phenomena are a part of all people, not just people who adhere to formal religious doctrines. By spiritual, Frankl (1984) referred to one's striving to find meaning in life. This meaning can be found through love or suffering. In suffering, one is placed before a hopeless situation, facing a fate that cannot be changed. The challenge to find meaning is to transform a personal tragedy into a personal victory. Under harsh conditions it seems a paradox, or a cruel impossibility without the spirit. One transcends the situation, finding meaning in a situation that is bleak and tragic. His concentration camp stories held many unbelievable accounts of such victories.

Another example of gaining spirituality by finding meaning is found in a recent book, *Dead Man Walking* by Sister Helen Prejean (1994), where we see the spiritual journey of a murderer and death row inmate, Patrick Sonnier. Sister Prejean's goals for him are not merely that he admits what he had done wrong, but also to change his relationship with these events. Through this spiritual journey, or development, he finally feels genuinely not abandoned or alienated by God, despite his heinous crimes, but sees the look of God's love on Sister Prejean's face before his execution. He is able to see some meaning in his life, and his death gains an aspect of humanity through the process of spiritual growth.

PHILOSOPHICAL APPROACHES TO DEFINING SPIRITUALITY

Our world reflects the philosophy and science that we use to view it, and our society reflects a complex technology that permeates our philosophy and science. Today, we have multiple sources of media: published materials, radio, television, and personal computers. Computers are growing in affordability and capabilities at exponential rates. We are influenced quickly and often, and perhaps quietly as events outside of us change faster than we change. Because of this rapid change around us with the influx of technology, it is important to understand how spirituality has evolved within this complex technological context.

In the seventeenth century, Rene Descartes, a French philosopher and mathematician, promoted the notion of separation between thought (mind) and the subject matter of physical science (body). The acceptance of this dualism as the basis for scientific knowledge placed emphasis on the material, sensate realm, or what is referred to as philosophical materialism. Scholars have recently suggested that this dualism has forestalled our growth as individuals and as a collective because this "way of knowing" has neglected many aspects of being human, such as our spirituality (Fahlberg & Fahlberg, 1991).

King (1989) provided a different philosophical perspective in her prologue to *Women and Spirituality*, as feminist views that seek to change not only power structures, but also social values and consciousness. In following the tenets of philosophical materialism, the patriarchal worldview is one of separatism and pluralism, with a hierarchical focus that emphasizes the individuals in power (in our case, Western society with a male-oriented power base). King's worldview, on the other hand, is not static, but dynamic and changes to the needs of individuals and society. The emphasis is on spiritual health and wellness, versus organized hierarchic religions per se. Perhaps feminism and spirituality have the same quest at heart: to transcend present human existence, search for fulfillment, liberation toward freedom, and the courage to ask and answer hard questions.

Beyond philosophical materialism, Burkhardt's (1989) analysis of the concept of spirituality consists of four main categories: spirit/spirituality, spiritual dimension, spiritual well-being, and spiritual needs. *Spirit/spirituality* is both a process and a journey of an individual's life. It evolves around the overlapping themes of transcendence, universal truth, meaning of existence, and empowering, intimate relationships. The theme of *spiritual dimension* is connectiveness. It is the force that integrates aspects of the spirit. *Spiritual well-being* is a characteristic of state and gives information about the functioning of an individual's spirit/spirituality and spiritual dimension to meet that person's spiritual needs. *Spiritual needs* are vital requirements of the self, which is unique to each individual. When individuals describe their experiences of spiritual well-being, such words as joy, harmonious, mysterious, essential being, essence, and going inside the self are used. Psychologists have referred to this aspect of human development as self-actualization, the part of development beyond the integration of the ego (Fahlberg & Fahlberg, 1991). An integrated ego functions as a major component of one's personality that includes adjusting to reality, modifying anxiety, problem solving, and adapting to internal and external demands (Antai-Otong, 1995). But, unlike twentieth century psychologist Abraham Maslow (1954), who saw self-actualization as a final stage of development, spiritual well-being occurs across an individual's life span, with spirituality as a facet of optimal health and well-being.

SPIRITUALITY AND WOMEN'S WELLNESS

Spirituality is established as an integral part of a person's well-being. Any promotion of holistic health of an individual includes all aspects of that person. Without attention to the total person, including spiritual needs, decreased functioning or illness can occur. Spiritual health is intertwined with our physical and/or emotional well-being. The writings of Jourard have been cited in the literature on spirituality and health (Heriot, 1992; Burkhardt, 1989). Jourard believed that as one's spiritual wellness diminished, depression, diffuse anxiety, and boredom were experienced. If this became a chronic state for the individual, that person would become more susceptible to bacteria, viruses, and the effects of stress.

But illness comes to all. Fostering one's spiritual life and meeting one's spiritual needs cannot prevent what is a natural experience of entropy and time. Spirituality is not just a panacea to prevent life's ills; it can prepare us to navigate life's adversities with greater dignity and completeness. We become less a victim and more a participant in the stories of our own life. Recent studies reported that terminally ill individuals possess a greater hardiness and satisfaction in life resulting from the value found in spiritual concerns (Berggren-Thomas & Griggs, 1995).

Spiritual needs should be considered as a component of any health-promotion or disease-prevention program for any person. Chapman (1986) stated that any well-managed lifestyle program without considering spiritual needs lacks important depth. Spiritual health provides a motivational factor in the difficult task of changing behavior, so often a goal of a health promotion program (Chapman, 1986).

King (1989) has analyzed the feminist movement as a spiritual quest for wellness that would affect our culture and society in positive ways, for all people. When spiritual dimensions are included in new patterns and value systems, vital needs of the soul are met. Feminism is then woven together with spirituality, because feminism is an important political and socioeconomic movement that promotes the change of the whole woman. As women transcend their human experience to effect change, their spiritual self assists in this transcendence. As feminism vigorously dissects all aspects of culture that exclude women, women seek a new way that embraces a new spirituality that is world- and life-affirming. Ecology issues, such as the destruction of flora and fauna by large corporations for profit, would fall under the protective umbrella of an evolved spiritual feminism. As part of women's spiritual growth, the following aspects are included: protest/anger, challenge, changing experience, a new spirituality, a new theology, and prophecy and integration (King, 1989).

Anger is a spiritual protest in always being the "other," being defined by another. The source of this anger is the desire for authenticity, for fullness of life, and love for the earth and its people. As a result of this anger, women form networks with other very different women, and begin a process of consciousness raising. These aware voices express concern about patriarchy, androcentrism, and sexism (which are a false ordering of reality). *Patriarchy* is a term used to describe the situation of order, now and in the past, whereby women are dependent or subordinated to fathers, husbands, brothers, sons, or all men in positions of power, privilege, and influence. Patriarchy is rooted in our values, attitudes, thoughts, and daily life. It permits the perception of androcentrism (male as center) and the ordering of life by gender. It values a masculinity that is aggressive, competent, competitive, and emotionally unavailable. In its contemporary version, it is associated with the rape of nature, destructive aspects of science and technology, and military megalomania with potential for human extinction. The Exxon Valdez oil spill into the pristine waters of Prince Williams Sound in Alaska is a concrete reminder of the destructive aspects of pure androgeny. One decade after the huge loss of wildlife, a glistening oil sheen can be seen in the remaining footsteps as one walks along the sandy surfaces near the water's edge (Mitchell, 1999). Does the sense of empty desolation or anger these Alaskan images provoke arise from our distance from spiritual concerns? Is the unbalanced face of androgeny, lacking in feminine principles, reflected in this oily mirror? As this anger is about being fully human and promoting the profound life-giving powers of individual and social transformation, it is spiritual.

Traditional, organized religions have been the wellsprings at which to satisfy spiritual longings: a hunger for wholeness, a sense of meaning, and purpose to one's life. But male hierarchies of power have focused traditional religions around male myths, recorded by males, and given male interpretation models. The challenge to spiritual feminism is somehow to reform and transcend their consciousness to exclude the old Gods, and invent a new spirituality. Mary Daly (1974) popularized this idea in her book *Beyond God the Father*. Whether we change the overburdening myth of Eve or focus on the transformation of God as maternal, or pull forth the biblical wisdom of Sophia, the question remains: Can religion as traditionally understood have meaning for contemporary women?

The spiritual journal of contemporary feminism is closely linked to the examination of stories of both the female and feminine dimensions of women's experience. The voices of these many women give their innermost experiences of hopes, joys, failures, and transcendence. Women begin to understand themselves by expanding their awareness of their situation, their collective history, and their own assets. Together, these voices of experience give rise to multiple ways of seeing problems and solutions. King (1989) recorded the words in her book of one participant at a Third World conference for women on religion and social change, which illustrates this point in a quietly moving way:

> The women who came were unique and remarkable. They had suffered, yet, they had great strength. Many had acquired an education, or reached where they were now, against all odds. I shall remember the quiet vision of the Hindu women; the outrageous individuality of the Muslims; the continued humor and hope of the black South Africans; and the amazing courage of women from Central America. Here one felt "the other half" of humanity. What if one could bring their common sense, their ability to work together, and their non-hierarchical ways of thinking into play on a world scale? I became aware the greatest potential which we have yet to put into the balance in the attempt to save our world is perhaps the potential of women. Here were exemplified alternative ways of thinking and acting. (p. 67)

The women described have transcended the restricting confines of their particular cultures, and are not defeated in spirit. The description is positive and energized. It gives example of the spiritual wellness within this group. But it also reminds us of an aspect of spirituality in feminism that goes beyond the transformation of the individual. It is the potential for transcendence of a new community. This is the final goal for change and it is accomplished by the spiritual growth of women as they progress from dependence and/or subordination to a realization of self. The voices of women revealing experiences and providing exemplars give power and authority by their expression. It gives other women a spiritual identity, or road map to enable the growth of self that extends on and beyond the self to the community. Women's liberation is a spiritual journey, the owning of self and soul.

As feminists search for renewed spirituality, they look for models that go beyond the gender of God. This search requires an analysis of matriarchal, patriarchal, and the androgynous modes of religious thought. Their voices have inquired into the past and found the Goddess worshipers of ancient times, and are trying to give them contemporary relevance. She may be the closest image we have for a female God. We go to the past for images, to recreate a vision for the future, not to recreate the past. This type of worship may be satisfying for some women and provide some personal affirmation, thereby meeting spiritual needs. It can be limiting for the woman who is not so concerned with analysis of the particular theological issues that can be construed with this version of worship. It also has the potential to limit spiritual growth for all concerned, as do the patriarchal religious institutions that are currently a predominate part of our culture, a flip side of what is already a rigidly gender-assigned expression of God, and thereby resistant to authentic transcendence.

In introducing the message to be delivered by voices of a new theology, King (1989) notes that the primary treatise of this theology is one of liberation. Its role would be to expose theological traditions that continue sexist beliefs and perpetuate violence and alienation. The voices of this category belong to radical, feminist theologians. Some of these women believe that change within the traditional church can come from within due to their influence, and others take the stance of separation, thinking the historical problems of patriarchy and sexism are too entrenched within the church. Mary Daly is known for her radical position of separatism, while Rosemary Ruether is known for her moderate stance (King, 1989). Both women have multiple publications that may be useful for any woman to explore when her spiritual journey takes her to this crossroad of discernment: the place to worship her God that will feed her self and soul.

In concluding King's categories, voices of prophecy and integration remind us that we all want a better world. As women look at the world and see dissatisfaction in political structures, they see both the effects of these structures on their ability to find their own identities and the identities of their communities. The powers that be shape policy, behavior, and public ethos, which in turn plays out in all conditions of our self and our world. Aspects of spirituality are not separated from the body politics; spirituality is both personal and political. The call for woman's spiritual journey, the search for true self, is to return back to the community. Spirituality is the path from power within to power outside, in the political arena. Feminist spirituality affirms the inner relatedness of all things; it calls for the use of power differently, and envisions a unity between the spiritual and the political. It will find expression in campaigning for peace and nonviolence, or for protecting the natural and animal resources of our earth.

WOMEN'S SPIRITUALITY AFRESH

Native American Women and Tribal Images

Sams (1994) offered a Native American portrait of images of the feminine to illuminate parts of the self in women's spiritual journey: the stories of the 13 original clan mothers. The legacy of these images found in "woman's medicine" was passed to the author by her two Kiowa grandmothers: Cisi Laughing Crow, aged 120, and Berta Broken Bow, aged 127. The bases of these stories are the result of the traditions that were struggling to stay alive over the years as Indian nations were scattered during the previous century. At the core of each story is the connection to the earth mother. These stories are the bits and pieces of different tribes collected over the centuries by women. The 13 original clan mothers are talks with relations, wisdom keeper, weighs the truth, listening woman, looks for, storyteller, loves all things, she who heals, setting sun woman, weaves the web, walks tall woman, gives praise, and becomes her vision. Each mother tells the stories exemplifying her wisdom. The clan mothers are universal and uniquely individual at the same moment because of their ability to appear as all facets of womankind. They offer contemporary women insights in healing the pain experienced from the undervaluing of traditional female roles and present a vision of a new balance between female and male. The author has personally benefited from knowing these stories and desires to bring them forth into the community, to "bring inner peace and, therefore, world peace" (Sams, 1994, p 7). It is a recurrent theme within the writings of the female spiritual journey to return to the community with a strong sense of self, well integrated, to share spiritual insights.

In the beginning of time, the 13 original clan women were created by Grandmother Moon and Mother Earth to depict all that is beautiful in woman. The clan mothers originally walked the face of the earth to gather all women together in a sisterhood. All the individual components of each woman's dream combined and produced the seed of peace and love, which were planted in the female side of all human hearts. This holistic philosophy, which does not fragment or separate, gives the unseen ingredient to embarking on a spiritual journey that is satisfying for women and men.

Appalachian Women's Study

In her research on Appalachian women, Barker (1989) asked the question of what spiritual well-being meant for these women. The perspective of each of 13 women was obtained through interviews that attempted to capture their lived experiences. Analysis of the information, or data, obtained from these interviews revealed two major themes to further elucidate relationships and self. The relationship theme included the individual relationship with a deity or creative force, relationship with kin, relationship with others, and the relationship with nature. The theme of self named seven essential aspects of purpose, satisfaction, inner strength, responsibility, clear values, individual identity, and service that are within the realm of self.

Relationship with deity, or creative force, involved a personal connection with a sense of being cared for that transcends the possibilities of any human relationship. This relationship needed daily attention to nurture and develop vis à vis meditation, prayer, or bible study. The women described an empowering relationship that gives meaning to their lives, peace, and security. This experience spills over in positive ways to other relationships and encourages a clear perception of self with the feeling of joy and satisfaction. Aspects of the kinship relationship are characterized by a union that is interdependent, versus the women being dependent. Relationships to others, which are outside the kin relationships, are chosen, intentional, and give meanings that enhance that sense of fellowship and belonging to something outside of one's self. These relationships can be near or far, but importantly, the relationships are active, reciprocal, and satisfying. The final domain of relationships, one's relationship with nature, was strong with all the women. The mountains were seen as a source of shelter, strength, and continuity in a fast world of change; places to return, visit, and leave renewed. This attitude of respect is seen in their behaviors of tending a garden, preserving resources, and expressing the symbolism, or poetry, found in flowers, trees, and mountains. This connectiveness to nature correlates with attitudes and philosophies of Native Americans, whose spirituality is strongly connected to the earth. These women transpose their relationship with nature, kin, and others in a holistic, interconnective weave of life. No distinction or separation is made. For discussion's sake, the author distinguished aspects of self from the theme of relationships. In lived experience, they are interrelated.

STRATEGIES FOR CONTEMPORARY WOMEN

Spiritual Power of Shared Stories

Sigmund Freud used talk to treat people with neurosis/hysteria (curiously predominate in the female population), and called it psychoanalysis. He believed it produced a catharsis, or a release of negative emotions that would lead to health. Freud recognized a powerful avenue for self-growth and transcendence a century ago. People find aspects of the spirit satisfying in a personal, intuitive level, and good results are realized when spiritual needs are met. It is not incidental that one of Freud's proteges, Carl Jung, developed an interest in a person's search for the soul. The following paragraph is composed of pieces from Jung's last book, *The Undiscovered Self* (Jung, 1958).

The forlornness of consciousness in our world is due primarily to the loss of instinct, and the reason for this lies in the development of the human mind over the past aeon . . . the unconsciousness . . . has been ignored altogether. . . . This was not the result of carelessness or lack of knowledge, but of downright resistance to the mere possibility of there being a second menace to the ego that [its] monarchy [author's note: or patriarchy] can be doubted. The religious person, on the other hand, is accustomed to the thought of not being sole master in his own house. . . . Here we must ask: Have I any religious experience and immediate relation to God, and hence that certainty which will keep me, as an individual, from dissolving into the crowd? . . . The religious person enjoys a great advantage. . . . Since it is universally believed that man is merely what his consciousness knows of itself, he regards himself as harmless and so adds stupidity to iniquity. (Jung, pp. 84–95)

Jung saw the need to go beyond the ego, beyond consciousness to explore the spiritual. Only in this approach would individuals find meaning and connectedness instead of fruitless alienation.

The benefit of sharing stories, life reviews, or retelling of myths is frequently recorded in the literature as valuable ways to enhance spiritual growth (Heriot, 1992; Miller, 1995; Reed, 1991). Heriot (1992) noted in her study of the literature concerning spirituality and aging that sharing of deeply personal life experiences with others in a social environment unveiled new dimensions of the self. In other words, these older adults experienced growth of the self when divulging intimate stories to another. In addition, alienation and isolation from support groups have shown to increase the symptomatology with women experiencing premenstrual syndrome (Ornitz & Brown, 1992). Sharing stories of one's experience is an important variant in maintaining health. Narrative, obtained by in-depth interviews, is at present the only way researchers have to obtain information about the experience of spiritual journeys and changes. In her research on midlife women and the spiritual transformation that occurs with death of the mother, Robbins (1990) used lifelines, drawn by the individuals studied, that mark significant life events and provide an anchoring effect during interviews. These lifelines represent complex and diverse life patterns of each woman interviewed. These life patterns are further analyzed as Robbins applies psychological principles to explain the development and change of the self. Images within the self are created and recreated in the relationship to the mother. Over time, with some remodeling of the self, fundamental changes were made with some of the study women. Changes can be made because the self is dynamic and change-able with every insight. New patterns are formed. This transformation does not happen in a void. It necessitates a narrative that occurs within and without the dialogue though relationships, families, small groups, society, and culture. It is a spiritual journey, occurring in a spiritual dimension, that meets spiritual needs. It satisfies the self, that deep part of our being. It recalls the wise words of sixteenth-century metaphysical poet, John Donne:

> No man is an island, entire of itself;
> Every man is a piece of the
> Continent, a part of the main.
> Devotions, 17.

We do not grow spiritually in a void. Only when we reengage with the world after looking inward do we find the power to change and redefine what we are, within our particular elements of women related to women, vocalizing that experience, and giving it spiritual life.

Transcendent/Spiritual Power of Poetry

What language better to illustrate the suffering or joys of the spirit than poetry? It speaks a universal language by the use of metaphor and rhythm that can help the individual in her quest for spiritual wellness: the ability to become larger than one's own actions or one's own life circumstances. Poetry speaks the common and universal language of the heart and thereby creates a unity between the poet, the reader, and others who have come before and after. It creates the primary spiritual element of transcendence. The piece *The First Elegy* by German poet Rainer Maria Rilke, describes the pain of alienation, transcendence, and joy from a moment of spiritual awareness with nature. He glim-mers a hint of human connection at the end (Mitchell, 1989):

> Who, if I cried out, would hear me among the angels'
> hierarchies? And even if one of them press me
> suddenly against his heart: I would be consumed
> in the overwhelming existence. For beauty is nothing
> but the beginning of terror, which we are still just able to endure,
> and we are so awed because it serenely disdains
> to annihilate us. Every angel is terrifying

And so I hold myself back and swallow the call-note
of my dark sobbing. Ah, whom can we ever turn to
in our need? Not angels, not humans,
and already the knowing animals are aware
that we are not really at home in
our interpreted world. Perhaps there remains for us
some tree on a hillside . . .

Oh and night: there is a night, when a wind full of infinite space
gnaws at our faces . . .

Yes, the springtime needed you, often a star
was waiting for you to notice it. A wave rolled toward you
out of the distant past, or as you walked
under an open window, a violin
yielded itself to your hearing. (p. 151)*

As in the tradition of native Americans, nature is viewed as a harbinger of goodness and nurturing, more so than anything not of this world, even angels.

Women's poetry is particularly interesting in that it also offers women a language to express their own, unique realm of the spirit. It is important for a woman to express her own identity to obtain spiritual wellness. Sewell wrote (1991) in her introduction to a book of poetry celebrating women's spirituality that at a point in her life, she discovered that she and other women have no language. She was plagued with this sense of muteness, but how could she change those entrenched cultural linguistic patterns? Women have no "vocabulary in place, no easy syntax, no context of allusion" (Sewell, p. 1). Perhaps we start in the silences, Sewell suggests; ah, if one woman would open up and tell her own story, the world could not endure it, often said in the feminists' literature. Women's poetry speaks of the places in the silence. The oneness, not separation, with her body, and the way she takes metaphor from the natural world, with its cycles. She flows with nature, not against it; she does not try to conquer it. She goes within to explore the daily experience of life and its meaning to her. Our place has an emphasis on feelings and emotions. The importance of intimacy, relationships, direct/honest language, and the owning of the self is in the silence. She speaks with the integrity of self-ownership

---

*Source: From *The Selected Poetry of Rainer Maria Rilke*. Edited and translated by Stephen Mitchell. Copyright © 1982 by Stephen Mitchell. Reprinted by permission of Random House, Inc.

about the unity with life and the call to justice. She is the expression of women's spirituality and is named women's poetry. Poetry can address issues powerfully for women in its aesthetic media. For is it not, as Sewell concludes, love, that is the fruit of spirituality? Nature abhors a vacuum and spirituality does not grow in one. In her suffering and silence, women's poetic voice transcends to empathize with the suffering of others.

In concluding this section on poetry, a poem by Alice Walker, author of *The Color Purple*, a monument in itself about transcendence, will be illustrative of a woman's spirituality of love and protest:

A Few Sirens

Today I am at home
writing poems.
My life goes well:
only a few sirens herald disaster
in the ghetto
down the street.
In the world, people die
of hunger.
On my block we lose
jobs, housing and breasts.
But in the world
children are lost;
whole countries of children
starved to death
before the age
of five
each year;
their mothers squatted
in the filth
around the empty cooking pot
wondering:

But I cannot pretend
to know
what they wonder.
A walled horror
instead of thought
would be my mind.
And our children
gladly starve themselves.

Thinking of the food I eat
every day
I want to vomit, like
people who throw up
at will,
understanding that whether
they digest or not
they must consume.

Can you imagine?

Rather than let the hungry
inside the restaurants
Let them eat vomit, they say.
They are applauded
for this.
They are light.

But
wasn't there a time
when food was sacred?

When a dead child
starved naked
among the oranges
in the marketplace
spoiled
the appetite?

(Walker, 1984, p. 30–31)

Reconciliation: Reading Biblical Scripture Renewed

In a study of homeless women, it was discovered that 88% of the homeless women prayed, 70% attended some type of church or mission worship service on a regular basis, and 68% of these women reported reading the Bible (Shuler, Gelberg, & Brown, 1994). Shuler et al. (1994) also note that those women who did not perceive prayer, or religious practices helpful, had a higher incidence of "worries" and reported depressive symptoms, including depressed feelings, tearfulness, decreased concentration, sleep disturbances, and loss of appetite. Traditional practices continue to have meaning for some women and enable them to meet their spiritual needs.

Omartian (1991) used biblical passages in a creative approach to bring emotional healing to contemporary women. With her ideas, reinforced afresh with scripture, the expectation is to bring healing, hope, and growth to any woman who is emotionally unfulfilled. The goals of her book, *Finding Peace for Your Heart,* meet the earlier mentioned definition of what is a spiritual journey and what are spiritual needs. She viewed women who are emotionally unfulfilled as individuals overwhelmed with fighting depression and feeling a sense of unforgiveness, decreased self-esteem, anger, hopelessness, boredom, fear, anxiety, and rejection—the entire host of negative feelings. Adult women are two to three times more likely to acquire a chronic depressive illness, called by psychiatrists dysthymic disorder (Diagnostic and Statistical Manual of Mental Disorders: DSM IV, 1994). Being of the female gender is a risk factor for depression with a point prevalence in western industrialized nations as 4.5–9.3 percent for women and a 20–25 percent lifetime risk for women (Depression Guideline Panel, 1993). Of interest, the root word for dysthymia, the Greek word *thymos,* is related to the English word *soul.*

Omartian (1991) described emotionally unfulfilled, contemporary women as diminished vectors of human beings who need a simple grade of truth, which can be found in her seven steps to emotional health. Her awareness of the need to share these steps came from the letters she received after she wrote her first book, which shared her destructive life experiences and how she restored herself emotionally. This autobiography detailed her life as a child raised by a mentally ill mother, and how she survived emotionally. Omartian's encounter with the power of the shared story led to the writing of her second book, which was designed to help women find emotional and spiritual health.

The seven steps include the following: acknowledge God, lay a foundation, live in obedience, find deliverance, receive God's gifts, reject the pitfalls, stand strong. Radical feminist theologians can find fault with the language of "live in obedience" and "acknowledge God," recognizing this as the patriarchal female denying God of our Western heritage. The semantics of language can be a problem, as Clemmons (1991) found in working with alcoholic women and the Twelve Steps program. As not to alienate her clients, she paraphrased the twelve steps of Alcoholics Anonymous to a transpersonal view. For example, step three states: Deciding to surrender to a higher consciousness. Starting to transcend isolation. Beginning spiritual recovery (Clemmons, 1991, p. 107). The original phrasing is: Made a decision to turn our will and our lives over to the care of God as we understand Him (p. 101).

The relationship with God discussed in this spiritual journey is one that empowers. Each step in its own way interfaces with aspects of the spiritual journey. Another aspect of the spiritual journey, unfolding of the self, can be unearthed in steps: live in obedience, receiving God's gifts, knowing the pitfalls, and standing strong. Biblical quotations embrace the notion of self or soul and the experience, or standpoint, that will enhance its awareness within the person, or woman: And do not be conformed to this world, but be transformed by the renewing of your mind, that you may prove what is the good and acceptable and perfect will of God (Romans 12:2); or For you have delivered my soul from death (Psalms 116:8) (Omartian, 1991). The significant aspect of the journey is the beginning, to accept a need for the relationship with God, that deity outside of one's self, and the empowerment it can bring. Omartian selected the following scripture to illustrate: the prophet Jeremiah asked God, "Why then is there no healing for the wound of my people?" (Jeremiah 8:12); God answers, "they go from one sin to another; they do not acknowledge me," (Jeremiah 9:3), NIV. To see this passage afresh, healing is referred to as the need for spiritual wellness, and sin as those aspects of the world, such as materialism (concrete or philosophical), sexism, or any specific gender-related issue that prevents women from realizing their self-potential. However, empowerment with this relationship is possible, for as scripture points out to us: "If God is for us, who can be against us?" (Romans 8:13).

CONCLUSION

As I was walking my Scottish terrier one evening, I considered in my thoughts how my pet keeps me a little closer to cardiovascular health. Not only does he remember and remind me of his daily 20-minute walk each evening, but recent studies (Jennings, 1997; Beck & Meyers, 1996) have documented some straightforward and positive physiological effects of pet ownership, such as decreased blood pressure, not even to mention the result on one's psyche to live in the moment of having unconditional love! The wind was rustling leaves in the way it does in the early spring, bringing in the warmer air. Most people were inside; it was dark and I could barely see the sashay of the dog's fuzzy, black hips as we walked under the dim light. In a moment of quiet and updraft of wind, I heard the clear, melodic tinkle of wind chimes in the distance. I felt fortunate to have a neighbor who would purchase and hang those wind chimes outside for anyone to hear their beautiful song. And it occurred to me that this tiny example presented an occasion to understand the spiritual journey and spiritual health. The wind chimes are a metaphor of the self in a state of spiritual well-being, expressed with clarity and beauty, and shared freely with its community. Spiritual health is about the true, bona fide self intertwining with parts of the world outside. It is characterized by one simple word, *satisfying,* and it is not about power or possession. At some part of the day, time must be spent outside of one's self reflected on a relationship, be it with a deity, nature, or a creative force, that is bigger than one's self. It is an empowering relationship that positively nourishes and nurtures the growth of self/soul. And, for women, it seems particularly important to bring it back home, for the benefit of family, friends, and community.

SUMMARY

This chapter has attempted to define spirituality, give sociopolitical and philosophical background pertinent to the understanding of women's issues, and present eclectic approaches or strategies to pursue spiritual well-being. Some of the traditional approaches were not explored because of their availability, easy access, and—less positively— the negative taint of historical sexism. Other strategies are discussed in different chapters in this book, including dancing and music, which contribute to spiritual health. Each specific strategy is less important than the overall philosophical belief in spirituality as an important part of holistic health and wellness for women.

REVIEW AND DISCUSSION

See boxes "Patient Education" and "Continuing Questions/Challenges" for discussion topics for this chapter.

Patient Education

Attaining a spiritual dimension may help in several ways.
  Decrease depression
  Increase self-esteem
  Decrease feelings of hopelessness
  Decrease boredom, fear, anxiety
May find spirituality in poetry, in stories, in telling of own stories.
May find spirituality/religiosity in organized religions.

Continuing Questions/Challenges

How can people develop spiritual approaches to wellness if they are not "religious?"
Is spirituality something that comes from within or can it be learned?

REFERENCES

Antai-Otong, D. (1995). *Psychiatric nursing: Biological and behavioral concepts.* Philadelphia: W. B. Saunders Company.

Barker, E. (1989). Being whole: Spiritual well-being in Appalachian women. A phenomenological study. (Doctoral dissertation, University of Texas at Austin, 1989).

Beck, A., & Meyers, N. (1996). Health enhancement and companion animal ownership. *Annual Review of Public Health, 17,* 247–257.

Berggren-Thomas, P., Griggs, M. (1995). Spirituality in aging: Spiritual need or spiritual journey? *Journal of Gerontological Nursing,* 5–10.

Boston Women's Health Collective (1998). *Our bodies, ourselves for the new century.* New York: Touchstone.

Burkhardt, M. (1989). Spirituality: An analysis of the concept. *Holistic Nursing Practice, 3*(3), 69–77.

Chapman, L. (1986). Spiritual health: A component missing from health promotion. *American Journal of Health Promotion, 1,* 38–41.

Clemmons, P. (1991). Feminists, spirituality, and the twelve steps of Alcoholics Anonymous. *Woman and Therapy, 11,* 97–109.

Daly, M. (1974). *Beyond god the father.*

Depression Guideline Panel. (1993). *Depression in primary care, Vols. 1–2,* (Clinical practice guideline No. 5). Washington, D.C.: United States Government Printing Office.

Diagnostic and Statistical Manual of Mental Disorders: DSM IV. (1994). (4th ed.). Washington, D.C.: American Psychiatric Association.

Dossey, B.M., & Guzzetta, C.E. (1995). Holistic nursing practice. In B.M. Dossey, L. Keegan, C.E. Guzzetta, & L.G. Kolkmeier (Eds.), *Holistic nursing: A handbook for practice.* Gaithersburg, MD: Aspen Publishers, Inc.

Fahlberg, L., & Fahlberg, L. (1991). Exploring spirituality and consciousness with an expanded science: Beyond the ego with empiricism, phenomenology, and contemplation. *American Journal of Health Promotion, 5,* 273–281.

Frankl, V. (1984). *Man's search for meaning* (3rd ed.). New York: Simon & Schuster.

Heriot, C. (1992). Spirituality and aging. *Holistic Nursing Practice, 7*(1), 22–31.

Jennings, L. (1997). Potential benefit of pet ownership in health promotion. *Journal of Holistic Nursing, 15*(4), 358–372.

Jung, C. G. (1958). *The undiscovered self.* Boston: Little, Brown and Company.

King, U. (1989). *Women and spirituality: Voices of protest and promise.* New York: New Amsterdam.

Macmillan Dictionary of Quotations. (1989). New York: Macmillan Publishing.

Maslow, A.H. (1954). *Motivation and personality.* New York: Harper & Row.

Miller, M. (1995). Culture, spirituality, and women's health. *Journal of Obstetric, Gynecologic, and Neonatal Nursing, 24*(3), 257–263.

Mitchell, J. (1999, March). In the wake of the spill: Ten years after Exxon Valdez. *National Geographic, 195*(3), 96–117.

Mitchell, S. (1989). *The selected poetry of Rainer Maria Rilke* (Ed.) [English translation]. New York: Vintage International.

Omartian, S. (1991). *Finding peace for your heart: A woman's guide to emotional health.* Nashville, TN: Thomas Nelson Publishers.

Ornitz, A., & Brown, M.A. (1992). Family coping and premenstrual symptomatology. *Journal of Obstetric, Gynecological, and Neonatal Nursing, 22*(1), 49–55.

Prejean, H. (1993). *Dead man walking: An eyewitness account of the death penalty in the United States.* New York: Vintage Books.

Reed, P. (1991). Spirituality and mental health in older adults: Extant knowledge for nursing. *Family Community Health, 14*(2), 14–25.

Robbins, M. (1990). Midlife woman and death of mother: A study of psychohistorical and spiritual transformation. *American University Studies, VII*(8). New York: Peter Lang.

Sams, J. (1994). *The 13 original clan mothers.* San Francisco: Harper & Row.

Sewell, M. (Ed.). (1991). *Cries of the spirit: A celebration of women's spirituality.* Boston: Beacon Press.

Shuler, P., Gelberg, L., Brown, M. (1994). The effects of spiritual/religious practices on psychological well-being among inner city homeless women. *Nurse Practitioner Forum, 5*(2), 106–113.

Walker, A. (1984). *Horses make a landscape look more beautiful.* New York: Harcourt Brace Jovanovich.

CHAPTER 16

Music Therapy

Lenore K. Resick, Joan Such Lockhart, Sr. Donna Marie Beck,
and Shirley Powe Smith

Key Points

Use of musical or rhythmic interventions to improve physical and/or
emotional health
Various theoretical frameworks to explain the effect of music
Behavioral
Sociological
Psychoanalytical
Cognitive
Phenomenological
Quantum theory
Guided imagery
Biomedical theory of music therapy
Pathways and mechanisms of music therapy
Music is processed by the ear first (auditory pathway of music).
Music is then interpreted (cerebral pathway of music).
Several obstacles exist to the effectiveness of music therapy in each
of these pathways.
Auditory pathway (any structural or physiological problems in the
ear)
Cerebral pathway (any problems in the structure or physiology of
the brain)
Patients seem to do best when music is self-selected.

The power of music to integrate and cure . . . it is quite fundamental. It is the profoundest nonchemical medication.

—Sachs, 1991, p. 32

MUSIC: NURTURING THE MIND, BODY, AND SOUL

Music therapy is a holistic health discipline that was originally derived from the quasi-therapeutic uses of music by non–music therapists. Today's practice of music therapy consists of the following: (1) a trained music therapist, (2) a patient assessment that includes attention to the total person, and (3) an appropriate evaluation procedure. It is assumed that both the music and the therapeutic relationship with the client are also necessary components of this music therapy (Maranto, 1991).

Broadly defined, music therapy is the use of musical or rhythmic interventions to improve physical health and/or emotional health. Music may be used as a physical and emotional stimulus as well as a symbolic language. This relationship between music and health is both intimate and ancient. Since the beginning of time, music has played a significant role in the healing practices of most cultures. For thousands of years, indigenous healers throughout the world have used songs and chants as well as whistles and drums, rattles, gongs, and flutes to restore health and vitality to their patients (Winn & Walker, 1996). The ancient Greeks believed that music was the language of the gods and that it was a gift given to humans so that they could access the mystical realms and thereby retrieve the knowledge they needed for health and healing. Their god, Apollo, was the god of music and medicine, who was believed to embody this very important connection between music and health (Tame, 1984).

Since music was first played to soothe King Saul, there has been the recognition that music can indeed bring relief to the affected. The Greeks, including Plato, believed that health in mind and body could be obtained through the use of music (Diserens & Fine, 1939). Florence Nightingale used music in her care of the sick (Spellbring, 1991). Since those times, great strides have been made in the use of music in healing. These examples of the early use of music in healing describe an *interpersonal process* wherein musical experiences were used to improve, maintain, or restore the well-being of a person. This process essentially describes music therapy. It may be considered as a servant source or a means of communication in the process of providing opportunities for healing and promotion of well-being (Beck, 1995).

Today's connection between music and medicine is concertized in the profession of music therapy. The American Music Therapy Association (AMTA) clearly articulates a definition of music therapy and the professional education it requires. Settings in which music therapy may be used are also outlined. Music therapy is the use of music in the accomplishment of therapeutic aims: the restoration, maintenance, and improvement of mental and physical health (AMTA, 1998). It is a systematic process using music experiences and the relationships that develop through them as dynamic forces of change (Bruscia, 1984). Music therapists are highly qualified professionals who have completed approved degree programs and clinical training in order to receive the credential of board certification (MT-BC) or the designation of registered (RMT), certified (CMT), or advanced certified music therapist (ACMT). Today, over 5,000 music therapists are employed throughout the United States. They may be found in a variety of settings, such as hospitals, clinics, day-care facilities, nursing homes, hospices, rehabilitation centers, correctional facilities, and private practices. Music therapists work with individuals of all ages who require special services because of behavioral, social, learning, or physical disabilities (AMTA, 1998).

Initially, music therapy became an established allied health profession in 1950 following World War II. Musical interactions with the traumatized and physically disabled veterans provided a mode of communication in their rehabilitation process, and these interactions were considered to be "good for the soul." Music began to be applied in a more specialized way, with greater emphasis placed on the evaluation of the impact of music. It was found that by engaging in a music process, desirable changes in behavior and adaptation in the psychosocial and physiological dimensions of the veterans appeared to be improved (Gaston & Thayer, 1968).

Over the years, the practice of music therapy has become increasingly recognized in the contemporary health community. Most recently, scientific studies on the physiological and psychological effects of music as a therapeutic modality have established a sound theoretical basis for the use of music as therapy. Nearly half a century of research reveals data to support its use. Its goals are nonmusical in nature, including the reduction of psychophysiological stress, pain, anxiety, and isolation (Hanser, 1985). Today music therapy is viewed as one of the foremost complementary modalities in health care.

There is a meeting point, whether intentional or unintentional, that lies between art and science. The art of listening to music keeps the heart's powers occupied so that the musical sounds awaken within us our deepest feelings and inspirations about life. Hence music may be defined as a "servant before the face of God." It has a priestly function as well. It speaks of the ineffable for it represents the *loci de secerdotio et de finibus*. Music is an art form of unity of motion. Music's sacredness with its underlying tension and conflict is reminiscent of life itself. Art, particularly in the form of music, is a special way to convey the holy, serving the whole person, body and soul, as an indivisible unit (Van der Leeuw, 1963).

This brief introduction to music therapy provides an overview of some of the uses of music in the accomplishment of therapeutic goals. Restoration, maintenance, and improvement of mental and physical health are the foci of the goals.

In order to discover the value of musical sound, we must first listen attentively to the sounds within and the sounds without ourselves and those of the clients we encounter. Healing involves many internal and external factors. These internal and external elements influence health and healing (Van Kaam & Muto, 1993).

We know that anxiety and stress play a key role in our mental and physical health (Hanser, 1985). When we are inundated with a multiplicity of sounds, both consonant and dissonant, such phenomena may dispose us to stress that may contribute to disease. The dissonant sounds of life caused by continuous perceptions of threatening situations may generate stress reactions in which the adrenal glands secrete epinephrine, which affects glucose metabolism; norepinephrine, which increases cardiac output and blood pressure; and steroid stress hormones such as cortisol. The research by Droh and Spintge (1983) has shown that music significantly reduces pulse rate and plasma levels of epinephrine, norepinephrine, and cortisol in patients undergoing medical and dental procedures. It should be noted that the field of medicine has acknowledged the existence and causation of psychosomatic illness in the past. More recently, new theories may account for illness far beyond what we previously believed. Music therapy may play a key role in reducing stress by increasing the relaxation response (Maranto, 1991). It may help to alleviate pain perception (Chetta, 1981; Standley, 1986) and reduce anxiety. It may foster aspects of the social dimension in those who suffer from feelings of isolation and being out of control emotionally, mentally, and in the behavioral aspects of life (Parente, 1989). Music may assist persons in developing self-awareness, fostering creativity, clarifying personal values, and coping with a variety of psychophysiologial dysfunctions. Let us consider this dynamic musical process and its impact on the mind and body.

THEORETICAL PERSPECTIVES OF MUSIC THERAPY

A variety of theories has evolved over the past years to explain the therapeutic influence of music therapy on an individual's body, mind, and spirit. These theories not only attempt to provide an explanation surrounding the mechanism of music therapy, but also help to dispel the misconception of music's effects as being purely mystical or magical in nature.

According to Taylor (1997), most of the theories used to explain the therapeutic effects of music therapy in humans have assumed a psychological direction, such as the following: behavioral (Madsen, Cotter, & Madsen, 1968), sociological (Hadsell, 1974), psychoanalytical (Noy, 1966, 1967; Wang, 1968), cognitive (Bryant, 1987; Maultsby, 1977), phenomenological (Barclay, 1987), quantum theory (Eagle, 1985), and guided imagery and music. While these theories provide insight into the way music therapy changes how humans think and feel, they offer little explanation into the detailed physical changes that occur within the body due to music (Taylor, 1997).

Other researchers have offered theoretical frameworks that emphasize a physiological point of view (Taylor, 1997; Watkins, 1997). The biomedical theory of music therapy (BTMT), shared by Taylor more than 10 years ago and based on previous research by Gaston (1964) and other experts, uses a biological perspective to define music therapy (Taylor, 1997). In addition, this theory provides a framework for music research, and an explanation of music therapy's clinical application related to health. The BTMT consists of four hypotheses that focus on the neurophysiology of outcomes such as pain, emotion, communication and movement, and anxiety and stress (Taylor, 1997). In Taylor's theory, the human brain is viewed as the focal point for understanding the therapeutic effects of music therapy. Past research provides evidence that notes changes in brain functioning that can be observed and measured (Taylor, 1997).

The diversity of theories used in music therapy offers researchers a variety of perspectives to interpret the results of research and to determine the therapeutic health-related outcomes of music in humans.

UNDERSTANDING THE PATHWAY AND MECHANISM OF MUSIC THERAPY

It is essential that researchers understand the physical path that music takes as it enters the body, its mechanism of action when used as a therapeutic intervention, and the human response to music. This knowledge would enable researchers to anticipate potential physiological barriers to music therapy in various populations under study, develop ways to assess these obstacles effectively when recruiting potential subjects, and incorporate mechanisms to overcome these barriers in their research designs. This information may also assist consumers of music therapy research to interpret findings reported in the literature and to critique published research studies.

It is possible that some researchers, unfamiliar with the physiological pathway and mechanism of music, may implement designs that lack methodological rigor and result in misleading or insignificant results. For example, the researcher may be unaware of an existing physical barrier present in a subject's ear that may interfere with his or her hearing the music intervention. Therefore, the desired effect may not have an opportunity to occur. While significant outcomes of research studies are applied in clinical practice, conversely, irrelevant findings may be readily dismissed and misinterpreted as being ineffective. The potential value of music therapy in health and wellness among diverse populations may not be realized.

Understanding How Music Is Processed by the Body

Music is processed first by the ear, and then by the brain, where it is interpreted (Taylor, 1997). While the auditory pathway of music can be compared with the predictable route used in sound transmission, the path and effect of music in the brain are less clearly understood (Taylor, 1997).

Researchers need to understand the physiology of music, and to anticipate and assess potential barriers that may exist among various individuals. If the pathway that music takes through the ear or brain is blocked or interrupted, an individual may not respond as anticipated to a therapeutic music intervention. Therefore, researchers must develop creative strategies to overcome these obstacles and to maximize the true effect of music therapy .

The Auditory Pathway of Music

Music, as physical sound waves in the air, travels through the three major divisions of the ear: the external, middle, and inner. The funnel-shaped auricle (pinna) of the outer ear collects the sound waves produced by music, and directs them into the ear canal toward the tympanic membrane (eardrum). This causes the membrane to vibrate, which, in turn, triggers a chain reaction of three tiny ossicles (bones) in the middle ear to vibrate. These bones are called the malleus (hammer), incus (anvil), and stapes (stirrup) and help to intensify the sound waves.

As the footplate of the stapes vibrates in the oval window, it causes a wavelike movement of the perilymph in the scala vestibuli and endolymph in the inner ear, and vibration of the vestibular membrane in the cochlea. These pulsations cause movement of the basilar membrane and move the hair cells in the organ of Corti. This results in the release of neurotransmitters. Mechanical sound vibrations are changed into electrochemical nerve impulses that are carried by the 8th cranial nerve called the vestibulocochlear (auditory) nerve to the brain.

The path taken by music through the ear is an involuntary and spontaneous process (Taylor, 1997). While this auditory route of music as sound is obvious at birth, research suggests that the human fetus during the last 3 months of development is capable of detecting and reacting to music that is transmitted through the mother's abdomen through amniotic fluid (Woodward, Guidozzi, Hofmeyer, Dejong, Anthony, & Woods, 1992).

Obstacles to Music Therapy in the Auditory Pathway

The structures in the ear that facilitate the conduction of music as sound and the transmission of its electrical impulses also have the potential to serve as barriers to the effects of music. The researcher needs to assess these situations when implementing music therapy in various groups so that the maximum results of music can be realized.

For example, ear conditions such as impacted cerumen, foreign bodies, middle-ear infections, cholesteatoma, and otosclerosis can interfere with conduction of sound waves and the subsequent hearing of music. Sensorineural hearing loss, cranial nerve damage, or the loss of hair cells through aging or environmental means can interfere with the transmission of sensory impulses to the brain.

The Cerebral Pathway of Music

After being processed in the ear, sensory impulses follow a complex path via the vestibulocochlear nerve to the medulla, midbrain, thalamus, and auditory cortex of the temporal lobe. Since nerve fibers cross in the brain, each auditory cortex receives impulses from both ears (Marieb, 1998).

First, afferent impulses travel to the spiral ganglion and cochlear nuclei in the medulla (Marieb, 1998; Taylor, 1997). They subsequently move to the superior olivary nucleus, and upward along the lateral lemniscus to the inferior colliculus in the midbrain. Next, these electrical impulses travel along relays in the medial geniculate body in the thalamus to the auditory cortex in the temporal lobe. Impulses travel from the auditory cortex to various parts of the brain based according to their function. This mechanism is automatic until impulses reach the cerebral cortex, where conscious processing of music occurs (Taylor, 1997). Connections with the frontal lobes are thought to be an essential part of a complex interactive system that enables individuals not only to perceive and enjoy music, but to remember it. However, the manner in which an individual perceives and responds to music depends on the brain activity that is occurring at the time that music is introduced (Taylor, 1997).

Watkins (1997), in her physiological framework designed to explain the effects of music therapy, proposes that a connection exists between impulses coming from the ear and the classic stress response in the brain. This physical communication allows the body to be affected by both the endocrine and autonomic nervous systems. Watkin's framework also suggests that impulses travel from the ear to the medulla, midbrain, thalamus, and amygdala or cerebral cortex using two distinct routes. One pathway is called the core region, which provides only auditory messages, while the second pathway, called the belt region, offers information for other sense organs in addition to the ear. The core region acquires its input from the dorsal ventral nuclei, and the belt region develops its input from a variety of sources.

There is controversy among researchers of music therapy concerning the many neurophysiological changes that occur in the brain in response to music (Taylor, 1997). Particular areas of focus include hemispheric processing, cortical arousal, cognition, and biochemical activity. All of these points have important implications for the use of music therapy in health-related situations. For example, researchers are trying to clarify what occurs in the right and left hemispheres as music is processed, and to search for a music center in the brain (Taylor, 1997). Although the right hemisphere was previously thought to process music, current investigations offer evidence to lend doubt to this belief.

A second area of interest involves the use of music with individuals who are experiencing adverse situations, especially those that elicit negative feelings such as pain or anxiety (Taylor, 1997). Researchers have used music therapy as a focal point in these situations. It is thought that music arouses the individual by stimulating particular areas in the brain, such as the reticular activating system (RAS) in the brain stem.

The use of music to augment cognitive processing and to improve various impairments is a third issue that has been researched (Taylor, 1997). Finally, work is being conducted to study how music causes the release of various neurotransmitters in the brain.

Obstacles to Music Therapy in the Cerebral Pathway

Similar to the ear, a variety of physical changes in the brain can interfere with the processing of music as therapy. Damage to portions of the physical pathway that sound takes through the brain may result in difficulties with perceiving, enjoying, and remembering music. For example, brain impairment resulting from conditions such as cerebrovascular accidents (stroke), Parkinson's disease, dementia, and trauma have the potential to influence anticipated effects of music therapy. Researchers need to assess these factors and interpret findings in light of them. The following literature review will further expand the reader's views concerning future implications for music's use in the pursuit of wellness and health.

REVIEW OF THE MUSIC THERAPY LITERATURE

The benefits of music therapy across the life span (Starr, Amlie, Martin, & Saunder, 1977; Owens, 1979; Chetta, 1981; Davis, 1992; Hanser & Thompson, 1994; Kaminski & Hall, 1996; Gowensmith & Bloom, 1997) have been studied in a variety of settings (Taut, 1989), in relationship to mood (Gowensmith & Bloom, 1997; Stratton & Zalanlowski, 1984), and during wellness and states of acute (Guzzetta, 1989) and chronic illness (Curtis, 1986; Colwell, 1997; King, 1997). The literature suggests that music, used either alone or in combination with imagery, dance, or massage can reduce pain, anxiety, and tension and improve quality of life (Stevens, 1990; McKinney, Tims, Kumar, & Kumar 1996). Most of the studies recommended that, to be most beneficial, music should be self-selected according to the individual preference.

As discussed earlier in this chapter, the studies report that differences were found in psychological and physiological parameters in those receiving music as therapeutic intervention. Many of the early studies about the benefits of music therapy focused on the role of music in reducing anxiety (Rohner & Miller, 1980), tension and stress (Logan & Roberts, 1984), and increasing relaxation (Stratton & Zalanlowki, 1984; Logan & Roberts, 1984). Music has also been found to improve the immunological response to disease (DiFranco, 1988). The effect of music on anxiety has been measured through having patients anticipating surgery complete an anxiety inventory scale and monitoring corresponding blood pressures, pulses, and respiratory rates (Kaempf & Amodei, 1989). Relaxation and a decrease in anxiety measured through questionnaires and the monitoring of changes in vital signs suggest a positive response to music intervention (Thaut & Davis, 1993).

Measures to determine the effect of music therapy have included the monitoring of electromyographic biofeedback (Scartelli, 1984), circadian amplitude, body temperature, urinary corticosteriods (Rider, Floyd, & Kirkpatrick, 1985), vascular changes, pulse, muscle constriction, body temperature (Davis & Thaut, 1989), and breathing patterns (Blumenstein, Breslav, Bar-Eli, Tenenbaum, & Weinstein, 1995). The use of music was found to reduce blood pressure and heart rate, and sensitivity to noise in preoperative cardiac surgery patients (Byers & Smyth, 1997). Music was found to increase mood in patients after coronary bypass grafting surgery (Barnason, Zimmerman, & Nieveen, 1995). In mechanically ventilated patients, music increased mood and decreased heart rate and respiratory rate (Chlan, 1995).

Many studies suggest that music decreases the perception of pain and anxiety. In the findings of a study comparing the perception of pain in patients listening to music and patients listening to a low-pitched sound, the patients listening to music reported twice as much decrease in pain as those who listened to sound only (Beck, 1991). Music has been used in reducing anxiety in hospital surgical waiting areas (Moss, 1988; Steelman, 1990; Evans & Rubio, 1994; Winter, Paskin, & Baker, 1994; Robb, Nichols, Rutan, Bishop, & Parker, 1995; Augustin & Hains, 1996) and in coping with acute and chronic pain.

The literature suggests that music is effective as a noninvasive pain control method in the perioperative period (Heitz, Symreng, & Scamman, 1992; Wipple & Glynn, 1992; Eisenman & Cohen, 1995; Heiser, Chiles, Fudge, & Gray, 1997). Music helped the patient to relax in the immediate postoperative recovery period (Heiser, Chiles, Fudge & Gray, 1997) and reduced pain and increased sleep on the 2nd and 3rd postoperative days after coronary artery bypass surgery (Zimmerman, Nieveen, Barnason, & Schmaderer, 1996).

Following myocardial infarction, music has a significant impact on lowering the apical heart rates when combined with relaxation (Guzzetta, 1989). The literature suggests that the effectiveness of music intervention may be related to the anxiety level of the patient (Zimmerman, Pierson, & Marker, 1988) and the duration of the exposure to the music (Elliot, 1994). Studies focusing on music alone suggest that music is effective in reducing anxiety, promoting rest of patients and calming the family members (White, 1992) of hospitalized patients in critical care environments where noise is often unavoidable.

Specifically, in regard to women's health, the literature reports several studies on younger women that suggest the positive effect of music during preparation for childbirth and during birthing to increase relaxation and to decrease the experience of subjective pain (Clark, McCorkel, & Williams, 1981; Hanser, Larson, & O'Connell, 1983; Durham & Collins, 1986; Geden, Lower, Beattie, & Beck, 1989). During labor, women who listened to music as a diversion to pain and as a cue to the controlled breathing and the relaxation response learned in prepared childbirth classes experienced less pain than women who did not listen to music in the same setting (Hanser, Larson & O'Connell, 1983). In an earlier study, women who listened to music during labor reported a more positive experience, reported perceiving more support from hospital personnel, and reported less anxiety during birthing (Clark, McCorkle & Williams, 1981). These findings suggest that music during labor and birthing adds to the mother's experience of control and decreases the need for pain medication that may cross the placenta and depress the respiratory and heart rate of the neonate at birth.

Walters (1996) studied 39 women between the ages of 19 and 65 years who were awaiting gynecological surgery. Those women in the group exposed to vibrotactile or music intervention spent less time in surgery and in the postanesthesia unit and required less postoperative pain medication than those women in the control group who received no interventions. Davis (1992) conducted a study of 22 women ages 17 to 43 who were scheduled for a procedure that involved instrumentation of the cervix. Those women who were exposed to their choice of music through headphones, along with receiving instructions on relaxation techniques, experienced a significantly lower respiratory rate and lower overt pain score than did the control group who received no music nor relaxation intervention.

Music as an intervention has been used in the management of chronic medical problems such as asthma (Lehrer et al., 1994), pain from endometriosis (Colwell, 1997) and in combination with guided imagery and relaxation techniques in chronic stress and anxiety (Hammer, 1996). Music was found to relieve cancer-related pain and to enhance mood (Beck, 1991; Whipple & Glynn, 1992); and to reduce the distressing side effects of chemotherapy (Zimmerman, Pozehl,

Duncan & Schmitz, 1989; Sabo & Michael, 1996; Ezzone, Baker, Rosselet, & Terepka, 1998). In addition, the literature suggests that music had positive behavioral and psychological effects in persons recovering from stroke (Purdie, Hamilton, & Baldwin, 1997).

The positive effects of music have been documented in studies across the life span from the neonate to the older person. In utero, the fetus is capable of hearing the mother's heartbeat and maternal voice as early as 24 weeks of gestation (Starr, Amlie, Martin, & Saunder, 1977). Studies focusing on the effect of music on healthy newborns in hospital nurseries in regard to the initial transition hours after birth suggested that soft, soothing music may assist newborns in experiencing less high arousal states and facilitate neonatal well-being (Kaminski & Hall, 1996).

Music therapy has benefits when used with the critically ill or premature neonate. Collins and Kuck (1991) used an experimental design of a pretest and posttest on 17 neonates to study the effects of intrauterine and female singing sounds on the oxygen saturation and heart rate and behavior state of agitated intubated premature neonates. Their findings suggested that the oxygen saturation and behavior states improved significantly while the mean arterial pressure and heart rates did not indicate significant changes. Stanley and Moore (1995) studied the therapeutic effects of music and the voice of the mother on 20 premature neonates. The experimental group listened to music while the control group listened to the mother's voice. Although listening to the mother's voice seemed to prove more beneficial to these neonates, as evidenced by the posttest rise in oxygen scores, the mother's voice may not always be available, especially in cases of abandonment and geographic distances of specialized intensive care neonatal centers. Music may be more accessible in some cases and can also increase the oxygen saturation levels of the premature neonates.

Older persons experiencing anxiety, distress, and symptoms of depression experienced clinically significant improvement in symptoms that persisted over a 9-month follow-up period after a home-based program of listening to music and stress-reduction techniques taught by a music therapist (Hanser & Thompson, 1994). The difference between males and females in regard to the effects of music on heart rates after exercise was reported in a study done by Beckett (1990). Results of the study suggest that those who were exposed to music walked further and a significant difference was discovered in the recovery heart rate of the males who listened to the music.

Music therapy intervention lessens the agitated behavior of patients with Alzheimer's disease (Brotons & Pickett-Cooper, 1996; Denney, 1997) and music may be the only means to make contact with patients in end-stage dementia (Norberg, Melin & Asplund, 1986). Music also induced effective relaxation and reminiscence in elderly patients who listened to both secular and sacred music (Lowis & Hughes, 1997). In addition, music increased reminiscence and socialization, relieved depression, and increased memory (Sambandham & Schirm, 1995) and significantly increased positive nonverbal behaviors such as smiling, nodding, gesturing, and humming in physically restrained patients (Janelli & Kanski, 1997).

SUMMARY

Music has played a significant role in the healing practices of most cultures since the beginning of time. Research studies have suggested that music therapy has been a source of healing by nurturing the mind, body, and soul in addition to fostering self-care and wellness across the life span. Today music therapy is considered as one of the foremost complementary modalities in health care.

REVIEW AND DISCUSSION

See boxes "Patient Education" and "Continuing Questions/Challenges" for discussion topics for this chapter.

Patient Education

Music therapy is useful for several conditions
> Reduces pain
> Decreases anxiety
> Decreases tension and enhances relaxation
> Improves quality of life
> Improves the immune response
> Decreases blood pressure
> May assist with easing/facilitating labor and delivery
> May help with Alzheimer's disease (decreases agitation and increases some memory)

Continuing Questions/Challenges

How can music therapy become part of routine patient care?
How is music chosen for a particular patient?

REFERENCES

American Music Therapy Association Source Book. (1998). Silver Spring, MD: AMTA Publications.

Augustin, P., & Hains, A.A. (1996). Effect of music on ambulatory surgery patient's preoperative anxiety. *Association of Operating Room Nurses Journal, 63*(4), 750–758.

Barclay, M.W. (1987). A contribution to a theory of music therapy: Additional phenomenological perspectives on gestault-qualitat and transitional phenomena. *Journal of Music Therapy, 24,* 224–238.

Barnason, S., Zimmerman, L, & Nieveen, J. (1995). The effects of music interventions on anxiety in the patient after coronary artery bypass grafting. *Heart & Lung, 24,* 124–132.

Beck, D. (1995). The role of music in the deepening of the disposition of compassion. Doctoral dissertation, Institute of Formative Spirituality, Duquesne University, Pittsburgh, PA. pp. 266–268.

Beck, S.L. (1991). The therapeutic use of music for cancer-related pain. *Oncology Nursing Forum, 18*(8), 1327–1337.

Beckett, A. (1990). The effect of music on exercise as determined by physiological recovery heart rates and distance. *Journal of Music Therapy, 27*(3), 126–136.

Blumenstein, B., Breslav, I., Bar-Eli, M., Tenenbaum, G., & Weinstein, Y. (1995). Regulation of mental states and biofeedback techniques: Effects on breathing pattern. *Biofeedback and Self-Regulation, 20*(2), 169–181.

Brotons, M., & Pickett-Cooper, P.K. (1996). The effects of music therapy intervention on agitation behaviors of Alzheimer's disease patients. *Journal of Music Therapy, 33*(1), 2–18.

Bruscia, K. (1984). *Defining music therapy.* Phoenixville, PA: Barcelona Publishing Co.

Bryant, D.R. (1987). A cognitive approach to therapy as music. *Journal of Music Therapy, 24,* 27–34.

Byers, J.F., & Smyth, K.A. (1997). Effect of a music intervention on noise, annoyance, heart rate, and blood pressure in cardiac surgery patients. *American Journal of Critical Care, 6,* 183–191.

Chetta, H.D. (1981). The effect of music and desensitization on preoperative anxiety in children. *Journal of Music Therapy, 18*(2), 74–87.

Chlan, L.L. (1995). Psychophysiologic responses of mechanically ventilated patients to music: A pilot study. *American Journal of Critical Care, 4*(3), 233–238.

Clark, M.E, McCorkle, R.R., & Williams, S.B. (1981). Music therapy-assisted labor and delivery. *Journal of Music Therapy, 18*(2), 88–100.

Collins, S.K., & Kuck, K. (1991). Music therapy in the neonatal intensive care unit. *Neonatal Network, 9*(6), 23–26.

Colwell, C.M. (1997). Music as distraction and relaxation to reduce chronic pain and narcotic ingestion: A case study. *Music Therapy Perspectives, 15,* 24–31.

Curtis, S.L. (1986). The effect of music on pain relief and relaxation of the terminally ill. *Journal of Music Therapy, 23*(1), 10–24.

Davis, C.A. (1992). The effects of music and basic relaxation instruction on pain and anxiety of women undergoing in-office gynecological procedures. *Journal of Music Therapy, 29*(4), 202–216.

Davis, W.B. & Thaut, M.H. (1989). The influence of preferred relaxing music on measures of state anxiety, relaxation, and physiological response. *Journal of Music Therapy, 26,* 168–187.

Denney, A. (1997). Quiet music: an intervention for mealtime agitation. *Journal of Gerontological Nursing, 23*(7), 16–23.

DiFranco, J. (1988). Music: Relaxation. In F.H. Nichols & S. and S. Humernick (Eds.), *Childbirth education, practice, research and theory* (pp 201–215). Philadelphia: W.B. Saunders Company.

Diserens, C., & Fine, H.A. (1939). *Psychology of music.* Cincinnati, OH: College of Music.

Dossey, B.M., Keegan, L., & Guzzetta, C. (1995). *The art of caring.* Boulder, CO: Sounds True Publishing Co.

Droh, R. and Spintge, R. (1983). Anxiety, pain and music in anesthesia. Basel, Switzerland: Editones Roches.

Durham, L., & Collins, M. (1986). The effect of music as a conditioning aid in prepared childbirth education. *Journal of Gynecologic and Neonatal Nursing, 15*(3), 268–270.

Eagle, C. (1985). A quantum interfacing system for music and medicine. In R. Spintge & R. Droh (Eds.), *Music in Medicine* (pp. 319–341). Basel, Switzerland: Editiones Roches.

Eisenman, A., & Cohen, B. (1995). Music therapy for patients undergoing regional anesthesia. *AORN Journal, 62*(6), 947–950.

Elliot, D. (1994). The effects of music and muscle relaxation on patient anxiety in a coronary care unit. *Heart and Lung, 23*(1), 27–35.

Evans, M.M., & Rubio, P.A. (1994). Music: A diversionary therapy. *Today's OR Nurse, 16*(4), 17–22.

Ezzone, S., Baker, C., Rosselet, R., & Terepka, E.(1998). Music as an adjunct to antiemetic therapy. *Oncology Nursing Forum, 25*(9), 1551–1556.

Gaston, E.T. (1964). The aesthetic experience and biological man. *Journal of Music Therapy, 1,* 1–7.

Gaston, E. Thayer. (1968). *Music in therapy.* New York: MacMillan Publishing Co.

Geden, E.A, Lower, M., Beattie, S., & Beck, N. (1989). Effects of music and imagery on physiologic and self-report of analogued labor pain. *Nursing Research, 38*(1), 37–41.

Gowensmith, W.N., & Bloom, L.J. (1997). The effects of heavy metal music on arousal and anger. *Journal of Music Therapy, 34*(1), 33–45.

Guzzetta, C.E. (1989). Effects of relaxation and music therapy on patients in a coronary care unit with presumptive acute myocardial infarction. *Heart and Lung, 18*(6), 609–616.

Hadsell, N.A. (1974). A sociological theory and approach to music therapy with adult psychiatric patients. *Journal of Music Therapy, 11*, 113–124.

Hammer, S.E. (1996). The effects of guided imagery through music on state and trait anxiety. *Journal of Music Therapy, 33*, 47–70.

Hanser, S. (1985). Music therapy and stress reduction research. *Journal of Music Therapy, 22*, 193–206.

Hanser, S.B., Larson, S.C., & O'Connell, A.S. (1983). The effect of music on relaxation of expectant mothers during labor. *Journal of Music Therapy, 20*(2), 50–58.

Hanser, S.B., & Thompson, L.W. (1994). Effects of a music therapy strategy on depressed older adults. *Journal of Gerontology, 49*(8), 265–269.

Heiser, R.M., Chiles, K., Fudge, M., & Gray, S.E. (1997). The use of music during the immediate postoperative recovery period. *Association of Operation Room Nurses Journal, 65*(4), 777–778, 781–785.

Heitz, L., Symreng, T., & Scamman, F.L. (1992). Effect of music therapy in the postanalgesic care unit: A nursing intervention. *Journal of Post Anesthesia Nursing, 7*(1), 22–31.

Janelli, L.M., & Kanski, G.W. (1997). Music intervention with physically restrained patients. *Rehabilitation Nursing, 22*(1), 14–19.

Kaempf, G., & Amodei, M.E. (1989). The effect of music on anxiety. *Association of Operating Room Nurses Journal, 50*(1), 112–118.

Kaminski, J., & Hall, W. (1996). The effect of soothing music on neonatal behavior states in the hospital newborn nursery. *Neonatal Network, 16*(1), 45–53.

King, C.R. (1997). Nonpharmacologic management of chemotherapy-induced nausea and vomiting. *Oncology Nursing Forum, 24*(7) (Suppl.), 41–47.

Lehrer, P.M., Hechron, S.M., Mayne, T., Isenberg, S., Carlson, V., Lasoski, A.M., Gilchrist, J., Morales, D., & Rausch, L. (1994). Relaxation and music therapies for asthma among patients prestabilized on asthma medication. *Journal of Behavior Medicine, 17*(1), 1–24.

Logan, T.G., & Roberts, A.R. (1984). The effects of different types of relaxation music on tension level. *Journal of Music Therapy, 21*(4), 177–183.

Lowis, M.J., & Hughes, J. (1997). A comparison of the effects of sacred and secular music on elderly people. *Journal of Psychology, 131*(1), 45–55.

Madsen, C.K., Cotter, V., & Madsen, C.H. (1968). A behavioral approach to music therapy. *Journal of Music Therapy, 5*, 69–71.

Maranto, C. (1991). Applications of music in medicine. In M. Heal & T. Wigram (Eds.), *Music therapy in health and education*. St. Louis, MO: Magna Music Baton.

Marieb, E.N. (1998). *Human anatomy and physiology* (4th ed.). Menlo Park, CA: Benjamin/Cummings Publishing Company, Inc.

Maultsby, M. (1977). Combining music therapy with rational behavioral therapy. *Journal of Music Therapy, 14*, 89–97.

McKinney, C.H., Tims, F.C., Kumar, A.M., & Kumar, M. (1996). The effect of selected classical music and spontaneous imagery on plasma B-endorphin. *Journal of Behavioral Medicine, 20*(1), 85–99.

Moss, V.A. (1988). Music and the surgical patient. *Association of Operating Room Nurses Journal, 48*(1), 64–69.

Norberg, A., Melin, E., & Asplund, K. (1986). Reactions to music, touch and object presentation in the final stage of dementia: An exploratory study. *International Journal of Nursing Studies, 23*(4), 315–323.

Noy, P. (1966). The psychodynamic meaning of music, Pt. I. *Journal of Music Therapy, 3,* 126–134.

Noy, P. (1967). The psychodynamic meaning of music, Pts. II–V. *Journal of Music Therapy, 4,* 7–23, 45–51, 81–94, 128–131.

Owens, L.D. (1979). The effect of music on the weight loss, crying, and physical movement of newborns. *Journal of Music Therapy, 16*(2), 83–90.

Parente, A.B. (1989). Feeding the hungry soul: Music as a therapeutic modality in the treatment of anorexia nervosa. *Music Therapy Perspectives, 6,* 44–48.

Purdie, H., Hamilton, S., & Baldwin, S. (1997). Music therapy: Facilitating behavioral and psychological change in people with stroke: a pilot study. *International Journal of Rehabilitation Research, 20,* 325–327.

Rider, M.S., Floyd, J.W., & Kirkpatrick, J. (1985). The effect of music, imagery, and relaxation on adrenal corticosteroids and the re-entrainment of circadian rhythms. *Journal of Music Therapy, 22*(1), 46–58.

Robb, S.L., Nicols, R.J., Rutan, R.L., Bishop, B.L., & Parker, J.C. (1995). The effects of music on preoperative anxiety. *Journal of Music Therapy, 32*(1), 2–21.

Rohner, S.J., & Miller, R. (1980). Degrees of familiar and affective music and their effects on state anxiety. *Journal of Music Therapy, 27*(1), 2–15.

Sabo, C.E., & Michael, S.R. (1996). The influence of personal message with music on anxiety and side effects associated with chemotherapy. *Cancer Nursing, 9*(4), 283–289.

Sachs, O. (1991). Music and health and well being. *Journal of the American Medical Association, 26,* 32.

Sambandham, M., & Schirm, V. (1995). Music as a nursing intervention for residents with Alzheimer's disease in long-term care. *Geriatric Nursing,16*(2), 79–83.

Scartelli, J.P. (1984). The effect of EMG biofeedback and sedative music, EMG biofeedback only, and sedative music only on frontalis muscle relaxation ability. *Journal of Music Therapy, 21*(2), 67–78.

Spellbring, A.M. (1991). Nursing's role in health promotion. *Nursing Clinics of North America, 26*(4), 805–813.

Standley, J. (1986). Music research in medical/dental treatment: Meta-analysis and clinical applications. *Journal of Music Therapy, 23,* 50–55.

Stanley, J.M., & Moore, R.S. (1995). Therapeutic effects on music and mother's voice on premature infants. *Pediatric Nursing, 21*(6), 509–574.

Starr, A., Amlie, R.N., Martin, W.H., & Saunder, S. (1977). Development of auditory function in newborn infants revealed by auditory brainstem potentials. *Pediatrics, 60*(6), 831–839.

Steelman, V.M. (1990). Intraoperative music therapy. *Association of Operating Room Nurses Journal, 52*(5), 1026–1034.

Stevens, K. (1990). Patients' perceptions of music during surgery. *Journal of Advanced Nursing, 15,* 1045–1051.

Stratton, V., & Zalanlowski, A.H. (1984). The relationship between music, degree of liking, and self-reported relaxation. *Journal of Music Therapy, 21*(4), 184–192.

Tame, D. (1984). *The Secret Power of Music.* Rochester, VT: Destiny Books.

Taylor, D. (1997). *Biomedical foundations of music as therapy.* St. Louis, MO: Magna Music Baton.

Thaut, M.H. (1989). Music therapy, affect modification and therapeutic change: Towards an integrative model. *Music Therapy Perspective, 7,* 55–61.

Thaut, M.H., & Davis, W.B. (1993). The influence of subject-selected versus experimenter-chosen music on affect, anxiety, and relaxation. *Journal of Music Therapy, 30*(4), 210–223.

Van Kaam, A., & Muto, S. (1993). Principles and practice of spiritual healing for health providers. *Advances, 9*(4), 56–68.

Van der Leeuw. G. (1963). *The Sacred and the Profane. Beauty: The Holy Art* [Trans. D.E. Green]. New York: Holt Reinhart Co.

Walters, C.L. (1996). The psychological and physiological effects of vibrotactile stimulation, via a Somatron, on patients awaiting scheduled gynecological surgery. *Journal of Music Therapy, 33*(4), 261–287.

Wang, R.P. (1968). Psychoanalytic theories and music therapy practice. *Journal of Music Therapy, 5,* 114–116.

Watkins. G.R. (1997). Music therapy: Proposed physiological mechanisms and clinical implications. *Clinical Nurse Specialist, 11,* 43–50.

Whipple, B., & Glynn, N.J. (1992). Quantification of the effects of listening to music as a noninvasive method of pain control. *Scholarly Inquiry for Nursing Practice: An International Journal, 6*(1), 43–57.

White, J.M. (1992). Music therapy: An intervention to reduce anxiety in the myocardial infarction patient. *Clinical Nurse Specialist, 6*(2), 58–63.

Winn, T., & Walker, W. (1996). Music therapy and medicine: A creative coalition. *Music Therapy Perspectives, 14,* 44–49.

Winter, M.J., Paskin, S., & Baker, T. (1994). Music reduces stress and anxiety of patients in the surgical holding area. *Journal of Post Anesthesia Nursing, 9*(6), 340–343.

Woodward, S.C., Guidozzi, F., Hofmeyer, G.J., Dejong, P., Anthony, J., & Woods, D. (1992). Discoveries in the fetal and neonatal worlds of music. In H. Lees (Ed.), *Music education: Sharing musics of the world* (pp. 58–66). New Zealand: University of Canterbury.

Zimmerman, L.M., Nieveen, J., Barnason, S., & and Schmaderer, M. (1996). The effects of music interventions on postoperative pain and sleep in coronary artery bypass graft (CABG) patients. *Scholarly Inquiry for Nursing Practice: An International Journal, 10*(2), 153–174.

Zimmerman, L.M., Pierson, M.A., & Marker, J. (1988). Effects of music on patient anxiety in coronary care units. *Heart and Lung, 17*(5), 560–566.

Zimmerman, L., Pozehl, B., Duncan, J., & Schmitz, R. (1989). Effects of music in patients who had chronic cancer pain. *Western Journal of Nursing Research, 11*(3), 298–309.

CHAPTER 17

Drama and Dance Therapy

Penny Lewis

Key Points

- Dance and drama therapy (movement therapy) gains access into the imaginal realm.
- Healing (balance among mind, body, soul) occurs during involvement in imaginal realm.
- Various dance and drama therapy techniques
  - Rechoreography of object relations: rechoreography of mother/ child-embodied relationship by the woman and her dance therapist
  - Embodied psyche: use of imaginal realm to learn about inner complexes, becoming aware of any dysfunctions
  - Dreamwork as theater: woman role-plays different characters and symbols from her dreams
  - Embodied art and sand play work: Jungian technique in which woman moves or shapes sand in a box or arranges small symbolic figures in the sand, and she is transformed by understanding the symbolic meanings
  - Authentic movement and drama: identified by Mary Whitehouse; experience of being transformed by the imagination that emerges through movement
  - Theme-based improvisational movement and drama: similar to authentic movement and drama, but based on specific suggestion of a theme (suggested by the therapist)
  - Ritual dance: using dance within groups, as rituals, for the purpose of transforming oneself

---

Movement and dance therapies are important components of the holistic approach to health care.

—Boston Women's Health Collective, 1998

THE EMBODIED FEMININE

Health is viewed as the capacity to be fully present in the moment, capable of healthy boundaries, and capable of intimacy with oneself, others, and the transpersonal. In order to achieve this level of health and wellness, a woman must have full access to the many aspects of her embodied feminine self. This embodied feminine self refers to a way of knowing that is rooted in bodily experience and comes from an intuitive, experiential, relational, cyclic, qualitative, mysterious, naturally embodied consciousness (Lewis, 1998). These many aspects of the embodied feminine principle may be viewed from a universal archetypal perspective. Archetypes, a concept introduced by C. G. Jung, are universal images, themes, movements, and sounds that can come together in patterns of behavior to which every woman has access through a connection to a deeper layer of her unconscious known as the collective unconscious (Jung, 1953, as cited in 1977). In Figure 17–1 Greek Goddesses are utilized to personify these various aspects of the embodied feminine.

THE MOVEMENT TOWARD AND THE SUSTAINING OF HOLISTIC HEALTH THROUGH THE IMAGINAL REALM

The means by which health within the mind-body-soul paradigm can be achieved and maintained is through the use of the imaginal realm. The left hemisphere of the brain is typically thought to provide rational analytical assessments. Time is seen as quantitative, linear. Most events have a cause-and-effect relationship to one another. This portion of the brain basically ascribes to two tenents: "what you see is what there is" and "if it can't fit into an existing logical scientific model, it doesn't exist." This realm encompasses reductive thinking. Juxtaposed to the left hemisphere is the right hemisphere, or imaginal realm. This hemisphere includes the realm of imagination, creativity, mystery, intuition, synchronicity, and qualitative time. It is the natural realm of the embodied feminine. The language of this realm is symbol and metaphor. In this realm is the threshold to the unconscious filled with unacceptable split-off parts of the self, personal historical

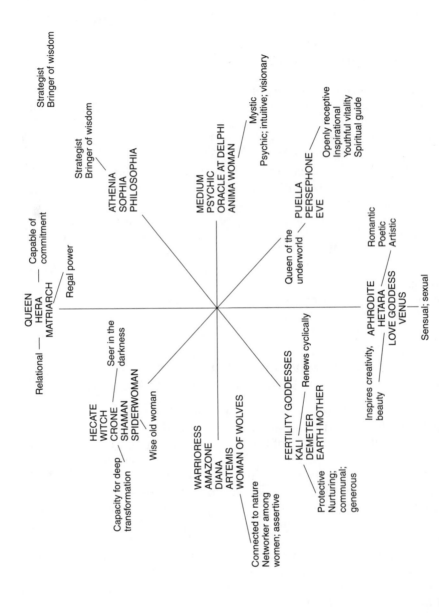

Figure 17–1 Female Archetypes and the Embodied Feminine

events too painful to remember, and all the informed archetypically potential of a woman's wholeness waiting for the right time to come forward (Lewis-Bernstein, 1986b; Lewis, 1988d, 1993a).

THE USE OF THE ARTS IN HEALING LIFE STAGE TRANSFORMATION AND CONTINUED WELLNESS

Jung, as did Freud, understood that dreams come from the unconscious. In addition, Jung realized that the arts, which embraced creativity and the imaginal realm, also come from the same source. Thus painting, drawing, story writing, stream-of-consciousness journaling, poetry, improvisational sound, movement, and drama all come from and access the imaginal realm through the unconscious. It is vital, when employing the arts to access healing, transformation, and wellness-maintaining processes, to remain in the right brain rather than to switch over to the left brain and interpret. Rather than interpret, it is important to enter and stay in the imaginal realm during times of healing, centering, and spiritual connection (Lewis, 1988d, 1989b, 1990a).

The embodied arts of drama and dance-movement are most powerful because, as a result, a woman can experience the healing process during her involvement in these arts. Embodied experience is basic to how women learn best, as such experience is fundamental to feminine nature. Art, poetry, story writing, and journaling can be used as well if a woman wishes first to distance herself to gain a safe perspective on what is emerging from the imaginal symbolic realm. She can then personify different aspects through drama therapy or role play.

In this way a woman can come to understand the meaning of an art symbol or dream image through experiencing it in role-play rather than suppressing it by left brain intellectual interpretation. She can come to her own inner knowledge. In doing so she can maintain the mystery and transformative power of these deep experiences of wholeness and soulful connection.

DANCE AND DRAMA THERAPY TECHNIQUES FOR WOMEN'S HEALTH AND WELLNESS

Through the embodied arts, a woman can help heal from physical and emotional trauma, including physical and/or psychological illness; she can heal from pre- and postoperative conditions; and she can come to terms with life stage processes such as childbirth, midlife, menopause, and dying. The embodied arts can also help women who want to increase their vital life force, maintain energetic balance and wellness, augment their immune systems by decreasing stress, and seek a greater transpersonal connection through the experience of the archetypal (Gersie et al., 1996; Holmes et al., 1991; Berrol & Katz, 1985, 1990; Berrol, 1992; Berrol, Ooi-Wee-Lock, & Katz, 1997; Lewis-Bernstein, 1980; Lewis, 1993b; Newburger, 1987; Thacker, 1984).

Women with chronic pain, cancer, high blood pressure, attention deficit hyperactive disorder, and high-performance personalities have been involved in dance and drama therapy programs since the 1970s, using such techniques as embodied guided visualizations, disease and pain personifications in Gestalt movement therapy (Berrol & Katz, 1985; Gersie et al., 1996; Holmes et al., 1991; Lewis-Bernstein, 1980), body scanning, and sense relaxation.

Dance and drama therapy have served women with depression, substance abuse and other addictions, as well as those in recovery from trauma and anxiety, employing such techniques as the choreography of object relations (Lewis-Bernstein, 1983a; Lewis, 1987, 1988a, 1992, 1993a, 1997), the embodied psyche, dreamwork as theater (Lewis, 1993a, 1993c, 1997), authentic movement and drama (Lewis-Bernstein, 1982, 1986a; Lewis, 1993a, 1996b, 1996c), and the embodiment of the arts (Lewis, 1997, 1998, 1990a, 1993a). Classic group approaches in dance therapy, such as the Chace approach (Lewis-Bernstein, 1986a), have aided women seeking to maintain wellness as well as those with severe psychological distress such as psychosis and dementia (Lewis, 1987, 1993b). Group approaches in drama therapy, such as sociodrama (Sternberg & Garcia, 1989; Fox, 1987) and playback-theater (Salas, 1993), have assisted individuals in experiencing the benefit of interpersonal relationships. Additionally, recovery groups that use these embodied approaches, such as psychodrama (Moreno, 1946, 1959; Blatner, 1988) and theme-based improvisation (Landy, 1994; Lewis, 1993a), move women from an experience of isolation into their natural relationally supportive sense of community. Spiritually ritual dance, sacred dance, authentic movement in dance therapy and the embodied archetypal, soul storytelling, authentic drama, and dreamwork as theater in drama therapy (Lewis-Bernstein, 1973–1974, 1981b; Lewis, 1993a, 1997) have all aided women who seek a greater connection to the transpersonal, and a deeper understanding of their personal path and expanded consciousness.

Rechoreography of Object Relations

Healthy infant and toddler care is delivered on a relational sensor-motor level. Mahler (1968), Kestenberg (1967), Stern (1985),

Winnicott (1971), and others discussed body movement concepts such as attunement, rhythmic synchrony, holding and handling by the mother as means of conveying to the infant relatedness, appropriate boundaries and a sense of trust, safety, and identity. All of these relational aspects are crucial to the development of the foundation for healthy functioning, the formation of a sense of self and healthy self-esteem. They are learned on a body movement level rather than only talking about them. Based on this theoretical approach, the developmentally housed rechoreography of the mother/child-embodied relationship by a woman and her dance therapist is often a sine qua non of transformation (Lewis-Bernstein, 1983a, 1987; Lewis, 1993a, 1996a).

This transformation requires a woman to imaginally enter her body (usually to her solar plexus) in search of her core self. Sometimes women describe this imagined entry as dark inside, making them unable to find anything. The therapist may ask if she is aware of any feelings and sometimes the woman will describe experiencing fear or anger. Any feelings indicate the presence of the core self or inner child. The therapist then asks if she can role-play the woman's adult self. While no one has yet refused this request of this author/therapist, most are unsure of where the therapist is heading. The therapist then asks questions directly to the source of the feeling, such as "I don't blame you for feeling afraid or angry. How long has it been since you have felt related to, really seen and cared for?" Invariably female clients will begin to respond reflecting their core self. For example, they may say, "Too long to remember." Or "Why should I talk to you; you haven't paid any attention to me." The therapist, in the role as the woman's adult self, might respond, "Yeah, I've been treating you just as you were treated as a child," or "Well I didn't want you to be hurt any more so I hid you far away inside me, but I guess I forgot you. But now I realize without you I have no idea what I truly need and want. What do you want right now, little one?" The response might be, " I want your attention" or "I want you not to go away and ignore me again." This begins the communication between the adult, and the core self. Women frequently keep journals and write down the dialoguing. Others will wait until they have a quiet moment such as in the car or before the day begins to check in with their inner child.

If a woman experienced abuse as a girl, she may need to literally start from the beginning of self-formation and learn healthy parenting from an attuned developmentally knowledgeable female dance or drama therapist. For example, one woman lay on the floor in the therapist's office. The therapist sat next to her and supported her back with her hand gently following the shape of her breath with synchronized sucking rhythms (Amaghi, Loman, Lewis, & Sossin, 1999; Lewis, 1994). Embodying her fetal self, the woman began to speak, "I feel empty." The therapist responds in a soothing tone, "Yes, little one, that is because there was no one to feed you, but we will fill you with love and care and you will feel full."

"I need to see myself" was this woman's first comment at the beginning of the next session. The therapist brought her a mirror and encouraged her to look into her own eyes. "I am worried. I need space; I am empty." The woman continued to use the mirror off and on as she progressed into the movement space. She was aware of her inner judge that she and the therapist had explored in earlier sessions. She was able to tell it to leave her alone. Her inner mother then appeared in this imaginal process and her body movement changed from rocking merging patterns to movements that are associated with the teething phase of development, which psychologically is in service to separating and experiencing the difference between one's own boundaries and those of the other (Amaghi et al., 1999; Lewis-Bernstein & Cafarelli, 1972; Lewis, 1988a, 1988b, 1990b). She growled and snapped and clawed the rug as she struggled to claim the needed differentiation from imagined inner mother. Her work in this relationally oriented dance and drama therapy continued until she had, through the embodiment of her infant self, grown within her a healthy core self and had replaced her negative inner mother with a healthy one. It was only then through first experiencing a connection to herself that she was able to begin an intimate relationship with another.

Embodied Psyche Technique

Concepts from Jungian psychology and dance and drama therapy are synthesized in the **embodied psyche technique**, which has proven successful in short-term work with substance abusers and those in recovery from childhood pain. The technique is useful in assisting to understand how an individual's psyche uniquely works (Lewis, 1996a; Lewis & Johnson, 2000).

In this technique individuals are introduced to their inner complexes within the imaginal realm. Inner child(ren), childhood survival patterns, inner parents internalized from childhood, any addictions, and inner masculine or feminine aspects are all drawn, sculpted in clay or embodied by group members, and then are personified and interviewed in relation to the mediating inner adult or ego. Power- and control-hungry survival mechanisms, negative inner parents, and addictions are seen to isolate the ego from a connection to the self, rendering it unable to ascertain personal needs and wants. Power is obtained through the siphoning off of psychic energy belonging to the inner child(ren) and ego. The more weight negative or outmoded complexes have, the more control they have over the individual's psyche. The adult ego, disconnected from the self, is then unable to make accurate interventions on its behalf.

Embodying the psyche with the woman, the therapist, or group members enacting various complexes enables the individual to come to a clearer awareness of any dysfunction. This process enables her to co-create strategies toward, for example, reclaiming her power back from an addiction or outmoded survival pattern whose main strategy is always to cut off any connection with the core self (inner child). Through embodied enactment, a woman learns how she can reclaim power within herself in a manner that provides her with an immediate experience of healthier functioning (Lewis, 1993a).

One woman assigned other women in a group to play her inner child, her survival mechanism of people pleasing, her addiction to sweets, and her mother as currently internalized from her childhood. Each complex was first enacted by the woman while being interviewed by the person who was to play the part. The other women then got into their roles and she arranged them. Her inner child was huddled on the floor with her people pleaser, food addiction, and inner mother all barring her adult ego (role played by her) access to her inner child. Her inner child began to attempt to communicate to the adult self, saying, "I feel so lonely. Please help me." The food addiction then said to the adult, "Oh don't listen to her. If you feel empty of a sense of self have some food. Besides, if you connect to your child self you will feel filled with a sense of self and I will be out of a job." The inner mother added, "Yes dear, don't focus on your inside. You must attend to doing something that I can brag about to my friends. Externals are what count." Then the people pleaser said, "And besides, no one will like you if you pay attention to yourself. Don't listen to your inner child; listen to others' needs and wants. If you don't, they will not want to have anything to do with you and then you will never get the love and acceptance you wanted." The process of this woman's reclaiming her connection to her child resulted in her claiming her own inner strengths. She then added more women to her drama: her inner truth seeker, her wise woman, and her caring, nurturing woman from the archetypes of Athena and Demeter, who helped her send the people pleaser and addiction away and rescue her inner child. She now had a template of what splits herself off from herself and a map of how to reclaim herself.

Dreamwork As Theater

Dreams provide avenues into the unconscious that can be of invaluable service to a woman seeking healing, spiritual connection, and ongoing health and wellness. However, it is important to distinguish what type of dream is emerging from the unconscious. Most dreams are symbolic and metaphoric. By using the creative language of the unconscious, they convey information from the unconscious into consciousness for the benefit of the dreamer. Dreams symbolically can identify parts of the self that have remained unavailable to the ego. They can be "red flags" brought forth to tell a woman that she is in a toxic situation or relationship or generally going in a destructive direction in her life. When an individual is in therapy or analysis, the unconscious often presents the dreamer with symbolic information pertinent to her therapy. Typically these dreams emanate from the personal unconscious. Occasionally, however, they emerge from the transpersonal collective unconscious. These dreams are what Jungian therapists refer to as "big dreams", whose purpose is to expedite the growth process by providing profoundly compelling experiences often of a deeply spiritual nature (Lewis, 1993a, 1993c, 1996a; Lewis & Johnson, 2000).

In addition to symbolic dreams, women can also have flashbacks during the dream cycle. These flashbacks are typically not symbolic but are the reexperiencing of actual prior traumatic events. Occasionally a woman will have nightmares that are partially symbolic and partially from a real recollection. The specific symbolism used typically is created at the time that the abuse was suppressed, and can be of archetypal proportions.

Women who are psychically inclined also have visions that either address communion with those in spirit or information given to them from that realm. These phenomena may aid a medial woman in knowing something previously unknown, in receiving spiritual wisdom, or in connecting or reconnecting with spirits who have a relationship with the dreamer.

Because there are very different types of phenomena that can occur during dream cycles, it is very important to be able to distinguish among them. For example, many women, upon first encountering their inner masculine, may dream that a strange man is chasing them. In the dream they fear that they might be raped or killed. In interviewing the pursuer, the woman discovers that this inner male is angry with her for not paying any attention to him, so he decided to make his presence known. Communicating with this aspect in the imaginal realm results in his softening and becoming more compellingly attractive to the dreamer. A union frequently ensues that is filled with all the romance and loving pleasure that could be hoped for. Flashbacks, even if couched in a layer of symbolism, have a very different feel to them. The woman describing the dream will frequently use the survival mechanisms that she used during the time of the abuse. She may become numb, frozen, withdrawn inside herself, or even leave her body.

With dreams that are symbolic in nature and emerge from the personal unconscious, the technique of dreamwork as theater can be used. This technique keeps the dream and the dreamer in the imaginal realm. The dreamer can then understand the dream through the experience of it and can frequently use the dream as a vehicle of transformation. The therapist who uses this technique avoids interpretation because interpretation creates a disconnection by shifting the experience into the left hemisphere, where analytic rationality labels it, often reducing it to "an interesting tidbit, " consequently minimizing its importance.

In dreamwork as theater, similar to the embodied psyche technique, a woman is asked to role-play different characters and symbols in the dream. The therapist then interviews the dreamer in character or the dreamer can interact herself, role-playing different characters or symbols in the dream. At times dialogues ensue between two characters or aspects of the dream. If the dream is too scary, the therapist further separates the dreamer from the dream by having the woman pretend that the dream is a movie in the process of being filmed. The dreamer is told that the actors and crew just took a break, and that the therapist is a newsperson interviewing the dreamer, who is cast in the role of the dream/movie character. At times the dream appears to have a beginning and a middle, but no ending. After interviewing the characters, the therapist suggests to the client that she imagine an ending. Since the woman's responses and story endings emerge from her imagination, she can't be "wrong" as the dream has come from the same source. This technique works only if the woman creates an ending rather than by being guided by the left brain, which focuses on what logically "should" occur (Lewis, 1993a, 1993c).

Embodied Art and Sand Play Work

Embodied art and sand play work is a dance and drama therapy technique based upon the premise that the purpose of art expressions is not only to inform, but also to transform the artist (Lewis, 1993a, 1993b). All forms of drawing, painting, sculpting, poetry, and writing can inform the artist by her interviewing the symbols through role-play and moving or transforming the themes.

Sand play is a Jungian technique in which an individual moves or shapes sand in a box or arranges small symbolic figures in the sand. Usually an individual allows her imagination to select from figures that range from animals (magical, domesticated, or wild), human figures (all ages and character types), environmental objects (trees, containers like walls, stones, shells), doll house furniture, vehicles, sacred icons, and other small objects of symbolic significance. Often the result is a symbolic representation of her psyche or a map of her psychological and spiritual journey. These figures are then given imaginal life, and the small sand space is treated as a world in and of itself. The figures are interviewed and converse among themselves, with the sand play arranger playing all the parts. Because the sand play arranger stays within the imaginal realm, she can experience the transformative power as she comes to understand the symbolic meaning through the experience of living in it (Lewis, 1993a).

Authentic Movement and Drama

Authentic movement and drama is an embodied dance and drama therapy technique that was first identified by dance therapist Mary Whitehouse (in Lewis-Bernstein, 1986a). It is an experience of being moved not by conscious volition but by the realm of the imagination that emerges from the unconscious. Whitehouse wrote, "It is a moment when the ego gives up control, stops choosing, stops exerting demands, allowing the Self to take over moving the physical body as it will" (1986a, p. 69). The Self is the Jungian archetype that moves an individual toward wholeness and toward her unique path in life. It resides in the imaginal realm of the unconscious.

Authentic movement and drama is employed with individuals and with groups (Lewis, 1993a, 1996b, 1996c; Lewis & Johnson, 2000). Some movers prefer silence, others prefer white noise such as ocean or wind recordings, while others prefer the many New Age tapes available. With those individuals who are unfamiliar with authentic movement, the therapist will offer guided imagery to assist them into a deeper imaginal state.

Some individuals feel various sensations and are moved in response to them. Most, however, create imagined environments and move within them. These environments can encompass recreations of the past that emerge from the unconscious realm to be consciously known or reclaimed by the mover, or they may be new experiences that are unfolding for the individual to embody and integrate into her personality. Once individuals have recovered from any childhood trauma or addictions, their authentic movement will assist in life stage transition, archetypal connection, and expanded spiritual connection. Archetypal movement and themes frequently are manifested at this time, as Jung described (Lewis, 1989, 1993a, 1997, 1998).

Theme-Based Improvisational Movement and Drama

Theme-based improvisational movement and drama is akin to authentic movement and drama. The only difference in theme-based improvisational movement and drama is that a suggestion is made by the therapist, which is then taken by the person into the imaginal realm. For example, the therapist frequently offers the suggestion to join aspects of the self that have remained polar opposites. When individuals live out of one side they leave in a shadow what they do not claim. In this case, a woman may become resentful because she is not allowed to or is not able to show anger and power.

If an individual employs a metaphor in her description of her life or current events, this metaphor can become an improvisational stimulus. For example, patients may complete the sentence, "My life is like a ———, " and then dance the metaphor, bringing it into the imaginal realm.

Theme-based improvisation can also take on dramatic qualities for a woman, as when a suggestion is made for her to personify a part of her body that may have just gestured as a response to something. These improvisational soliloquies help draw the person into greater self-awareness (Lewis, 1993a, 1995).

Ritual Dance

Ritual dance contributes to the archetypal universal pool of transformational movement. Typically carried out in communities in circle formation, this dance therapy technique can subtly but profoundly transform the participants (Lewis, 1995, 1996a).

Rituals can occur without groups as well. An example of an individual dance therapy session, which employed rituals can be seen with one woman in her late 40s. She and the therapist had previously discussed how her mother had felt shame and disdain for all aspects of feminine sexuality. This woman learned to put on weight to block herself from her feelings and to protect herself from the all-powerful males around her. Menarche came and went in hidden shame. There was no pubertal rite of passage, no acknowledged ritual for her. In this ritual dance therapy session, the therapist, in collaboration with the woman's pubertal self and her adult self, planned and performed a pubertal ritual. Drum music was played as they danced in pelvic-initiated sexual rhythms (Amaghi et al., 1999; Lewis-Bernstein, 1977; Lewis & Loman, 1996; Lewis, 1998). As this woman and her therapist danced, sensually provoked laughter erupted spontaneously. Pelvises were tilted forward in prideful presentation. Strong thighs were used to stomp powerfully in embodied assertiveness.

An example of ritual dance within a group context can be seen in one ongoing authentic movement and drama group in which one woman was in the throes of midlife crisis. Her adult life stage process entailed beginning to connect with herself and acknowledge her many gifts, during which time she began to experience her true value and power. It was at this point in her process that this example of her authentic movement and drama work is drawn. The group began, as always, with everyone "checking in" with one another, allowing the therapist to have a sense of what individuals were bringing with them into the work. Where appropriate, suggestions were made to focus on a particular dream image, childhood experience, or the next step in their personal journey. At this time the woman described said she again was feeling disempowered and victimized by life. The authentic movement component of the session began with the lights dimmed. This woman curled up in a fetal position in the middle of one of the double rooms. From the other double room another group member could be heard. She began employing a group authentic movement technique, which had been clearly contracted for by all the members. This technique allowed for each member to imagine the other members to be any figure in their imaginal realm (Lewis, 1993a). Thus it is understood among them that one member can, for example, represent someone's mother while to another she could represent a wise spiritual being. In the group, this woman began to imagine the vocal expressions as both those of her internal and external selves. She began to rock and to moan. The moan developed into her saying, "I'm so alone." She had clearly disconnected from herself and others.

At this point the therapist began to focus attention on this woman in the group. The therapist moved over to her and crouched into a fetal position in empathic reflection next to her. Feeling physical and emotional support next to her, the woman began to rock and finally to sob. In a childlike voice she said, "They're bad." The therapist responded, "Big and bad." "They're big and bad," she chimed louder. Then both the therapist and the woman moved their hips from side to side in rhythmic synchrony to a chant, "Big and Bad." This movement chant began to transform organically from referring to others as "big and bad" to referring to the therapist and the woman as "big and bad." The movement became stronger, more assertive, and powerful, and the woman added, "Big bad thighs . . . mega thighs." The therapist added, "Thunder thighs." At this point it became clear that this woman had moved from feeling powerless to feeling powerful. The rhythmic side to side movement had changed from the horizontal to the vertical plane. The tonal quality of the voices deepened and the woman finally yelled, "I'm getting out of here," referring to her former state of disconnection.

Both the therapist and the woman danced to the corner of the room where another woman was engaged in authentic movement. Without conversing, these two women and the therapist then began to spontaneously move in synchrony together, kneeling and making gathering motions on the floor with their arms as if we were scooping up something. Then, cupping their hands, they brought the imagined substance up through their torsos and out the top of their heads. The movement sequence finished with their arms reaching upward and outward with their heads tilted toward the sky. They began chanting words each time they brought their hands back to their torsos and moved them upward. Some of these archetypal words of the feminine were: "woman . . . womb source . . . power within . . . wellspring . . . wisdom . . . communion." This is an archetypal movement. This ritual movement has been carried out in many cultures in different eras (Lewis, 1989, 1993a).

WOMEN'S HOLISTIC HEALTH: A WOMEN'S DANCE AND DRAMA THERAPY SELF-EXPLORATION SPIRITUAL RETREAT

An example of the integration of these techniques can be seen in a workshop, which brought women, ranging in age from their 20s to their 70s, to an island in Greece for a spiritual journey of self-exploration. They employed daily embodied sand play, dreamwork as theater, and authentic and archetypal improvisational movement.

Each morning was spent doing dreamwork, followed by a descent to the shores of the Aegean to do sand play. Authentic movement occurred in the afternoon. In the evenings the archetypes of the assertive instinctually related Cretan Snake Goddess; the nurturing creatively fertile Demeter, the earth mother; Persephone, the receptive girl transformed into spiritual guide; and the compassionate loving Virgin Mary were sequentially explored employing improvisational movement and drama. This movement and drama delved into the women's mythic stories, drawing the women into their own relationship to the archetypal themes that moved them in their evolution toward wholeness (Bolen, 1984).

Group Dreamwork As Theater

A Dream from the Personal Unconscious

Inspired by the former evening's work, one woman dreamt that she found a formless, skinless mass of flesh on the shore. She wanted to throw it back into the sea. I encouraged her to reenter into the imaginal realm of the dream and to take what she had found and heal it. She suggested saline solution while I suggested a womblike vessel. Although she felt safe with me when I suggested that the group of six women create a group womb, she became anxious. I then pointed out that each one of us had brought our histories with all important groups from the past, including our families of origin, into the group. Perhaps, then, a way of being fully present in the moment with each other would be, for her and the other women, to take time to look deep into each other's eyes and connect soul to soul. By the time this woman looked into my eyes she had automatically embodied that wounded undeveloped creature she had found on the beach. Her eyes expressed fear. I responded, "You are afraid, but I only want to love you and care for you in a way that you can heal." Other women echoed this in their own words. We then all created a circle and this woman crawled into it. We all spontaneously gestured and chanted a lullaby and the women spoke to her with loving tones. She, in turn, moved her hands over her body as if to bathe herself in love. I then suggested that she imaginally internalize us by saying, "Take us inside you into your own womb to help you continue the loving healing of this core inner self."

A Dream from the Archetypal Collective Unconscious

Another woman in the group dreamed, "I am in an underpass. Two men approach me. I see a way out above. I ascend and see a magnificent open landscape. The sky is red and gold with a sunset. A voice says, 'Wake up!' I then think that I have woken up, but I am actually still in a dream state. Three giant dwarfs come into my bedroom. I am expecting them. They bring me a box. Then I wake up from my alarm."

As the therapist, I am struck by the archetypal themes: being in the underworld; the ascent into nature; the ending reflected by a setting sun; the wake-up call into consciousness; the presence of the unification of opposites ("giant dwarfs"); three being the number of movement toward wholeness; and, of course, the magical box. Without mentioning any of my thoughts so as not to violate the power of the dream with analytical reduction, I asked her if she wanted to explore the dream. She responded by saying, "I'll try." I questioned what "trying" meant to her by asking her to role-play the voice in her that suggested she "try." Playing this voice, she said in response to my question, "I am here like cotton around ——— (the dreamer) you to protect you from living fully. After all you might not be up to what life requires of you and it might be painful. So if you don't engage fully in life, it will be safer for you. The dreamer then disenrolled from her inner "try don't be fully engaged in life" survival pattern, and was able to tell it to leave her dreamwork. She then entered her dream and opened the box. Three women in the group role-played the dwarfs who were peering over her shoulder. As she looked inside, I asked, "What's in there?" "It's imagination!" she exclaimed. "Look at all the colors; it's sparkling in there. Look at the possibility." I suggested that she climb in the box to experience it. She then invited us all in. Many of us climbed inside gleefully, beginning to experience something powerful and feeling deeply moved, but having difficulty expressing our feelings in words. She said, "Life is a dream; it's all a dream; it's what we make of it." The dreamer, a Buddhist, knew that this reality was an illusion, but this was the first time she had understood this premise though the actual experience of it.

Embodied Sand Play

The following are sand play worlds from two women both in the second adult midlife stage. This stage is often (though not always) a time in a woman's life when her children, if she has had children, are grown, and her focus and care for the community often extend beyond her immediate surroundings to a more profound connection to the family of humankind, the planetary well-being, and an ever-deepening spiritual connection.

The first woman arranged stones and figures in the sand to construct a sand play world entitled "The Wailing Well," where she placed a figure of a woman with her daughter and another woman walking toward the well with two pails strapped to a shoulder yoke. Monumentally larger in proportion was a statue of the Minoan Snake Goddess. A buried urn was placed in the center to represent the archetypal wellspring at the center of the mandala. "We women mourn at the well," She spoke as one of the figures. But like Demeter at Eleusis we are also rejuvinated and replenished through access to the connection to the womb of the Great Mother (Bolen, 1984).

The second woman also created a feminine mandala entitled "A Woman's Community." "This is," she reported as the community builder in the sand play world , "an un-man made community which taps into the great ocean." (The hole had been dug to receive the water from the incoming tide.) She continued, "We use consensus rather than a hierarchical system of power over."

Authentic Movement and Drama

In authentic movement and drama, women move together in a playfully freeing way. They become spontaneously clumped together sounding childlike nonsensical and at times irreverent tones while invoking themes of mother-daughter bonding and girls at play.

Archetypal Dance and Drama

Daily female archetypes were invoked through Greek Goddesses for theme-based movement-drama experiences. The Minoan Snake Goddess was used to stimulate a journey into the women's unconscious. I suggested, "Snakes often appear in our symbols when something new is emerging from deep in our psyche. When we, as women, grasp the snake, we can begin to claim that which wants to evolve, transform and be integrated into our conscious life." I then led them through a guided visualization into those untamed places that frequently represent the primordial unconscious, including the jungle, the swamp, the forest, the ocean, or the magical realm. I then suggested that they allow an image of a snake to emerge and I encouraged them to interview the imaged snake and then finally to embody the snake, that is to become the snake in consciousness and movement.

After a period of time I suggested that their snake skin was getting ready to be sloughed off and that something new was emerging underneath. For when a woman starts to claim an aspect of herself that has resided undeveloped in her unconscious, it frequently will begin to transform, becoming more civilized and more humanlike. I then suggested that each woman draw this emerging part of herself and write a poem reflecting this aspect of herself.

Another evening, Persephone, the daughter of the Earth Mother Goddess, Demeter, was invoked. Persephone was abducted by the God of the Underworld and eventually transformed from being a victim to becoming the Queen of the Underworld. Through this process she moved from unconsciousness into one who had psychic abilities and became a charismatic guide into death.

Many women have suffered victimization in their lives through their reexperience of being abused by their family, individuals outside, and/or the culture. The capacity to let go of this view of being a victim and, instead, to claim the power of womanhood with all its wisdom and ability to venture into the cyclic realms of death and rebirth, is key for some. In the movement drama experience, women let go of whom they were in service to, claiming greater wholeness. Each in her own way fertilized herself with her own new potential and then lay down on the floor and surrendered to the pull of symbolic death. Each was shrouded, ritually experiencing her life force leave her body as she floated into a gestating pregnant timelessness. After a period of time, she experienced reanimation and gradually arose renewed with a greater access to divine wisdom.

SUMMARY

Women understand the world and access their inner wisdom through embodied experience. The use of the embodied approaches of dance and drama therapy in service to a woman's heath and wellness is basic to the fundamental nature of being a woman. Within a mind-body-soul paradigm health is viewed as the capacity to be fully present in the moment, capable of healthy boundaried intimacy with oneself, others, and the transpersonal. Dance and drama therapy can help a woman heal from physical and emotional trauma, more fully claim herself, undergo life stage experiences and transitions, support growth, and expand spiritual connection throughout her life span. Additionally these approaches can help a woman stay healthy via reducing stress, strengthening her immune system, and maintaining an ongoing connection to her body, her emotional expression, and her intuitive, soulful knowing.

REVIEW AND DISCUSSION

See boxes "Patient Education" and "Continuing Questions/Challenges" for discussion topics for this chapter.

Patient Education

Therapy can help healing from both physical and emotional trauma.
Therapy can help increase one's vital life force, maintain energetic balance, augment the immune system by decreasing stress, and achieve greater transpersonal connections.
Therapy can lessen chronic pain and lower blood pressure.
Therapy can help with attention deficit hyperactive disorder.
Therapy can help women with depression and addictions.
Therapy can help women with psychosis and dementia.

Continuing Questions/Challenges

How does the "general public" respond to the idea of movement therapy?
Are there particular patients for whom dance/drama therapy is effective?

REFERENCES

Amaghi, J., Loman, S., Lewis, P., & Sossin, M. (Eds.). (1999). *The meaning of movement: Developmental and clinical perspectives as seen through the Kestenberg movement profile.* Newark, NJ: Gordon & Breach Publications.

Berrol, C., Ooi-Wee-Lock, & Katz, S. (1997, Fall–Winter). Dance/movement therapy with older adults who have sustained neurological insult: A demonstration project. *American Journal of Dance Therapy, 19*(2).

Berrol, C., & Katz, S. (1990). The functional assessment of movement and perception. Unpublished assessment.

Berrol, C. (1992, Spring-Summer). The neurophysiologic basis of the mind-body connection in dance/movement therapy. *American Journal of Dance Therapy, 14*(1).

Berrol, C., & Katz, S. (1982). Dance-movement therapy with adults with traumatic brain injury. *American Journal of Dance Therapy, 19.*

Berrol, C., & Katz, S. (1985). Dance movement therapy in the rehabilitation of individuals with head injuries. *American Journal of Dance Therapy, 8.*

Blatner, A. (1988). *Acting-in: Practical applications of psychodramatic methods.* New York: Springer Publishing Co.

Bolen, J.S. (1984). *Goddesses in every woman: A new psychology for women.* San Francisco, CA: Harper & Row.

Boston Women's Health Collective (1998). *Our bodies, ourselves for the new century.* New York: Touchstone.

Fox, J. (1987). *The essential Moreno:Writings in psychodrama, group method and spontaneity* by J.L. Moreno, M.D. New York: Springer Publishing Co.

Gersie, A. et al. (Eds.). (1996). *Dramatic approaches to brief therapy.* London: Jessica Kingsley Publishers, Ltd.

Grotstein, J. (1981). *Splitting and projective identification.* New York: Jason Aronson.

Holmes, P. et al. (Eds.). (1991). *Psychodrama: Inspiration and technique.* London: Tavistock/Routledge.

Johnson, D.R. (1982). Developmental approaches in drama therapy. *Arts in Psychotherapy, 9,* 172–181.

Jung, C.G. (1977). *The Collected Works of C.G. Jung* (Vols. 12, 13, 14, 16, 18). New York: Bollingen Foundation. (Original work 1953.)

Kestenberg, J. (1967). *The role of movement patterns in development,* Vol. 1. New York: Dance Notation Bureau Press.

Landy, R. (1994). *Drama therapy: Concepts, theories, and practices.* Springfield, IL: Charles C Thomas.

Lewis-Bernstein, P., & Cafarelli, E. (1972). An electromyographical validation of the effort system of notation. In *Writings on Body Movement and Communication* (Vol. 2). Columbia, MD: American Dance Therapy Association.

Lewis-Bernstein, P., & Bernstein, L. (1973–1974). A conceptualization of group dance movement therapy as a ritual process. In *Writings on body movement and communication* (Vol. 3). Columbia, MD: American Dance Therapy Association.

Lewis-Bernstein, P. (1980, Spring). A mythic quest: Jungian movement therapy with the psychosomatic client. *American Journal of Dance Therapy, 3*(2), 44–55.

Lewis-Bernstein, P. (1981a). Moon goddess, medium, and earth mother: A phenomenological study of the guiding archetypes of the dance movement therapist. *Research as Creative Process.* Columbia, MD: American Dance Therapy Association.

Lewis-Bernstein, P., & Leah Hall. (1981b). Cross cultural puberty rituals and Jungian dance therapy: A comparative study. Presented at the *12th Annual American Dance Therapy Association Conference, 1st International Conference,* Toronto, Canada.

Lewis-Bernstein, P. (1982). Authentic movement as active imagination. In J. Hariman (Ed.), *The compendium of psychotherapeutic techniques.* Springfield, IL: Charles C Thomas.

Lewis-Bernstein, P., & Singer, D. (Eds.). (1983a). *Choreography of object relations.* Keene, NH: Antioch University.

Lewis-Bernstein, P. (1983b). Ancient and modern embodied rites of transformation. Presented at the 18th Annual American Dance Therapy Association Conference: The Healing Power of Dance Therapy, Pacific Grove, CA.

Lewis-Bernstein, P. (1984). The somatic unconscious and its relation to the embodied feminine in dance-movement therapy process. In *Theoretical approaches in dance-movement therapy* (Vol 2). Dubuque, IA: Kendall/Hunt.

Lewis-Bernstein, P. (1986b) Embodied transformational images in dance-movement therapy. *Journal of Mental Imagery, 9*(4).

Lewis-Bernstein, P. (1986a). *Theoretical approaches in dance-movement therapy* (Vol. 1, rev.). Dubuque, IA: Kendall/Hunt.

Lewis-Bernstein, P. (1986c). The somatic countertransference. Paper presented at the American Dance Therapy Association Conference, Chicago.

Lewis, P. (1987). The expressive arts therapies in the choreography of object relations. *Arts in Psychotherapy Journal, 14,* 321–331.

Lewis, P. (1988d). The transformative process in the imaginal realm. *Arts in Psychotherapy Journal, 15,* 309–316.

Lewis, P. (1988a). *Theoretical approaches in dance-movement therapy* (Vol. 2). Dubuque, IA: Kendall/Hunt.

Lewis, P. (1988b). The unconscious as choreographer: The use of tension Fl rhythms in the transference relationship. In C.P. Geffen (Ed.), *Moving in health* (Monogr. 4). Columbia, MD: American Dance Therapy Association.

Lewis, P. (1988c). The dance between the conscious and unconscious: Transformation in the embodied imaginal realm. In *Moving dialogue.* Columbia, MD: American Dance Therapy Association.

Lewis, P. (1989b) The soul and spirit in the work: The transformative power of the archetypal. Paper presented at the Second International Dance Therapy Conference, Toronto, Canada.

Lewis, P. (1990a). Recovery from codependency through the creative arts therapy. Paper presented at the National Coalition of Arts Therapy Associations Conference, Washington DC.

Lewis, P. (1992). The creative arts in transference/countertransference relationships. *Arts in Psychotherapy, 19,* 317–323.

Lewis, P. (1993a). *Creative transformation: The healing power of the arts.* Wilmette, IL: Chiron Publishers.

Lewis, P. (1993b). The use of Chace techniques in the depth dance therapy process of recovery, healing and spiritual consciousness. In A. Sandel et al. (Eds.), *Foundation of dance/movement therapy: The life and work of Marian Chace.* Columbia, MD: Marian Chace Memorial Fund.

Lewis, P. (1993c). Following one's dreams: Dance therapy as transformation. In *Following our dreams dynamics of motivation: 28th ADTA conference proceedings.* Columbia, MD: American Dance Therapy Association.

Lewis, P. (1994). The clinical interpretation of the Kestenberg movement profile. Keene, NH: Antioch University.

Lewis, P. (1995). Depth drama therapy and the stages of midlife. *16th Annual National Association of Drama Therapy.* New Haven, CT: Yale University.

Lewis, P. (1996a) Depth psychotherapy and dance-movement therapy. *American Journal of Dance Therapy, 18,* No. Z.

Lewis, P. (1996b). Authentic sound movement and drama: An interview with Penny Lewis, Annie Geissinger, interviewer. *A Moving Journal. Providence, 3*(1).

Lewis, P. (1996c). Authentic sound, movement, and drama: An interactional approach. In M. Robbins (Ed.) *Body oriented psychotherapy* (Vol. 1). Somerville, MA: Inter Scientific Community for Psycho-Corporal Therapies.

Lewis, P. (1997). Transpersonal arts psychotherapy: Toward an ecumenical worldview. *Arts in Psychotherapy Journal, 24*(3).

Lewis, P. (In process). An embodied relational model: The use of the somatic counter-transference and inter subjectivity within the affective-imaginal realm. In M. Robbins (Ed.), *Body oriented psychotherapy* (Vol. 2). Somerville, MA: Inter Scientific Community for Psycho-Corporal Therapies.

Lewis, P. (1998) Healing early child abuse: The application of the Kestenberg movement profile. In J. Amaghi et al. (Eds.), *The meaning of movement: Developmental and clinical perspectives as seen through the Kestenberg movement profile.* Newark, NJ: Gordon & Breach.

Lewis, P., & Johnson, D. (Eds.) (2000). *Current approaches in drama therapy.* Springfield, IL: Charles C Thomas Publishing.

Lewis, P. & Loman, S. (Eds.). (1990b). *The Kestenberg movement profile: Its past, present applications and future directions.* Keene, NH: Antioch University.

Mahler, M. (1968). *On human symbiosis and vicissitude of individuation.* New York: International University Press.

Moreno, J.L. (1946, 1959). *Psychodrama* (Vols. 1, 2). New York: Beacon House.

Newburger, H. (1987, Spring). The covert psychodrama. *Journal of Group Psychotherapy, Psychodrama and Sociometry, 40*(1).

Salas, J. (1993). *Improvising real life: Personal story in playback theater.* Dubuque, IA: Kendall/Hunt.

Stern, D. (1985). *The interpersonal world of the infant.* New York: Basic Books.

Sternberg, P., & Garcia, A. (1989). *Sociodrama—Who's in your shoes?* Westport, CT: Praeger Publishers.

Thacker, J. (1984, Spring). Using psychodrama to reduce "burnout" or role fatigue in the helping professions. *Journal of Group Psychotherapy, Psychodrama and Sociometry, 37*(1).

Winnicott, D.W. (1971). *Playing and reality.* New York: Penguin Books.

CHAPTER 18

Therapeutic Touch

B. Jane Cornman

Key Points

TT is a consciously directed process of energy exchange.

Hands are used as focus for facilitating healing (may or may not actually touch the patient).

The most common effect of TT is the relaxation response.

TT helps to rebalance the flow of energy in the body.

There are three parts of the TT process.

1. Centering
   - Focused attention
   - Peaceful state of consciousness
2. Assessing
   - Moves hands 2 to 6 inches from skin surface
   - Gathers information about patient's energy fields
   - TT practitioner is "listening" with her hands
3. Treating
   - Directs or modulates energy
   - Restores balance in energy
   - Treatment lasts from 5 to 20 minutes

This chapter is dedicated to Dora Kunz.

Nurses refer to the "hands on" phenomena of nursing as touch therapy, therapeutic touch, healing touch, therapeutic massage, body work, or a variety of other labels. Despite the different names, the intent is always the same: to care for another through some mode of physical touch or energy field manipulation.

—Dossey, Keegan, Guzzetta, & Kolkmeier, 1995, p. 537

A 33-year-old woman named Emma finds herself in the emergency room (ER) of a local hospital close to the town where she has gone hiking with friends. A bad fall on some rocks just a small detour from the trail to see the view has resulted in her ankle being extremely swollen and a rainbow of colors. The doctor thinks she may have broken a bone. The nurse asks her permission to do therapeutic touch on her ankle as well as applying a cold pack to the area while they wait for the x-ray. The nurse explains that therapeutic touch is a technique used to help reduce the pain and swelling from injuries. Emma agrees to try therapeutic touch. Let's leave Emma and the ER nurse for a moment to explore this technique.

DESCRIPTION OF THERAPEUTIC TOUCH

Therapeutic touch, a healing method used by thousands of nurses and other health professionals, was developed over 25 years ago by Dora Kunz, a healer, and Dolores Krieger, a member of New York University's nursing faculty (Krieger, 1993; Wager, 1996). Therapeutic touch (TT), is a "consciously directed process of energy exchange during which the practitioner uses the hands as a focus for facilitating healing" (Nurse Healers-Professional Associates, 1992, p. 9). The applications of TT are varied in terms of patient age, conditions, and settings. The most common effect of TT is the relaxation response, and it has also been used and studied as a way to reduce pain and accelerate healing.

The term *therapeutic touch* is in some ways confusing since the practitioner does not, in fact, have to physically touch the patient to have a beneficial effect. The method is derived from the "laying-on of hands," but recognizes the ability to direct energy with or without actual physical contact. While TT may or may not involve the practitioner's making actual physical contact with the recipient's body, this technique will always involve making contact with the energy field of the recipient (Krieger, 1975). A review of the theories upon which TT is based will help explain this premise.

Therapeutic touch can be conceptualized within Martha Rogers' (1970) science of unitary human beings and Kunz and Peper's (1995) human energy field model, where both frameworks view energy fields as fundamental units of all beings and their environments. This view is consistent with many Eastern philosophies that believe the universe is "composed of interacting systems of energy, derived from a unified source. There is an underlying unity to all consciousness of which an individual is a localized expression" (Wager, 1996, p.10). Human beings are open and complex systems of energy that are in constant flux as they interact with the environment of energy that surrounds them. As human beings, our essence really does not end at our skin, but instead we extend beyond the mere physical boundaries of our body. Our physical health, as well as our thoughts and feelings, affect our own energy field. Since these systems of energy interact, we can affect and are affected by others' energy fields. TT recognizes the interconnectedness of all energy systems, including those of the nurse and the patient, acknowledging a universal energy that has order and wholeness (Kunz, 1995; Malinski, 1996).

When we are healthy, our life energy flows through us in a balanced, harmonious way (Kunz, 1995). Disease or feeling ill means that our energy is not in a state of balance; the pattern and organization are disrupted. Yet organisms do have an intrinsic movement toward balance, order, and healing. In TT, the practitioner attempts to find areas of imbalance in a person's energy field. By using her hands as a focal point, the TT practitioner rebalances that energy to facilitate the field's natural movement toward harmony. A crucial component is the practitioner's intentionality to help the person. TT is, as Krieger states, "an act of compassion," not just a set of hand maneuvers that can result in a more balanced state of health (Buenting, 1993).

One study that demonstrated the importance of intentionality was conducted by a research team in Mexico City (Dossey, 1997). The team examined the electroencephalograms (EEGs), or brain wave tracings, of persons in two different locations. There was no correlation among the EEG patterns of the individuals when they just sat quietly. "When they allowed a feeling of emotional closeness or empathy to develop between them, the EEGs begin to resemble each other, often to a striking degree" (Dossey, 1997, p. 180). Even moving the persons further apart did not diminish the statistical correlation. There seemed to be a non-local connection, yet no type of energy or signal could be measured between the distant individuals.

Returning to Emma, the injured hiker, she asks, "what do I have to do while you do therapeutic touch?" The nurse reassures Emma that, in fact, she can just sit quietly. The nurse explains that she will take a few minutes to focus and quiet herself and will then be moving her hands slowly and rhythmically a few inches away from Emma's skin. We will examine the steps of TT as Emma and the ER nurse begin the treatment.

THE THERAPEUTIC TOUCH PROCESS

Centering

The first and most significant part of the TT process is termed *centering*. In centering the practitioner brings her attention inward beyond the chattering mind to that quiet, still, peaceful state of consciousness. This focused attention brings the practitioner's own energy to a harmonious state, which is maintained throughout all the phases of TT. This centered state is one explanation for TT's being referred to as a "healing meditation" (Krieger, Peper, & Ancoli, 1979). By connecting with one's own inner core of wholeness and having the intention to help, one becomes a knowing participant in the universal healing energy that can assist in the rebalancing of the person's energy. Both the practitioner and the patient can benefit from the treatment since they both have the opportunity to experience a place of order and wholeness.

Assessing

The second phase of TT is the *assessment*. While remaining in a state of centeredness, the practitioner uses her hands to gather information about the energy fields of the patient, by moving the hands 2 to 6 inches from the skin surface. This scanning of the whole body, head to toe, front and back, gives cues to differences in the quality of energy flow in all areas. The practitioner is "listening" with her hands to detect a variety of cues. She may discern a loss of energy, a disruption in the flow, an accumulation, or a blockage (Krieger, 1979). At times she perceives a temperature differential such as heat or cold, or pressure differences or other subtle sensations such as tingling. Practitioners may sense cues differently. Where one practitioner feels cold, another may sense a void or absence of energy. Some practitioners may experience visual or emotional impressions. With practice, over time the practitioner becomes more sensitive and knowledgeable about identifying variations in energy (Macrae, 1987; Schmidt, 1995). These variations can be signs of imbalances present in the patient's energy field.

Treating

The third phase of TT is the *treatment*. In this phase the practitioner uses the assessment and the information obtained from the patient to direct and/or modulate the energy with the goal of restoring balance. During the treatment the practitioner responds to the various cues from the assessment. For instance, she may attempt to strengthen the energy in areas that seem depleted, to reinstate flow where it feels blocked, or to establish rhythm in areas that feel out of synchronization (Krieger, 1993; Macrae, 1995). The treatment may include "unruffling the field," which is a smoothing motion to clear disruptions in the field. This motion seems to facilitate the rebalancing of the energy. The treatment can last from 5 to 20 minutes. The length of treatment is individualized, based on changes or cues the practitioner senses in the energy field. By staying centered and assessing any changes, the practitioner knows when to stop (Krieger, 1979; Wright, 1987).

Doing TT is considered a natural human potential that can be learned by virtually everyone. It is a natural part of a nursing intervention, which already involves assessment, touch, and promotion of healing.

APPLICATIONS OF THERAPEUTIC TOUCH TO WOMEN'S HEALTH CONDITIONS

The following section includes descriptions of how TT is used to treat or ameliorate certain health conditions. Not all the conditions are unique to women or were studied exclusively with women, but they are certainly conditions that apply to women. Other conditions are exclusive to women, such as pregnancy and premenstrual syndrome (PMS).

Relaxation

Krieger (1993) ranks relaxation as the most reliable response to TT, observed within 2 to 4 minutes from the beginning of a treatment. The practitioner can note physical changes in the patient, including reduced respiratory rate, facial flushing, and increasing temperature in the extremities. Relaxation facilitates the body's response to disease by enhancing the immune response and stimulating the production of endorphins, natural pain relievers. A study by Quinn and Strelkauskas (1993) reported positive changes in immunological measures in both recipients and practitioners of TT.

Krieger et al. (1979) were among the first researchers to document the relaxation response to TT. In their exploratory study they measured the EEG, the EMG (electromyogram, or muscle tension), and GSR (galvanic skin response) for three patients as well as for Dr. Krieger, the practitioner conducting the TT. "Each patient reported relaxing during TT and the physiological indices indicated that the subjects were indeed relaxed" (p. 661). The predominant, rapid, synchronous beta in Dr. Krieger's EEG is what led to TT's first being termed a healing meditation.

Heidt (1981) studied the effect of TT on anxiety levels of hospitalized cardiovascular patients. Ninety patients were divided into three groups to receive TT, casual touch (taking pulses), or no touch (nurses sat and talked with the patient). State of anxiety was measured by a standardized measure of anxiety (A-State Self-Evaluation Questionnaire) that was administered pre- and postintervention. The group that received TT reported a significant decrease in their anxiety compared with those who received casual or no touch.

Quinn (1984) extended the study by Heidt to test whether or not TT, done without physical contact, could relieve anxiety. She divided 60 cardiovascular patients into two groups. One group received TT but without any physical touch during the process. The other group received mimic TT, which is a series of hand movements that, if observed, look just like a TT treatment, but the practitioner does not focus on the process, instead concentrating on a series of numbers. In this study, Quinn did support her hypothesis that "physical contact should not be necessary between practitioner and subject to produce the effect of anxiety reduction" (p. 79).

However, in a later extension and replication using a new and larger sample, adding physiological measures of anxiety, and testing an additional condition, Quinn (1989) was unable to achieve significant anxiety reduction in the patients who received TT. Important lessons were learned from this study. Limiting the TT treatments to 5 minutes could have interfered with the efficacy of the intervention, as this time limit does not allow the practitioner to decide on the length of appropriate treatment based on the individual response. Also, having the researcher give both the TT and mimic treatments may have interfered with the outcome of the study. In Quinn's earlier study (1984) TT was administered by experienced practitioners and mimic TT was administered by nurses with no TT experience.

The majority of evidence in research studies and clinical reports supports the notion that individuals receiving TT do experience a relaxation response. The qualitative study by Samarel (1992) of patients' experiences of receiving TT treatments proposes that far more than relaxation may be taking place. Responses were obtained from 20 participants. The descriptions of the recipients included "I felt internal peace," "I was feeling loved," "I was able to let go," and "I am whole." The patients experienced receiving TT as a process of personal growth that "occurred on all dimensions of being: physiological, emotional, and spiritual" (p. 655).

Pain Control

Krieger (1993) stated that after relaxation, relief of pain is the second most reliable result from TT. In the treatment of acute pain, Keller and Bzdek (1986) studied the effects of TT on tension headache pain. Sixty participants were randomly divided between treatment and placebo groups. The placebo group received the mimic TT treatments developed by Quinn (1984), in which the practitioners do hand movements that are indistinguishable from TT, but focus their attention on subtracting 100 by 7s. The treatment group received actual TT. Participants completed a widely utilized pain questionnaire before, immediately after, and 4 hours after treatment. Both groups reported reduction in pain but in the placebo group "the effect did not occur as often, was not as great, and did not last as long as the effect of TT" (Keller & Bzdek, 1986, p. 104). Ninety percent of the TT group experienced a sustained reduction in headache pain ($P < 0.0001$). Twice the average pain reduction was sustained for 4 hours following TT compared with the placebo treatment.

Meehan (1993) studied the effects of TT on reports of pain in postoperative patients using a protocol similar to that in Quinn's 1989 study. Meehan did not find that patients in the TT group experienced significantly reduced postoperative pain compared with those in the placebo group. Secondary analysis suggested that TT may decrease the need for analgesic medication, but the results were nonsignificant. This study had a problem similar to that identified in Quinn's 1989 study. That is, the restriction of limiting treatments to 5 minutes rather than allowing a range of up to 20 minutes, depending on the need of the individual patient, may have influenced these nonsignificant results.

The treatment of chronic pain is much more challenging to both traditional and alternative health care due to its complexity, in both its cause and how it manifests in each individual. From an energetic perspective, one challenge of chronic pain is the recurrent pattern of pain that has been habitually established in the person's energy field. The longer the pattern has been present, the harder it is to change that pattern (Kunz & Peper, 1995). Wright (1987) wisely described the multifaceted approach necessary to treat individuals with chronic pain, including altering "energy field pattern, medication use, alterations in work, activities of daily living, leisure activities, and relationships with care giver, family, and friends" necessary to treat individuals with chronic pain (p. 711).

The most difficult challenge is to assist the individual in changing her self-image; that is, changing her identification of self as a person in pain. Wager (1996) described the erosion of self-confidence, feeling hopeless for a future free of pain, and the negative impact on one's relationships with others. TT is used to help the individual mobilize her own inner resources. It is useful in relieving anxiety, which is often closely related to the experience of pain; promoting relaxation; and helping the person to feel less isolated (Wright, 1987), in the hopes of helping to alleviate pain.

Wound Healing

TT has been reported to accelerate healing in a variety of circumstances, ranging from orthopedic injuries to dermal wounds (Jurgens, 1989; Wirth, 1990; Wirth et al., 1993). Wirth's 1990 study is particularly impressive given its rigorous standards of a randomized double-blind, placebo-controlled protocol to study the effect of noncontact TT on the wound healing rate of full-thickness dermal wounds. The precisely uniform size wounds were made by a physician using a skin biopsy instrument. Half of the 44 study participants received TT treatments to the wound, but without their knowledge. All participants were instructed to put their arm through a circular opening in a laboratory room door. The TT practitioner administered treatments to half of the participants for five minutes each day for 16 days. The control group did not receive TT treatments, but went through the same procedure of putting their arm through an opening in a laboratory room door without knowing that the adjoining room was vacant. Neither group was aware of the presence or absence of the practitioner, since the TT treatments were administered without physical contact. On both day 8 and day 16 of the study, the treated group's wounds measured significantly smaller than those of the nontreated group. More than half of the treated group's wounds completely healed by day 16 and none of the untreated group's wounds healed at that time. Because of the double-blind design, as well as the isolation of the TT practitioner from the participants, Wirth believed that these procedures "added confidence to the results by precluding the role of suggestion, expectation, and the placebo effect" (1990, p. 20).

Pregnancy

Krieger (1993) studied pregnant women and their partners taking Lamaze childbirth preparation classes. Half of the 60 couples were only trained in the Lamaze method. The husbands in the other 30 couples were taught TT in addition to Lamaze. These husbands gave their wives TT two to three times per week for the last 3 months of the pregnancy. For those couples who used TT as part of childbirth preparation and labor, "a concerned satisfying relationship of mutual dependent caring developed within the family" (Krieger, 1993, p. 139). Those couples scored significantly higher on marital satisfaction scales postpartum as compared with couples who did not use TT. In addition, many of the husbands using TT reported feeling more personally connected to their unborn child.

Labor and Delivery

The use of TT with patients in labor and delivery is reported anecdotally in the professional literature. Krieger (1993) suggested that the mother, the father, and the caregiver all use TT techniques, as she believed that such techniques can reduce pain and anxiety and facilitate the normal birthing process. Stern (1985) described the use of TT during labor to promote relaxation and decrease discomfort (Buenting, 1993). Jurgens (cited in Cornman, Jurgens, & Eldridge, 1992) reported using TT with a 38-year-old professional woman, Gloria, who was having her first child. Gloria had been sent home from the birthing center at 10 PM by her midwife when she was 80% effaced and 3 cm dilated, but was not progressing. After centering, Ms. Jurgens assessed Gloria's energy field, finding low energy flow. Gloria verbalized her fear of giving birth at "this age." Jurgens combined her TT treatment of moving the energy down and through the pelvis and out the feet as Gloria envisioned the cervix relaxing and opening, similar to how a lotus would unfold. By 1 AM Gloria was heading back to the birthing center in active labor. Of course, there is no way to know whether TT made the difference, but this is a common response related by nurses using TT with patients during labor.

Having TT treatments following my own cesarean section at age 45 helped not only to bring a sense of relaxation sorely needed, but also to provide the experience of wholeness and connection. This goal seemed elusive, given the sleep deprivation due to breast-feeding a newborn while recovering from major abdominal surgery. It was especially helpful to experience the centered and grounding presence of the two nurses who treated me with TT at this time. Given my own lack of energy, the boost that I received from their treatments reminded me of how my energy had felt in the past and would feel more consistently in the future.

Premenstrual Syndrome

There is a wide range and intensity of symptoms experienced by an estimated 10% to 80% of women in the United States due to PMS (Shephard & Shephard, 1997). The alternative health community offers many forms of treatment, from acupuncture/acupressure to herbs and homeopathy. TT, too, can be considered a vital component of one's self-care program in relation to PMS. Krieger (1993) suggested that TT can successfully treat symptoms of PMS, including irritability, anxiety, lethargy, fatigue, depression, water retention, and breast engorgement.

Caring for the Terminally Ill Patient

The role of TT in the care of terminally ill patients is at least twofold. First, there are numerous reports of symptom relief for individuals suffering from end stage cancer, acquired immune deficiency syndrome (AIDS), and Alzheimer's disease (Cornman et al., 1992; Newshan, 1989; Wager, 1996; Woods, Craven, & Whitney, 1996). While TT does not cure the underlying disease, it does seem to decrease pain, provide relaxation, and alleviate anxiety, all of which are welcome in the care of the seriously ill. Second, TT also seems to help many individuals who are dying experience the final transformation with peace and a sense of acceptance.

My own work with a patient who was dying from AIDS provides an example of the usefulness of TT. After weekly TT sessions, he was able to discuss frankly his fears about death and what would become of his elderly mother, who had outlived her husband by many years and would probably survive her son as well. Because his pain from neurological damage would subside after TT, he had some energy to discuss, plan, and problem-solve ways to address both his and his mother's needs in practical ways.

A nurse reported that when her father was dying after a long illness due to advanced adenocarcinoma of the liver and lungs, her own experience with TT helped her to be a source of strength for her father and her family (Cornman et al., 1992). "The centering, the openness and the detached caring learned through meditation and the technique of therapeutic touch . . . assisted Dad in attaining a sense of peace and control. The night that Dad died, my mother, five of the six siblings, a sister-in-law, and one grandchild were with Dad. We encircled Dad and sent him healing and peaceful thoughts. The energy being directed at this time was directed with the thought of letting Dad go physically, of sending him off with peace. The home had a sense of peace, joy, of release, of birthing in the moment of physical death" (Cornman et al., 1992, pp. 14–16).

Gayle Newshan (1989), while working as a nurse in pain management, wrote about her experiences of using TT with persons with AIDS. She wrote about the ways that TT is used with the complex symptoms of these patients in terms of respiratory and gastrointestinal symptoms, fever, pain, and anxiety. She recognized that each patient, each treatment, and each practitioner is unique, and therefore she offers her suggestions as guidelines or suggestions rather than as mandates.

Woods et al. (1996) reported on a study of 57 patients between the ages of 67 and 93 with a diagnosis of Alzheimer's disease. The objective was to determine whether TT could decrease the frequency of disruptive behaviors in these patients. Two of the six behaviors, vocalization and manual manipulation, did show a decrease after the intervention of contact TT. The authors stated that "therapeutic touch offers a noninvasive, clinically relevant modality that could be used routinely to decrease or prevent disruptive behaviors and increase the safety and comfort of those with Alzheimer's disease" (Woods et al., 1996, p. 95).

Wager (1996) provided an insightful summary of the ways TT assists in the care of the dying patient. She emphasized that besides helping with some of the symptoms that dying patients may experience, TT can help relieve their fear as well as provide comfort to the family and friends of the dying patient. TT also helps the practitioner from becoming overwhelmed by the emotions being experienced by patients and their support persons.

Transformation

A significant component of learning TT is that it is a means of self-transformation. Maria Arrington (1998) stated, "If you are like me, embarking on the study of TT was the beginning of massive changes in your way of interacting with the world. My whole world view changed. I began to understand more clearly how the world within me and without me was interrelated" (p. 1). Macrae (1995) described TT as a "synthesis of concentrative and insight techniques" (p. 275) of meditation. The act of centering "introduces a meditative quality into the background of one's activities of daily living" (Krieger, 1995, p. 265). This "cultivation of mindfulness" (Krieger, 1995, p. 265) is a cornerstone of the immense change in all aspects of their lives that practitioners report experiencing after learning and practicing TT over time.

In the process of TT, practitioners learn to stay centered during all phases, calming their minds while focusing on the process of helping the patients. While assessing, they "listen" without preprogramming by thinking "I should feel this or that." Their minds are still, quiet, and open in order to be able to perceive what is actually occurring. They recognize that the result of the treatment is not in their conscious control but that they facilitate the process. As Quinn (1979), one of Krieger's early students and a longtime TT researcher and practitioner, so aptly stated, "It seems important for the healer to be certain that he or she is acting as the transmitter of energy, and not the generator" (p. 664). The practitioner must leave her ego behind and not become attached to any particular outcome for the treatment. The practitioner's compassion and intention to help enable her to identify with a quality of wholeness and unity that is then available to the patient's energetic field. How that energy is used then becomes the prerogative of the patient's energetic field.

To illustrate this point, Macrae described one of her pediatric patients, a little girl with cystic fibrosis. Macrae (1979) listened to the girl's lungs with her stethoscope before and after TT treatments. She was disappointed that the patient's lungs sounded as "gunky" after TT as they did before TT. Later, however, when the girl's father was leaving, he mentioned that his daughter "ate like a horse" that evening for the first time in weeks (Macrae, 1979, p. 665). This anecdote is an example of the necessity of the practitioner to let go of her own expectations and accept and respect the patient's individual responses.

The detachment that the healer experiences from the outcome of TT is tied to the "conviction that each patient is first of all a human being with a point of wholeness within, which is unaffected by the pain and frailty. The healer has to have a sense of wholeness within herself so that she can reach that in the patient, whatever that person's suffering and no matter how great his pain. One can convey it to another only if one experiences the wholeness within oneself" (Kunz, 1995, p. 300).

This connection between the practitioner and the patient seems particularly congruent with the recognition of the nondualistic nature of our existence. As Wilber (1991) stated, an "equality consciousness" develops, referring to the exchangeability of self and other (p. 249), the deep compassion present in experiencing that all beings suffer and that self and other can be easily exchanged since both are equal.

The National Institutes of Health (NIH) established the Office for Alternative Medicine (OAM) in 1992 for the purpose of investigating the efficacy and safety of complementary health care practices. The OAM has recognized TT as the most evolved of energetic healing modalities due to its body of published research (Samarel, 1993). As of the summer of 1998, there were more than 80 studies, including qualitative and quantitative outcome studies, on TT (Ulan, 1998). In their comprehensive review of TT research to date, Mulloney and Wells-Federman (1996) concluded that in terms of quantitative research, continued replication and extension of studies are needed. Regarding qualitative investigations of TT, they recommend that such research be approached through an interdisciplinary effort given the enormous area of possible study. As a practitioner of TT, I am reminded of the balancing statement of Quinn (1989), who said, "There is a need to be cautious and creative in conducting this scientific study lest, like the butterfly that is pinned down for closer inspection, the phenomenon is destroyed in the attempts to understand it" (p. 87). In a culture that rewards outcomes, measurable results, and quantitative evidence, we are challenged to honor a healing modality that requires "being" as much or more than "doing." Dossey (1991) has described the difference between "doing" and "being" therapies. "Doing" therapies include such interventions as giving medication, doing surgery, or changing a patient's diet. "Being" therapies "utilize states of consciousness, such as imagery, prayer, meditation, and quiet contemplation, as well as the presence and intention of the nurse" (Dossey, Keegen, Guzzetta, & Kolkmeier, 1995, p. 14).

As an adjunctive therapy that is accessible to so many patients, in so many settings, and has such a transformative effect on practitioners, the future of TT seems bright and promising. It is an honor to be on the path.

REVIEW AND DISCUSSION

See boxes "Patient Education" and "Continuing Questions/Challenges" for discussion topics for this chapter.

Patient Education

Elicits relaxation response.
Decreases anxiety.
Helps to relieve pain.
Helps to facilitate wound healing.
Helps couple relationship during pregnancy.
Assists with labor and delivery.
Assists with alleviating PMS symptoms.
Assists with facilitating increased comfort in the terminally ill.
Facilitates positive self-transformation.

Continuing Questions/Challenges

Are there any risks in therapeutic touch?
Are there some people who are more amenable than others to therapeutic touch as an effective health care approach? If so, what explains this phenomenon?

REFERENCES

Arrington, M. (Summer, 1988). Learning and growing through TT intensives. *Cooperative Connection Newsletter of the Nurse Healers-Professional Associates, Inc. 19*(4), 1, 6.

Buenting, J.A. (1993). Human energy fields and birth: implications for research and practice. *Advances in Nursing Science, 15*(4), 53–59.

Cornman, B.J., Jurgens, A., & Eldridge, P. (1992). Therapeutic touch: Healing energy in research and practice. Unpublished manuscript, Seattle, Washington.

Dossey, L. (1991). *Meaning and medicine: A doctor's tales of breakthrough and healing.* New York: Bantam Books.

Dossey, L. (1997). *Be careful what you pray for . . . You just might get it.* San Francisco: Harper.

Dossey, B.M., Keegan, L., Guzzetta, C., & Kolkmeier, L.G. (1995). *Holistic nursing.* Gaithersburg, MD: Aspen Publishers, Inc.

Heidt, P. (1981). Effect of therapeutic touch on anxiety level of hospitalized patients. *Nursing Research, 30*(1), 32–37.

Jurgens, A. (1989). Personal communication.

Keller, E., & Bzdek, V.M. (1986). Effects of therapeutic touch on tension headache pain. *Nursing Research, 35*, 101–106.

Krieger, D. (1975). Therapeutic touch: The imprimatur of nursing. *American Journal of Nursing, 75,* 784–787.

Krieger, D. (1979). *The therapeutic touch: How to use your hands to help or heal.* New York: Prentice Hall.

Krieger, D. (1993). *Accepting your power to heal: The personal practice of therapeutic touch.* Santa Fe, NM: Bear & Co. Publishing.

Krieger, D. (1995). High-order emergence of the self during therapeutic touch. In D. Kunz (Ed.), *Spiritual healing* (pp. 262–271). Wheaton, IL: Theosophical Publishing House.

Krieger, D., Peper, E., & Ancoli, S. (1979). Therapeutic touch: Searching for evidence of physiological change. *American Journal of Nursing, 79,* 660–665.

Kunz, D. (Ed.), (1995). *Spiritual healing.* Wheaton, IL: Theosophical Publishing House.

Kunz, D., & Peper, E. (1995). Fields and their clinical implications. In D. Kunz (Ed.), *Spiritual healing* (pp. 213–261). Wheaton, IL: Theosophical Publishing House.

Macrae, J. (1979). Therapeutic touch in practice. *American Journal of Nursing, 75,* 664–665.

Macrae, J. (1987). *Therapeutic touch: A practical guide.* New York: Alfred A. Knopf.

Macrae, J. (1995). Therapeutic touch as meditation. In D. Kunz (Ed.), *Spiritual healing* (pp. 272–288). Wheaton, IL: Theosophical Publishing House.

Malinski, V. (1996). An invitation to dialogue on the theoretical basis of therapeutic touch. *Rogerian Nursing Science News, 8*(3), 1.

Meehan, T.C. (1993). Therapeutic touch and postoperative pain: A Rogerian research study. *Nursing Science Quarterly, 6*(2), 69–78.

Mulloney, S. S., & Wells-Federman, C. (1996). Therapeutic touch: a healing modality. *Journal of Cardiovascular Nursing, 10*(3), 27–49.

Newshan, G. (1989). Therapeutic touch for symptom control in persons with AIDS. *Holistic Nursing Practice, 3*(4), 45–51.

Nurse Healers-Professional Associates, Inc. (1992). *Therapeutic touch teaching guidelines: Beginner's level.* New York: Nurse Healers-Professional Associates, Inc. Cooperative.

Quinn, J.F. (1979). One nurse's evolution as a healer. *American Journal of Nursing, 75,* 662–664.

Quinn, J.F. (1984). Therapeutic touch as engery exchange: Testing the theory. *Advances in Nursing Science, 6,* 42–49.

Quinn, J.F. (1989). Therapeutic touch as energy exchange: Replication and extension. *Nursing Science Quarterly, 2,* 79–87.

Quinn, J.F., & Strelkauskas, A.J. (1993). Psychoimmunologic effects of therapeutic touch on practitioners and recently bereaved recipients: A pilot study. *Advances in Nursing Science, 15*(4), 13–26.

Rogers, M.E. (1970). *An introduction to the theoretical basis of nursing.* Philadelphia: F.A. Davis.

Samarel, N. (1992). The experience of receiving therapeutic touch. *Journal of Advanced Nursing, 17,* 651–657.

Samarel, N. (1993). Report to the membership and board of the National Institutes of Health office of unconventional medical practices workshop. *Cooperative Connection, 14*(1)1,3–5.

Schmidt, C.M. (1995). The basics of therapeutic touch. *RN, 58*(7), 50–54.

Shephard, B.D., & Shephard, C.A. (1997). *The complete guide to women's health.* New York: Plume/Penguin Books, Inc.

Stern, Z. (1985, Summer). The Healing Touch. *Child Birth Educator, 43*–47.

Ulan, D. (1998). Position statement on therapeutic touch (letter to the editor). *Cooperative Connection, 19*(4), 4.

Wager, S. (1996). *A doctor's guide to Therapeutic Touch.* New York: Berkeley Publishing Group.

Wilber, K. (1991). *Grace and grit: Spirituality and healing in the life and death of Treya Killam Wilbur.* Boston: Shambhala.

Wirth, D. (1990). The effect of non-contact therapeutic touch on the healing rate of full thickness dermal wounds. *Subtle Energies, 1*(1), 1–20.

Wirth, D. P., Richardson, J.T., Eidelman, W.S., & O'Malley, A.C. (1993). Full thickness dermal wounds treated with noncontact therapeutic touch: A replication and extension. *Complementary Therapies in Medicine, 1,* 127–132.

Woods, D.L., Craven, R., & Whitney, J. (1996). The effect of therapeutic touch on disruptive behaviours of individuals with dementia of the Alzheimer type (abstract). *Alternative Therapies, 2*(4), 95.

Wright, S.M. (1987). The use of therapeutic touch in the management of pain. *Nursing Clinics of North America, 22,* 705–714.

SUGGESTED READINGS

Horrigan, B. (1998). Dolores Krieger, Healing with therapeutic touch. *Alternative Therapies, 14*(1), 86–92.

Ledwith, S. (1995). Therapeutic touch and mastectomy: A case study. *RN, 58*(7), 51–53.

Resources for Therapeutic Touch

For information about practitioners, teachers, and workshops:
Nurse Healers-Professional Associates, Inc.
P.O. Box 444
Allison Park, Pennsylvania 15101-0444
412-355-8476

For information about invitational workshops for health
  professionals:
Pumpkin Hollow Farm
1184 Route 11
Craryville, New York 12521
518-325-3583

Orcas Island Foundation
Route 1, Box 86
Eastsound, Washington 98245
360-376-4526

PART III

Personal Perspectives As Exemplars

Ellen Olshansky

Part III presents two very "experiential" chapters, in which personal experiences of different ways of achieving wellness are described. Tina Brewer, in an interview, relays how quilting provides her with a form of art therapy that helps in improving health and well-being. Gerri Adreon describes how she developed new strategies to improve her own health after suffering a stroke. Two other chapters present examples of specific cultural aspects of women's health. The chapter on women's health and health care in Nicaragua provides one cultural group's particular issues with achieving and maintaining wellness. The chapter on storytelling provides examples of how storytelling functions to assist women in maintaining their health.

The intent of Part III is to provide insight into women's wellness through some actual experiences. In addition, Part III attempts to emphasize the importance of understanding cultural diversity as integral to understanding women's health and wellness.

CHAPTER 19

Exemplar: Health Care of Women in Nicaragua

Nicole Rawson, Leah Vota Cunningham, Patricia Fedorka,
Lenore K. Resick, and Melinda Kai Smith

> *Health and healing relationships and experiences predictably have*
> *different meanings to women from different cultures and subcultures.*
>
> —Ruzek, Olesen, & Clarke, 1997, p. 247

This chapter reviews the current health status of women in Nicaragua as revealed in the research literature, government publications, and personal experience and interviews with Nicaraguans. It discusses Nicaraguan health strategies that are either planned or in place, and illustrates how understanding and working within the social/cultural context is essential to improving women's health worldwide. The intent of this chapter, within the context of this book on integrated women's health, is to present one example of a cultural group of women, emphasizing the importance that that cultural group has on the health of the women within the group. It is important to keep in mind that this is one cultural group, and each individual culture has its own unique aspects that contribute to the health status of the women within that group. In addition, individuals within the group may differ in how they respond to or cope with the issues that arise from their cultural group.

> Maria lives in an 8 × 10-foot lean-to in a barrio in Managua with her five daughters, ages 7 years and under. Bananas and rice serve as breakfast, lunch, or dinner, with an occasional meal of beans, if they are lucky. The family sleeps on the

ground, using lice-infested old clothes and rags as their mattress and blankets. Their eyes are empty, their hair is full of lice, there is no smile, no connection, and there is much mistrust. What little money Maria has, she gets from her "companero," Juan, who makes small amounts of money for labor he does for people in the barrio. After spending most of his earnings on alcohol, he may give Maria a few cordobas for food. He stays with her on an intermittent basis. Maria is used to the violence and abuse at the hands of this drunken companero, who routinely beats her and demands sex. Last night he put out a cigarette on her forehead and hit her with a shovel. As if this isn't enough, she is urged to go to the Centro de Salud where it is discovered that she has venereal warts and syphilis. Life is hard. . . .

BACKGROUND/SETTING

Nicaragua, a Central American country located between Honduras and Costa Rica, is about the size of the North American state of Georgia. Located along the Pacific fault line and having two coastlines make Nicaragua susceptible to earthquakes, volcanic eruptions, and hurricanes such as the recent Hurricane Mitch (Pan American Health Organization [PAHO], 1998b). The years of the Samoza regime, and the subsequent Sandinista revolution and Contra wars left Nicaragua with an eroded infrastructure, an underdeveloped manufacturing and service sector, and a dependence upon foreign assistance. Twenty-two percent of the gross domestic product (GDP) in 1996 came from foreign assistance (U.S. Department of State, 1998).

In the last 3 years, Nicaragua's economy has remained strong and grown 3% to 5% each year (U.S. Department of State, 1998). Nicaragua's historically agricultural economy has a rapidly growing service sector. Currently, commerce, construction, government, banking, manufacturing, and transport account for 45% of the GDP. The rapidly growing service and manufacturing sector has contributed to an increase in the urbanization of the population. As a result, 61.5% of Nicaragua's population lives in the Pacific region, in and around the capital, Managua (Pan American Health Organization [PAHO], 1998a). Women constitute 27% of the work force in Latin America (PAHO, 1998a). The majority of migrants to urban areas are women in the 15- to 29-year-old age range (60%), most of whom work in commerce and service and increasingly in prostitution (Otis, 1992). Urban women earn 71% of the salary of their male counterparts (PAHO, 1998a).

The inflation rate of 12% and an unemployment rate of 17% to 35% has also strained Nicaragua's economy and pushed more families into poverty (Banco Central de Nicaragua, 1993; PAHO, 1994). In 1994, PAHO estimated that 47% of the population of Nicaragua was earning less than 412 U.S. dollars per year. Single women head one third of Nicaraguan households (World Bank, 1994 as cited in Zelaya et al., 1997). Even though women's opportunities to participate in the work force are increasing, women still maintain the burden of domestic tasks, resulting in a double or even triple workload compared with men (PAHO, 1998a).

The challenge for Nicaragua is to meet the basic social, economic, and health needs of its population, while simultaneously meeting the national needs for economic growth and development and political stability. Nicaragua's development is plagued by limited national resources and a dependence upon foreign assistance. This challenge provides the context within which the health and health care of Nicaraguan women is examined and understood.

HEALTH CONDITIONS IN NICARAGUA

Nicaragua's morbidity and mortality data reflect a developing country in transition. For example, diseases of the circulatory system (associated with more advanced strategies of socioeconomic development) were the number one cause of death for 1990–1995 (PAHO, 1998a). Deaths due to intestinal infections, respiratory infections, and conditions of the perinatal period still rank among the top five causes of death; a testimony to the continued lack of access to clean water, sanitation, and essential social and health services. Children between the ages of 1 and 5 years account for 45% of all deaths (Lane, 1995). These children's deaths are attributed mostly to malnutrition, respiratory infections, and diseases preventable by vaccination (MINSA, 1994).

Health of Women and Children

In developing countries, women have about 100 times the chance of dying from pregnancy and childbirth than do women in developed countries (Seipel, 1992). Maternal mortality estimates for Nicaragua vary from 93 to 155/100,000 live births (PAHO, 1998a). It is estimated that maternal mortality and morbidity can be underestimated by as much as 40% (Mauldin, 1994). A demonstration of the use of the Sisterhood Method for estimating maternal mortality (an informal survey method) resulted in a maternal mortality ratio estimate of 241/

100,000 live births in Region 1 of Nicaragua (Danel, Graham, Stupp, & Castillo, 1996). There is general agreement that regardless of the estimate, the major causes of maternal mortality (sepsis, hemorrhage, hypertension, and untoward consequences of abortion) can be prevented or detected early by improved access to preventive health services and emergency services (MINSA 1994).

The birth rate of 33.2/1,000 population, a fertility rate of 5 children per a woman's lifetime, and a shortened birth interval of less than 24 months in some rural areas collectively contribute to the high maternal risk status and morbidity rate (PAHO, 1998a). Social science research in Nicaragua reveals that boys and men are encouraged to be sexually active early, while girls and women are expected to remain chaste and faithful (Zelaya et al., 1997). As a result, the percentage of teen births is 28% of all pregnancies in Nicaragua, compared with 10% of all pregnancies worldwide (PAHO, 1998a). While male gender roles encourage sexual activity and productivity, the responsibility for using contraception and raising children is seen as the sole responsibility of the women (Zelaya et al., 1997). Educational efforts to promote a sense of sexual responsibility among men and to bring contraceptive use into the domain of mutual negotiation counter traditional cultural attitudes toward male and female gender roles and behaviors. In addition, the self-care model of health promoted by Western societies (Leininger, 1992) may not apply to women in Nicaragua, especially poor urban or rural women.

Currently, most births (73%) are attended by trained health personnel (UNICEF, 1995) and 46% take place in a health center or hospital (PAHO, 1998a). In rural areas, many women (48% to 68%) give birth at home, with 69% of these women being assisted by trained local birth attendants or "parteras" (UNICEF, 1995). Local traditional midwives already attending births in the community are given extra training from the Ministerio de Salud (MINSA). They are equipped to recognize, refer, and treat emergencies during labor and delivery, as well as to promote breast-feeding, and to recognize and refer for symptoms of neonatal syphilis. A 1987 report stated that "parteras" were effective in reducing maternal mortality by referring women for malpresentation, obstructed labor, and placenta previa (Pascoe & Stein, 1987). The success of these midwives' ability to work with the health care system, while continuing to provide services to women in their communities in culturally appropriate ways, demonstrates how important it is to work with existing cultural attitudes and social structures in order to effect health changes.

In 1991, the Ministry of Health declared the maternal mortality rate an epidemic (Lane, 1995; MINSA, 1991). Women and children were declared priority populations, and programs were put into place emphasizing prenatal care, family planning, and care during childbirth and the puerperium, as well as early detection and prevention of cervical and breast cancer (PAHO, 1998a). Prenatal services are offered at all health posts and health centers free of charge, yet only 72% of all women in Nicaragua use prenatal services (Profamilia, 1993; Wellstart International, 1995). A study done by Profamilia (a private institution delivering family planning services in Nicaragua) demonstrated that increased education and living in urban areas was associated with higher use of prenatal services. The report concluded that urban women were located closer to health services, and had more monetary resources to spend on health care (Profamilia, 1993). Rural women may need to walk more than 1 to 3 hours to get to a health post where staff or equipment may be lacking. Other factors such as other children at home, lack of knowledge of benefits of prenatal care, and viewing pregnancy as normal and not an illness have been identified as influencing women's decisions to not seek prenatal care (York, Williams, and Munro, 1993).

While women have a purported access to free prenatal services, they arrive at their first prenatal visit significantly at higher risk as a population due to the high fertility rates, shortened birth intervals, and high percentage of teen pregnancies (PAHO, 1998a). In addition, women's health status is often undermined by exposure to chronic malnutrition and exposure to environmental conditions (toxins, infectious diseases), within a social context that does not necessarily place women and children as a priority (WHO, 1996). Research has revealed that in order to affect perinatal outcomes significantly, the general health status of women and teens prior to pregnancy needs to be addressed (Reynolds, 1999).

Examining the population pyramid for Nicaragua in 1998 reveals that the age group from 15 to 64 is the largest and the fastest-growing age group (PAHO, 1998a). The average life expectancy in Latin America is 73.2 years for women (6.4 years longer than that for men). When women reach the age of 50 worldwide, their average life expectancy ranges from 27 to 32 additional years (WHO, 1996). As a result, over the next decade, women in their midlife and aging years are going to constitute a large proportion of the population in Nicaragua. Currently, programs addressing menopause, cancer screening and prevention, and care for the elderly in Nicaragua are still in their infancy (MINSA, 1994). Data and statistics on the meaning of menopause for Nicaraguan women, the symptoms of menopause, and the morbidity associated with aging in Nicaragua are just beginning to be collected (MINSA, 1994).

Nicaragua's infant mortality rate of 52/1,000 births in 1996 has been steadily decreasing since 1990 (PAHO, 1998a). Reasons for this successful drop in infant mortality rates, despite decreased funding of the health care system, include improved access to health care services due to the increased urbanization of the population (Sandiford, Morales, Gorter, Coyle, & Smith, 1991), and improved economic opportunities for and literacy of women (Garfield & Williams, 1992). Despite the aforementioned improvements, Nicaragua's infant mortality rate is still above the Latin American and Caribbean average of 40/1,000 births and the United States rate of 8/1,000 births (PAHO, 1998a). The major causes of infant mortality were listed as prematurity, puerperal infections, respiratory infections, intrauterine hypoxia, and deaths associated with the perinatal period or congenital anomalies (MINSA, 1995; PAHO, 1998a). Many of these deaths theoretically could have been prevented through access to and use of adequate prenatal care, more births attended by trained delivery attendants, and improved access to emergency perinatal services.

Infection and diarrheal diseases in the first year of life continue to remain a leading cause of death for children under the age of 1 year (PAHO, 1998a). While 95% of women initiate breast-feeding in Nicaragua, many infants receive formula and other supplementation as soon as 2 months of age (UNICEF, 1994). Only 45% of infants are exclusively breast-fed at 1 week of age, and only 2% exclusively breast-fed at 5 weeks of age. This low rate of exclusive breast-feeding and early introduction of foods and liquids contributes to diarrhea and malnutrition (Picado, 1994). In addition, only 40% of infants receive their first breast-feeding in the first hour of life (UNICEF, 1994). Picado (1994) demonstrated that Nicaraguan women perceived exclusive breast-feeding as insufficient for the infant and draining on the mother. In 1993, Nicaragua signed the International Code for "Breast-feeding Initiative" to combat the low levels of breast-feeding, popularity of supplementation, and lack of control/enforcement of regulations of infant formula production and marketing in Nicaragua (UNICEF, 1994). The initiative includes health personnel training, public information campaigns, legal reforms, and intersectorial cooperation at the central and local levels (UNICEF, 1994). The International Code also includes a "Baby Friendly Hospitals Initiative," which requires hospital personnel to be educated about and support early breast-feeding and "rooming in" for mothers and babies. Evaluations of the "Baby Friendly Hospitals Initiative" reveals an increase in staff knowledge of breast-feeding, increase in education of women about benefits of breast-feeding, and increase in initiation of first-hour breast-feeding (MINSA, Bureau of Nutrition, 1996).

The high maternal and infant mortality rates reflect a primary health care system struggling to carry out vaccination, screening, and prevention programs while the population struggles with decreased economic opportunities, increased levels of illiteracy, and lack of access to clean water and sanitation. While access to primary and secondary health services for women markedly improved maternal-infant morbidity and mortality profiles throughout the 1970s and 1980s, lack of adequate supplies, personnel, supervision, and community involvement has limited health systems' efforts to improve the health status of women and children in Nicaragua. As a result, Nicaragua still has one of the highest infant mortality rates in Central America (Lane, 1995).

Despite the intention to spend more resources on the two priority populations of women and children, the per capita spending on health care has fallen (Lane, 1995; Sales, 1993) and the UNO government felt "forced" to initiate fee for service and private pay health care delivery models (Garfield, Low, and Caldera, 1993). In addition, the current Aleman government has been overwhelmed by the demands of the destruction from Hurricane Mitch and the increased cases of cholera and other water and sanitation issues in the affected coastal areas. All of these factors undermine the central concepts that guide Nicaragua's health care system: primary health care as a right for Nicaragua's citizens.

Human Immunodeficiency Virus/Acquired Immune Deficiency Syndrome and Sexually Transmitted Diseases

Despite a high rate of sexually transmitted diseases (STDs) and other economic and cultural factors, the acquired immune deficiency syndrome (AIDS) epidemic in Nicaragua is not as widespread as in the United States and other Latin American countries. However, AIDS is expected to have a significant social and economic impact on Nicaragua by the end of the decade (Low et al., 1993; Siegel et al., 1996). The increase in number of AIDS cases is thought to reflect the transmission of human immunodeficiency virus (HIV) into Nicaragua by returning refugees and repatriates, as well as an increased in-country transmission rate (Low et al., 1993). The epidemiological profile of AIDS in Nicaragua reflects a heterosexual transmission pattern, which means women and their children will constitute a large proportion of the HIV-infected population. During the Contra wars, many young men fled the country, and Nicaragua was isolated socially and economically due to embargoes and lack of tourism. During this time, Nicaragua depended upon its own blood supply for transfusions, and intravenous drug use was rare. It was not until the Sandinistas came to power and Nicaraguans returned from other Latin American countries and the United States that the first cases of HIV were identified (Low et al., 1993). Since 1987, the number of HIV cases has doubled every 12 months, but has leveled off after 1995 (Organizacion Panamericana de la Salud/Organizacion Mundial de la Salud [OPS/OMS] Nicaragua, 1996). Of the 96 cases of HIV infection and 114 cases of AIDS reported since 1987, the majority were transmitted heterosexually (>50%), about 20% homosexually, 15% bisexually, and most rarely, via perinatal or blood transfusion (OPMS, 1996; PAHO, 1998a).

There are many factors in Nicaraguan society that increase the likelihood of an AIDS epidemic and increase the risks for women to contract HIV. These factors include misconceptions about transmission, a high rate of STDs, low use of condoms, machismo values (which promote early and multiple sexual experiences for males), and a lack of economic opportunities, which sometimes forces young girls and women into prostitution (Egger et al., 1993; Low et al., 1993).

In a country where diarrhea, respiratory infections, and skin conditions are common problems, it is possible for HIV to go undiagnosed or underdetected. Furthermore, physicians lack the experience and training to interpret these conditions as manifestations of HIV. Rather than seek professional care, people often treat and medicate themselves for infections, which are possibly HIV-related (Egger et al., 1993). Reported prevalence rates of HIV/AIDS may be inaccurate due to a statistical reporting system that is still in its infancy and death reporting that is incomplete. Despite these factors and statistics, the AIDS epidemic is relatively rare compared with other countries, and accounts for only 1% of all cases in Latin America.

There is a high rate of STDs in Nicaragua. Many women are not routinely screened for STDs due to lack of laboratory and material resources. Treatment is often based on clinical reports of symptoms (personal experience). Appropriate medications are not available or affordable in the marketplace. For many years, infections caused by *Neisseria gonorrhoae* and *Chlamydia* were treated with penicillin. The extensive use of antibiotics in Nicaragua has increased the levels of susceptibility to pathogenic bacteria, and highly resistant strains have emerged (Castro, Bergerton, & Chaberland, 1993). Coupled with a lack of epidemiological surveillance programs, the development of resistant strains and treatment failures is not surprising.

Reproductive Health and Rights

Although Nicaragua has a relatively advanced record on general political issues such as pluralism, democracy, and abolition of the death
penalty, the position regarding reproductive rights remains relatively
conservative (Molyneux, 1988; Zelaya et al., 1997). It is not uncommon for a woman to have had 8 to 12 children, as well as several abortions (Pascoe & Stein, 1987). Nicaraguan women, many of whom participated in the revolution, have increasingly gained control over
aspects of their lives and have sought to gain control over their fertility
(Pascoe & Stein, 1987). A family code was established in the 1987 constitution giving men and women equal rights. Contraception and sex
education, however, were minimally promoted. Reasons for this lack
of attention were poverty, the influence of the Catholic church, perceived underpopulation, machismo, and fear of repressive population
control (Wessel, 1991). Intentions to promote women's rights and status in the culture during the Sandinista years were cast aside with the
increasing emphasis on maintaining the Sandinista government in
place and fighting the Contra wars (Wessel & Campbell, 1997).

Sterilization was the most common and sometimes only birth control method offered, and often this option was only offered to women
at high risk or those who had experienced previous complications of
pregnancy. Contraceptives as a method of family planning, child spacing, or prevention of unwanted pregnancy was not an option offered
to women until recently. Most contraceptives were provided by hospitals, but with decentralization these services were moved to the health
posts and health centers. Because of the reluctance of women to go to
health centers for care, the irregularity of contraceptive supplies at the
health centers, outdated oral contraceptives, and lack of health work-
ers trained in contraceptive services, many women were unable to obtain quality family planning services (Wessel, 1991). In addition, gender and social inequality result in poor, rural, and young women being
less likely to insist on contraceptive use (Zelaya et al., 1996). Traditionally, contraceptive use is regarded as the women's responsibility
(Zelaya et al., 1996). Underlying this disparity in contraceptive use and
fertility rates between poor, rural, and young women and their older,
urban counterparts are the educational and economic gaps between
the two groups. In other words, less educated women with fewer economic opportunities will depend upon men to provide for them in
exchange for sexual favors, and feel less likely to be able to insist upon
condom or contraception use. Currently, the Ministry of Health, non-

governmental organizations such as Profamilia, and private physicians or pharmacies offer everything from male and female sterilization, intrauterine devices (IUDs), pills, injections, condoms, vaginal tablets, and Norplant implants (Profamilia, 1993). The largest distributor of female sterilization and IUDs is the MINSA, with pharmacies and private doctors providing pills and injections (Profamilia, 1993).

Overall contraceptive prevalence was estimated to be 49% in 1990 (UNICEF, 1995), which implies that only 50% of all people eligible for family planning services were using them. In their National Health Survey, Profamilia (1993) found that 94% to 99% of women ranging in age from 15 to 49 years had heard of contraceptive pills, IUDs, and injections. Of the women interviewed, 53% of unmarried and 70% of married women reported using a method at one time. Actual use of contraceptives during "the moment of contact" varied from 54% of the time among married women to 1% of the time among adolescents (Profamilia, 1993). Knowledge of contraceptive methods and use of methods was higher in urban than rural areas. As their number of children increased, women's use of contraceptives became more frequent, with sterilization becoming more popular. Reasons stated for using contraception were to limit family size (68% of women surveyed), or for family spacing (30% of women surveyed) (Profamilia, 1993). Of those women not using contraceptives, married women cited subfertility, postpartum status, breast-feeding, and infrequent sexual activity as reasons, or other reasons as contraindicated health reasons, side effects, or didn't like methods available. Only 1% stated religious objections to contraceptives. Reasons for discontinuing a method were undesirable side effects and desiring a pregnancy. Only 25% of urban and 4% of rural women stated cost or partner objection as a reason for discontinuation of their birth control methods.

Self-induced or illegal abortion remains a significant (yet underreported) cause of maternal mortality in Latin America (PAHO, 1994; Pathfinder International, 1994), reflecting a need for improved family planning services. Abortion was declared illegal under the criminal code of 1974, although this code has never been fully enforced. Therapeutic pregnancy termination could be obtained in certain circumstances if requested and permitted by the spouse or next of kin and approved by a medical panel. For the majority of women seeking pregnancy termination, self-induced or illegal abortion appears to remain the primary option. In 1989, several European-funded women's clinics performed first-trimester abortions for a moderate fee, provided legal and mental health services, and raised the consciousness of many women regarding women's rights. The more conservative current government has "imposed severe restrictions on abortions" resulting in women seeking "unsafe or self-induced abortions" (Zelaya et al., 1997, pp. 44, 45). In fact, abortion and infection remain two of the main causes of perinatal morbidity in Nicaragua today (PAHO, 1998a).

Violence

The occurrence of physical, emotional, and sexual assault against women in Nicaragua is difficult to ascertain. Research on the prevalence of or attitudes toward violence against women is minimal. In one survey in Leon, Nicaragua, of 360 women, 52% reported a history of battery, and 27% stated they were currently being battered (Wessel & Campbell, 1997). Wirpsa asserts that "There has been a rise in alcoholism, and violence against women and children has reached epidemic proportions" (Wirpsa, 1995, p. 8). Contributing factors are believed to include increasing economic pressures, male unemployment combined with "machismo" cultural values, and lack of support and economic opportunities for women (Wessel & Campbell, 1997).

Deighton (as cited in Stephens, 1990) stated that in Nicaragua "[o]ne of 'machismo's' characteristics is the assumption of male privilege and power in the family: the man is 'master' of his 'own' woman—to the point even of physical violence" (p. 71). Bunch (in Lykes, Brabeck, Ferns, & Radan, 1993) observed that "although violence against women is pervasive, it is seldom seen as a human rights issue" (p. 526). According to the women's legal office in Managua (a project developed by La Asociacion de Mujeres Niccaraguense—Association of Nicaraguan Women [AMNLAE], a women's rights group), virtually all of the cases they see involve physical abuse (Stephens, 1990). According to Stephens (1990), a recent analysis of the situation concluded that "in our [Nicaraguan] society, it is so common for a man to hit his wife that it tends to be seen as a natural part of their life together" (p. 73). And a Nicaraguan proverb states "he who loves you, beats you" (p. 73). Research is currently being conducted in the areas of violence toward women, with the establishment of referral and treatment services as part of the research (Wessel, 1991).

SUMMARY

The change from the hierarchical, hospital-focused, centralized health care system of the 1940s to 1970s to a primary health care–

oriented system resulted in great improvements in the status of health for women and children during the 1970s and 1980s, despite civil war and political upheavals. Nicaragua has, in the last 30 years, increased access to health care from 40% to almost 80% in rural areas and 90% in urban areas (UNICEF, 1995). In studies of life expectancy and mortality rates, researchers have found that increases in access to and development of primary and secondary health services has led to the largest declines in morbidity and mortality rates in Latin America (Sandiford et al., 1991; Bahr & Wehrman, 1993).

However, women in Nicaragua continue to be at risk of death from pregnancy and childbirth. As providers for their families, they are often forced to take lower-paying jobs in urban settings or agricultural production, which may increase their exposure to environmental toxins (Lane, 1995; PAHO, 1998a), may interrupt breast-feeding, and may not provide enough money to feed themselves or their families adequately. Access to sanitation, clean water, and basic health care is especially difficult for rural people and the urban poor. As Nicaragua continues in its socioeconomic development, women become more at risk for cancers, heart disease, diabetes, and other chronic conditions of the "first world" that may be exacerbated by pregnancy and childbirth. Trying desperately to meet basic physiological health needs makes attention to mental health, violence, and women's rights a luxury the health care system of Nicaragua cannot always afford.

REFERENCES

Bahr, J., & Wehrman, R. (1993). Life expectancyand infant mortality in Latin America. *Social Science Medicine, 36*(10), 1373–1382.

Banco Central de Nicaragua. (1993). Informe annual [annual report]. Managua, Nicaragua: Author.

Castro, I., Bergerton, M., & Chaberland, S. (1993, November/December). Multiresistant strains of *N. gonorrhoae* in Nicaragua. *Sexually Transmitted Diseases,* 314–419.

Danel, I., Graham, W., Stupp, P., & Castillo, P. (1996). Applying the sisterhood method for estimating maternal mortality to a health facility-based sample: A comparison with results from a household-based sample. *International Journal of Epidemiology, 25,* 1017–1022.

Egger, M., Ferrie, J., Gorter, A., Gonzalez, S., Guiterrez, R., Pauw, J., & Smith, G. (1993). HIV/AIDS-related knowledge, attitudes, and practices among Managuan secondary school students. *Bulletin of the Pan American Health Organization, 27,* 360–369.

Garfield, R., Low, N., & Caldera, J. (1993). Desocializing health care in a developing country. *Journal of the American Medical Association, 270*(8), 989–993.

Garfield, R., & Williams, G. (1992). *Health care in Nicaragua: Primary care under changing regimes.* New York: Oxford University Press.

Lane, P. (1995). Economic hardship has put Nicaragua's health care system on the sick list. *Canadian Medical Association Journal, 152,* 580–582.

Leininger, M. (1992). Self-care ideology and cultural incongruities: Some critical issues. *Journal of Transcultural Nursing, 4*(1), 2–4.

Low, N., Egger, M., Gorter, A., Sandiford, P., Gonzalez, A., Pauw, J., Ferrie, J., & Smith, G.D. (1993). AIDS in Nicaragua: Epidemiological, political, and sociocultural perspectives. *International Journal of Health Care, 23*(4), 685–702.

Lykes, M., Brabeck, M., Ferns, T., & Radan, A. (1993). Human rights and mental health among Latin American women in situations of state-sponsored violence. *Psychology of Women Quarterly, 17*(4), 525–544.

Mauldin, W. (1994). Maternal mortality in developing countries: A comparison of rates from two international compendia. *Population and Development Review, 20*(2), 413–421.

Ministerio de Salud. (1991). Health Master Plan 1991–1996, Executive Summary. Managua, Nicaragua: Author.

Ministerio de Salud. (1994). Boletin Epidemiologico. [Epidemiology Bulletin]. Managua, Nicaragua: Author.

Ministerio de Salud, Bureau of Nutrition. (1996). Informe de Evaluacion Initiativa Hospitales Amigos de la Ninez y la Madre. [Evaluation of Baby Friendly Hospital Initiatives]. Managua, Nicaragua: Author.

Molyneux, M. (1988, Spring). Abortion; The International Agenda. *Feminist Review, 29,* 23–132.

Organizacion Panamericana do la Salud and Organizacion Mundial de la Salud (1996). Datos Basicos Nicaragua (on-line). Available: ops.org.ni

Otis. (1992).

Pan American Health Organization. (1994). *Health conditions in the Americas* (1994 ed.). Washington, DC: Author.

Pan American Health Organization. (1998a). *Health in the Americas* (Vol. 1). Washington DC: Author.

Pan American Health Organization (1998b). Infectious diseases posing greatest epidemiological risk following Hurricane Mitch in Central America [on-line]. Available: HYPERLINK http://www.paho.org/english/ped/pedep07.htm. http://www.paho.org/english/ped/pedep07.htm.

Pascoe, M., & Stein, A. (1987). Midwifery work exchange project in Nicaragua. *Journal of Nurse Midwifery, 32,* 101–104.

Pathfinder International. (1994). America Latina, Pioneros de la planificacion familiar [Latin America, pioneers in family planning]. Waterton, MA: Author.

Picado, J. (1994). Breast feeding duration in low-income urban neighborhoods of Managua, Nicaragua. Unpublished Master's Thesis, Cornell University.

Profamilia. (1993). Encuesta sobre salud familiar Nicaragua 1992–93 [Survey of family health 1992–93 Nicaragua]. Managua, Nicaragua: Author.

Reynolds, H. (1999). Preconception care: An integral part of primary care for women. *Journal of Nurse Midwifery, 43,* 445–458.

Ruzek, S.B., Olesen, V.L., & Clarke, A.E. (1997). *Women's health: Complexities and differences.* Columbus, OH: Ohio State University Press.

Sales, P. (1993). Primary health care in Nicaragua five years later. *Social Science Medicine, 37*(12), 1585–1586.

Sandiford, P., Morales, P., Gorter, A., Coyle, E., & Smith, G. (1991). Why do child mortality rates fall? An analysis of the Nicaraguan experience. *American Journal of Public Health, 81,* 30–37.

Seipel, M. (1992). Promoting maternal health in developing countries. *Health and Social Work, 17,* 200–206.

Siegel, G., Bonilla, G., Pao, R., Villatoro, E., Forsythe, S., Gaillard, E., & Calderon, R. (1996). The epidemiological, social, and economic impact of HIV/AIDS in three Central American countries: A country specific and regional analysis. *International Conference on AIDS, 11*(2), 49.

Stephens, B. (1990). A developing legal system grapples with an ancient problem: Rape in Nicaragua. *Women's Rights Law Reporter, 12*(2), 69–88.

UNICEF. (1994). Codigo International de Comercializacion de Sucedaneos de la Leche materna y su Application en Nicaragua. [International Code of Commercialization of Breastfeeding Supplements and its Application in Nicaragua]. Managua, Nicaragua: Author.

UNICEF. (1995). *The state of the world's children.* London: Oxford University Press.

United Nations Economic Commission for Latin America and the Caribbean. (1990). The water resources of Latin America and the Caribbean—Planning, hazards, and pollution. Santiago, Chile: Author.

U.S. Department of State. (1998). Background notes: Nicaragua, March 1998.Washington, DC: Author.

Wellstart International. (1995). Lactancia materna en Nicaragua: Diagnostico de practicas y promocion. Washington, DC: Author.

Wessel, L. (1991). Reproductive rights in Nicaragua: From the Sandinistas to the government of Violeta Chamorro. *Feminist Studies, 17,* 537–549.

Wessel, L., & Campbell, J. (1997). Providing sanctuary for battered women: Nicaragua's casas de la mujer. *Issues in Mental Health Nursing, 18,* 455–476.

Wirpsa, L. (1995, May 26). Poor seek way out of Nicaraguan crisis. *National Catholic Reporter,* 7–8.

World Health Organization. (1996). Research on the menopause in the 1990s. (WHO Technical Report Series 866). Geneva, Switzerland: Author.

York, R., Williams, P., & Munro, B. (1993). Maternal factors that influence inadequate prenatal care. *Public Health Nursing, 10,* 241–244.

Zelaya, E., Pena, R., Garcia, J., Berglund, S., Persson, L., & Liljestrand, J. (1996). Contraceptive patterns among women and men in Leon, Nicaragua. *Contraception, 54,* 359–365.

Zelaya, E., Flor, M., Garcia, J., Berglund, S., Liljestrand, J., & Persson, L. (1997). Gender and social differences in adolescent sexuality and reproduction in Nicaragua. *Journal of Adolescent Health, 21*(1), 36–46.

SUGGESTED READINGS

Morgan, L. (1989). The importance of the state in primary health care initiatives. *Medical Anthropology Quarterly, 3,* 227–231.

Purath, J. (1994, July). Health care for Hispanic clients. *Nurse Practitioner,19*(7),71.

CHAPTER 20

Quilting as an Exemplar of Art Therapy

Ellen Olshansky
(from an interview with *Tina Brewer*)

Though effective in helping patients deal with chronic physical pain, art finds a wider application in the treatment of emotional pain.

—Loecher & O'Donnell, 1997, p. 57

One way of assisting women in achieving wellness is through the use of art as therapy. Art therapy represents a particular holistic health approach that uses creativity to enhance health and, in particular, a sense of psychological well-being. Art therapy exists in many forms, including painting, sculpting, and sketching, to name a few. This chapter presents an example of one form of art therapy, that of quilting, which focuses on promoting women's wellness. The format of this chapter is different from that of the previous chapters in the book because it is more similar to a journalistic report of an interview rather than a review of current research. This chapter is based on an interview with Tina Brewer, an African American woman who has made numerous beautiful quilts and has organized groups of women quilters. She is known nationally for her quilting and is often asked to speak to groups about her quilts. In addition to being an extremely talented artist, Brewer is also a contributor to the health of women through her quilting and through her quilting groups. I met her at a presentation she did for a women's group and I was impressed with her artistic abilities, her creativity, and her sensitivity to women's issues. Of particular interest was her description of how quilting can serve a therapeutic function for women in assisting them to achieve a significant level of wellness. This chapter focuses on the health benefits to women, as described by Brewer, from quilting and, in particular, quilting among a group of women. In this respect, the "therapy" involves not only the actual artwork itself, but also the interaction among the women in the group based on doing the artwork. I asked Brewer if she would consent to being interviewed for this book chapter and she graciously agreed. She invited me to the restaurant that she and her husband own in Pittsburgh. Upon entering the restaurant, one of the first things I noticed was that several of her quilts were hanging on the walls of the restaurant, adding a warmth to the environment. The following is an account of the conversation I had with Brewer.

Brewer described both the process of actually doing the quilting and the process of "coming together," as women from diverse backgrounds were able to share ideas and feelings together in a group where the commonality was involvement in quilting or a project related to quilting. She spoke of "getting rid of the pecking order" in that all the women were valued based on their contributions to the group rather than on their social class, status, or titles within the larger society. Interestingly, some of the women didn't even always quilt. Some darned socks or simply came to join in discussion. The quilting, then, served as the catalyst for bringing the women together, whether or not they actually engaged in quilting and regardless of who they were in the larger society. Brewer's expertise in quilting attracted other women to the group, often in the hopes of learning to quilt, but the more important aspect was that the group served as a "safe haven" for the women to engage in conversation with one another within a context of egalitarianism. For Brewer, herself, quilting provided her with space and time for her own thoughts, as the rest of her life was constantly busy with other obligations. For women as a group, Brewer spoke of celebrating these women who are passionate about life.

Brewer noted that, "Quilting is a way of breaking down barriers, of encouraging friendships and peer relationships." She described the diversity of the various quilting groups that she had organized. Each group was racially and ethnically diverse, socioeconomically diverse, and academically diverse. The focus within the groups was much less on the individual separate identities that each individual woman brought with her to the group, but instead on how the women felt within the group and on the common issues of concern to women. At the beginning of each group, the women were encouraged to talk about why they chose to attend the group, focusing on group cohesion and how the women, together within the group, could attend to the needs of individuals. Brewer emphasized the importance and the strength of encouraging diversity within the group. Clearly the relationships that formed among the women within the groups were key in serving as a way of promoting health, in the form of increased sense of self within relationships. The therapeutic aspect of the quilting group was evident in the positive effect it had on the self-esteem of the individual women. While this concept was not actually "tested" out through systematic research, the feelings and reactions of the women within the group give credence to such a hypothesis that would be quite worthwhile to test systematically.

Of particular interest was Brewer's comment on how quilting has helped her in dealing with issues of social injustice, and, in particular, racism. She described how, for her, the process of quilting allowed her to gain a better understanding and insight into the injustice of slavery and, ultimately, to achieve a sense of forgiveness and ability to move on in her life. She described her experiences in seeing racism within society and not understanding it, and, especially, not knowing what to do or how to move on beyond the anger associated with racism. The fact that quilting is a very slow process facilitates the ability eventually to understand complex issues that do not appear to have any rational basis of understanding. Some of her quilts represent African Americans experiences of slavery. While slavery, indeed, is not something to be condoned, Brewer described how she needed and wanted to move beyond the injustice of slavery so that she could focus on positive aspects of her life. She does not presume to be able to explain slavery, as any explanation for slavery should elude us all, but she can move on in her life in positive ways.

By quilting in groups, women who join such groups are given an opportunity for a designated time in which the women can relate to and communicate with one another. The Wednesday night quilting group provided such an opportunity. Women were able to talk about issues of concern to them, receive validation for many of their concerns, and give validation and encouragement to others in the group. Another important aspect of the group is that it serves as a coming together of a diverse gathering of women, from various cultural and socioeconomic backgrounds as well as from various interests and quilting ability. Brewer even described how the women often incorporated the work of one another as they continued constructing their own quilts.

The process of quilting as an art form reflects the complexity of society as well as of one's life. Brewer described the layers of quilting that are done, as the quilter sews on pieces of fabric, which symbolize particular aspects of one's life or of the society in which we live. These layers, overlapping with one another, reveal such complexity. The layers also represent the quilter's ongoing development and construction of ideas throughout the quilting process. By becoming involved in understanding the meanings of each of these layers, a woman is encouraged to understand the complexity of life, both of her own and of others significant to her. In many ways the women are able to construct new meanings for aspects of their lives and to come to terms with some of the difficult and painful aspects of their lives. Ms. Brewer noted that not everyone has to see the meanings in the same way and, in fact, some people may simply see quilts as an art form without any particular meaning. The important point is that for those women who are able to construct meaning through their quilts, a certain kind of therapy or coming to terms with particular issues can occur.

In another chapter of this book the benefits of storytelling are described, particularly as related to women of African descent. Brewer, in her description of quilting as a form of therapy, also emphasized the importance of storytelling and how storytelling is achieved through quilting. She also noted that within African culture there is a strong oral tradition in which storytelling plays a central and key role. Each community has a storyteller to pass along cultural traditions. The quilts themselves often tell a story, with much symbolism used within the quilts. The process of quilting allows a person to engage in the story and to tell the story through art as a medium. The fact that quilting is often done in groups provides another medium for storytelling. The context of the group is a place for a woman to tell her story and to hear the stories of others.

It was a privilege and honor to talk with Tina Brewer about the quilting that she does, as well as the women's quilting groups she organizes. Her energy and enthusiasm for her work were immediately apparent. Her work and her approach to her work most definitely contribute to a greater understanding of how art can have therapeutic value in promoting women's wellness.

REFERENCE

Loecher, B., & O'Donnell, S.A. (1997). In S. Faelten (Ed.), *New choices in natural healing for women: Drug-free remedies from the world of alternative medicine.* Emmaus, PA: Rodale Press, Inc.

CHAPTER 21

Storytelling as a Tool for Providing Holistic Care to Women

Joanne Banks-Wallace

The importance of storytelling to cultures is recognized throughout the world; the therapeutic benefits of storytelling were first noted in the nursing literature more than 60 years ago (Bacon, 1933; Howard, 1991). In recent years, there has been a renewed interest in storytelling as a tool for educating students (Irvin, 1996), as a therapeutic intervention (Wenckus, 1994), and as a means of strengthening staff-client relationships (Mayers, 1995). The purpose of this article is to discuss storytelling as a tool for assisting nurses in providing holistic care to women.

FUNCTION OF STORIES AND STORYTELLING

Stories are ubiquitous in our lives, filling our cultural and social environments (Polkinghorne, 1988). A story may be defined as the depiction of an event or series of events encompassed by temporal or spatial

Joanne Banks-Wallace is an Assistant Professor at The University of Missouri, Sinclair School of Nursing, Columbia, Missouri.
Source: Reprinted with permission from J. Banks-Wallace, Storytelling as a Tool for Providing Holistic Health Care to Women, *MCN: The American Journal of Maternal/Child Nursing,* Vol. 24, No. 1, pp. 20–24, © 1999, Lippincott Williams & Wilkins.

boundaries. Stories provide cohesion to shared beliefs and transmit values at a cultural level. Stories also provide a means of preserving the common characteristics of a culture and passing them on to subsequent generations. As conveyors of cultural values, stories provide guidelines to help people cope with milestones or transitions and assist people in finding their way in the world. In addition to culture-specific values and concerns, stories articulate the more universal yearnings or struggles of humans. In this capacity, they help us answer more existential questions about the meaning of life in general and of our lives in particular (Gates, 1989; Livo & Rietz, 1986).

Creating stories provides a means of thinking about our lives. The process of structuring experiences into stories is known as "story-ing" (Livo & Rietz, 1986; Robinson & Hawpe, 1986). Story-ing helps us to make sense out of our behavior and the behavior of others. The narrative scheme serves as a lens that brings elements previously viewed as disconnected and independent into focus as parts of a unified collage. Explanations of why one behaves in a certain manner focus on the events in an individual's life history that have had an influence on a particular action, including the future goals that a particular action is projected to achieve or affect (Polkinghorne, 1988). This assists us in analyzing who we are and where we are going. Storytelling allows us to share stories and our thoughts about them with others.

Storytelling is an age-old tradition that continues to serve many functions in the world today. It is the process of sharing stories with others using an oral medium or sign language. Storytelling was a very important method of transferring information within a society prior to the establishment of written records (Livo & Rietz, 1986). The significance of this function diminished considerably following the advent of mass media, but recently, there has been a resurgence of interest in storytelling within the United States. The storytelling process and the stories themselves provide insight into various cultures and offer a means of passing on important aspects of a culture from one generation to the next (Gates, 1989).

Storytelling provides a means of expressing our hopes, fears, and dreams (Klingler, 1997). Baker and Greene (1987) state that the primary purpose of storytelling is to nurture the spirit-self. They view storytelling as a "sharing experience" which requires a willingness to be vulnerable and express our deepest feelings. The process of storytelling establishes a common experience between the teller and listener, or "storytaker," creating a connection between them.

CULTURAL SIGNIFICANCE OF STORIES AND STORYTELLING

Story development and storytelling are both done within particular cultural contexts (Livo & Rietz, 1986; Mishler, 1986). All cultures maintain language systems and pass on to subsequent generations knowledge of the connections between signifying sounds and the things that they signify. Individual cultures also maintain collections of typical narrative meanings in their myths, histories, folklore, and fairy tales. Storytelling is used in this capacity to share or validate cultural values and customs. Thus, it provides a context in which to examine and express life experiences. Understanding the full range of accumulated meanings is essential for members of a particular culture and others desiring to interact competently within a given culture (Howard, 1991; Polkinghorne, 1988).

In the introduction to *Talk That Talk: An Anthology of African American Storytelling,* Gates (1989) underscores the cultural significance of storytelling:

> Telling ourselves our own stories—interpreting the nature of our world to ourselves, asking and answering epistemological and ontological questions in our own voices and on our own terms—has as much as any single factor been responsible for the survival of African Americans and their culture. The stories that we tell ourselves and our children function to order our world, serving to create both a foundation upon which each of us constructs our reality and a filter through which we process each event that confronts us every day. The values that we cherish and wish to preserve, the behavior that we wish to censure, the fears and dread that we can barely confess in ordinary language, the aspirations and goals that we most dearly prize—All of these things are encoded in the stories that each culture invents and preserves for the next generations, stories that, in effect, we live by and through. And, the stories that survive, the stories that manage to resurface under different guises and with marvelous variations, these are a culture's canonical tales, the tales that contain the cultural codes that are assumed or internalized by members of that culture.

The author is most familiar with African American traditions of storytelling. There is substantial evidence, however, that storytelling serves similar roles among many cultural groups, including Native Americans (Sarris, 1993), lesbians/gays (Zurlinden, 1997), and women (Berry & Traeder, 1995).

The significant role that storytelling among women plays in the re-definition of womanhood and development of self-identity has been noted by feminist scholars. Berry and Traeder (1995) argue that naming and articulating our experiences through storytelling is a critical aspect of regaining a sense of self-worth as women. Cannon (1988) posits that storytelling has been an especially important vehicle for women of African descent to cultivate their history and carve out a space in the midst of an environment that is racist, sexist, and classist.

CULTURAL INFLUENCES ON STORY-ING AND STORYTELLING

The process of structuring experiences into a story is governed by culturally specific rules that influence what information about an experience will be represented and how it is stored in memory (Livo & Rietz, 1986). The conventional ways of relating a series of events, or telling a story, are known as "story grammars." They are the framework that allows us to link characters, motives, plots, and resolutions into an "intelligible" story. Listeners, or "storytakers" (Robinson & Hawpe, 1986) expect storytellers to observe these conventions. Likewise, storytellers expect storytakers to know these conventions. Smith (1978) argues that the manner in which information is bound together determines whether or not it will be considered a coherent story within a particular cultural context.

The culturally appropriate rules for story-ing and "storytaking" are not formally taught. Instead, the memory structures used to recognize and store stories are developed as a result of repeated exposure to oral stories (Heath, 1982). Knowing the appropriate ways that stories are told within a particular culture is an important aspect of being able to comprehend the meaning of a specific story. Studies by Heath (1982) and Gee (1985) indicated that racial and economic class differences among school children were accompanied by variations in story-ing and storytelling. The degree to which children's ways of developing and sharing stories matched the dominant methods within the school system greatly influenced the ease with which children adapted and blossomed within the school environment. Gee (1985) concluded that academic settings make it more difficult for certain children to get the assistance that they need to do well by labeling some storytelling methods as more desirable and others as deficient. Situations like this have led some scholars to suggest that analysis of stories needs to include an interpretation of how the stories reflect and express broader cultural frameworks (Mishler, 1986; Sarris, 1993). They also demonstrate the need for practitioners to develop multilingual skills with respect to story creation, storytelling, and listening.

STORYTELLING IN CLINICAL PRACTICE AND RESEARCH

Storytelling is gaining ground as a tool for both clinical practice and research. Theoretical papers and anecdotal discussions comprise the bulk of support regarding the therapeutic potential of storytelling. These sources have provided evidence that creating, telling, or listening to stories may be valuable as a means of helping children (Hahn, 1987) and adults (Larkin & Zahourek, 1988) develop skills or serve as a relaxation or diversion technique for hospitalized clients (Bacon, 1933).

Clinical and research evidence supporting the value of storytelling is small but promising. Moody and Laurent (1984) used folk tales and storytelling as a tool for improving the health of Seminole Indians with diabetes. They designed their project in conjunction with an advisory panel composed of members of the Seminole nation. The long-term outcomes have not yet been reported in the literature.

Rogler, Malgady, Costantino, and Blumenthal (1987) examined the therapeutic use of folk tales or "Cuento." They used traditional and revised folk tales to help second-generation Puerto Rican children work through mental health issues. A significant reduction in trait anxiety was noted after children participated in the folk tale therapy. Unfortunately, the interventions were designed so that the clinician-researchers rather than the children made the decisions regarding how and when traditional folk takes would be altered. This pattern is also common when storytelling has been used as a therapeutic tool in clinical practice. Drawing upon Richard Garner's mutual storytelling technique, clinicians are assigned the task of determining whether a story could be changed to allow for the possibility of other options. If the clinician decides that a story should be changed to reflect more positive possibilities, he or she assumes the majority of the responsibility for constructing the new version of the story (Larkin & Zahourek, 1988). Other clinicians have identified what they call "archetypical" stories. These "universal" stories are thought to serve as a means for identifying and working through the existential crises common to mankind (Chinen, 1989). Mutual storytelling and universal stories are useful tools for assisting people to live healthier lives; however, as commonly used, they continue to leave the power and control for healing or maintaining health within the hands of the practitioner rather than the client. A notable exception is Hahn (1987), who promotes therapeutic storytelling that expects clients to retain maximum control of the story. Maintaining control over one's stories is particularly important for people belonging to groups whose health is negatively influenced by institutionalized oppression. The author's study on the function of storytelling among women of African descent (Banks-Wallace, 1998) further supports the importance of people maintaining control over their stories. It also provides evidence of the therapeutic potential of storytelling in the context of research.

Newbern's (1992) analysis of stories taken from a larger study of self-care practices among elderly Southerners corroborates the therapeutic potential of storytelling in conjunction with research. She found that storytelling and reminiscence provided richer insight into the lives of people than traditional interviews or patient histories. They provided a means of understanding relationships between specific events, values, and choices made over a period of time. In addition, stories served as a vehicle for understanding the problems of a particular group. Newbern (1992) noted that telling one's own stories resulted in a sense of accomplishment for the elderly. They realized that they could pass on to future generations their knowledge and experience through their stories. Finally, reminiscence provided opportunities for people to construct meaningful stories about their lives, recreating themselves in the process.

Clinical Implications

Storytelling may serve many useful purposes in clinical practice. Some of these are (1) as an aid in designing appropriate plans of care, (2) as a tool for enhancing client-practitioner communication, and (3) as a vehicle for staff development.

Storytelling as an Aid in Designing a Plan of Care

Storytelling provides an opportunity for the practitioner to more fully understand the context in which a woman is making decisions about her health. The author calls this "contextual grounding." This refers to the use of stories as a means of clarifying one's understanding of the world and his or her place within it (Banks-Wallace, 1998). It is influenced by the historic and contemporary experiences of individuals and the social-political-cultural groups to which they belong. Contextual grounding, in turn, affects how people view themselves and others as well as the choices they make of the way they respond to a given situation.

As a doctoral student, I wrote a story entitled "Silenced Induced Illness," which chronicles my experiences related to having an abortion as a teenager. The purpose of writing the story was to examine how social-cultural and familial values influenced the decision to have an abortion and the process of healing. In particular, the story sought to illustrate how historic and contemporary factors affecting African American families had an impact on the responses of a particular family in relation to an unplanned teenage pregnancy.

The story has been shared numerous times with young college students who have come forward, desperately seeking a means of dealing with their decision to have an abortion. The majority of these students have been women of color or women from families in lower social-economic groups. Many of them were the first generation to go to college in their family. These women all expressed conflicts between ending a potential life and disappointing their family. Each woman talked about the sacrifices that had been made to get her to college as well as the importance of her graduation and success for her family. The weight of this responsibility is often not understood by health care providers.

Having clients share stories about their lives in general and the meaning of a particular health issue within their overall life may greatly enhance the ability of practitioners to develop appropriate plans of care. Standardized treatment protocols provide guidance based on presenting symptoms or diagnostic criteria; however, they do not provide a means of integrating interventions into the larger context of clients' lives. Storytelling may serve as a bridge, allowing practitioners to plan care that takes into full account a client's resources, barriers, and competing concerns.

Storytelling can precede the initial history and physical examination or can be incorporated into these tasks. For example, the practitioner can begin a visit with a new client by asking her to share information about her daily life, pressing concerns outside of the health issue, or goals that she is currently working toward. This will provide insight into the amount of energy or resources that are available for dealing with a particular health concern. During the physical examination, the practitioner can encourage the woman to talk about previous findings during examinations and her thoughts about how practitioner visits fit into her overall health regime. The stories a client shares can provide valuable information regarding her understanding of her body and ability to care for herself. The stories shared early in the visit coupled with stories told during the physical examination will provide the practitioner with a more thorough set of information from which a plan of care can be developed.

Enhancing Client-Practitioner Communication Through Storytelling

Storytelling can be used to improve communication between clients and practitioners. Two importance uses of storytelling are for sharing philosophic frameworks guiding care and for teaching clients how to care for themselves.

Practitioners often overlook the importance of sharing their philosophic framework with clients. As a result, they miss an opportunity to create a sense of connection or community. Two stories shared by a former nursing instructor illustrate the importance of sharing one's framework. The first story concerned her experiences regarding trying to make a decision about whether to proceed with a pregnancy after learning that the fetus she carried was severely deformed. The second story was about making the decision to leave an Eastern European country rather than continuing to risk religious persecution. Both of these stories highlighted her struggles to reconcile the needs/desires of her family with fundamental beliefs and values of her spiritual faith. Through sharing her stories, this instructor created a space for the students to know her as a human being and established a foundation for examining health issues within the social-political-spiritual context of people's lives. Storytelling in a clinical situation can serve a similar function of assisting clients in seeing practitioners as humans bound by particular traditions.

Storytelling can also be a tool for empowering women to be more active participants with respect to their health. The creation and sharing of stories provides an opportunity for a female client to select which aspects of experiences related to a health issue she wishes to emphasize (Mishler, 1986). This may help create a space for a more egalitarian collaborative client-practitioner relationship. The woman brings expertise about her life and investment in her own health into the partnership. The practitioner contributes clinical expertise and knowledge gained through personal experience. The knowledge that each has to offer is shared through mutual storytelling.

Storytelling can be a powerful tool for educating clients. Listening to clients' stories provides insights into the natural language that they use to describe and think about health issues. The stories also provide information about gaps in their understanding. Practitioners can use this information to create stories that convey essential information in a way that clients can understand and more readily remember. Finally, evaluation of client knowledge and incorporation of practices into a client's daily life can also be done through storytelling sessions at subsequent visits.

The use of storytelling as an educational tool can be expanded to include interaction among clients within a clinical setting. This can be done by setting aside a room within a clinic where clients can gather to share their experiences related to a particular health issue for which they are seeing the practitioner, such as breast cancer or the transition to motherhood.

Byllye Avery (1994), the founder of the National Black Women's Health Project, was one of the cofounders of Birthplace, an alternative birthing center located in Gainesville, Florida. She illustrates the potential therapeutic significance of facilitating storytelling among women in clinical settings:

> Through the work of Birthplace, we have created a prenatal caring program that provides each woman who comes for care with a support group. She enters the group when she arrives, leaves the group to go for her physical checkup, and then returns to the group when she is finished. She doesn't sit in a waiting room for two hours. Most of these women have no one to talk to. No one listens to them; no one helps them plan. They're asking: "who's going to get me to the hospital if I go into labor in the middle of the night, or the middle of the day, for that matter? Who's going to help me get out of this abusive relationship? Who's going to make sure I have the food I need to eat?" . . . We have to do what's necessary to survive. It's just a part of living. But most of us are empty wells that never get replenished. Most of us are dead inside. We are walking around dead.

Group storytelling in a clinical setting can provide support and education for clients. Listening to women in similar situations talk about how they chose to deal with a particular event provides opportunities to gain knowledge through others' experiences. This increases a woman's insight regarding the range of coping strategies available for dealing with a given issue. It may also create a sense of community for women who are feeling isolated or alone in their daily life. The creation and maintenance of places for women to share stories during office visits does not require a major investment in time or resources. The therapeutic and educational potential of storytelling groups in clinical settings warrants further consideration by women's health practitioners.

Storytelling and Staff Development

The changing demographics within our society makes it imperative that all providers develop competence in working with clientele of diverse cultural backgrounds. Folk tales and literary stories can be invaluable tools for assisting practitioners in recognizing the influence of socially constructed norms within cultural groups.

I have used "The Three Pigs" as a tool for helping nurses and students to understand how cultural values shape our perception of people and events. This is done by having participants first discuss the values and claims presented in the dominant version of this story. I then tell the story from the perspective of the wolf as told in "The True Story of the Three Little Pigs" (Scieska, 1989). Afterwards, we discuss insights gained from listening to the wolf's version of the story and the importance of understanding the perspectives of a client or population group. Participants also discuss barriers to gaining these perspectives and brainstorm solutions to overcoming these barriers.

Folk tales, literary tales, and local myths can be incorporated periodically into staff meetings. This will provide a nonthreatening means of raising consciousness about assumptions, values, or norms and their effects on client-provider interactions. In addition, storytelling can serve as a means of processing clinical experiences and evaluating the efficacy of a given care regimen for a particular population. Finally, storytelling can be used to enhance staff-clinician relationships. It may be especially valuable for helping resolve conflicts within and among groups of employees.

CONCLUSIONS

Storytelling can be an invaluable tool for planning and providing holistic care for women and may assist nurses in obtaining information that will enhance the development of an appropriate plan of care for clients. Storytelling also provides insight into language that can facilitate enhanced communication and more egalitarian client-practitioner partnerships. Group storytelling in clinical settings can provide opportunities for clients to benefit from the knowledge and experience of other clients. It may also facilitate the development of support networks among clients. Finally, storytelling can be used to promote professional growth among staff and clinicians.

REFERENCES

Avery, B. (1994). Breathing life into ourselves: The evolution of the National Black Women's Health Project. In E. White (Ed.), *The black women's health book: Speaking for ourselves* (rev. ed.) (pp. 4–10). Seattle: Seal Press.

Bacon, F. (1933). Getting well with books. *American Journal of Nursing, 33*(11), 1143–1146.

Baker, A., & Greene, E. (1987). *Storytelling: Art and technique* (2nd ed.). New York: R. R. Bowker.

Banks-Wallace, J. (1998). Emancipatory potential of storytelling in a group. *Image: Journal of Nursing Scholarship, 30*(1), 17–21.

Berry, C., & Traeder, T. (1995). *Girlfriends: Invisible bond, enduring ties.* Berkeley: Wildcat Canyon Press.

Cannon, K. (1988). *Black womanist ethics.* American Academy of Religion Academy Series 60. Atlanta: Scholars Press.

Chinen, A. (1989). *In the ever after: Fairy tales and the second half of life.* Wilmette, IL: Chiron Publications.

Gates, H. (1989). Introduction: Narration and cultural memory in the African American tradition. In L. Goss & M. Barnes (Eds.), *Talk that talk: An anthology of African American storytelling* (pp. 15–19). New York: Simon & Schuster.

Gee, J. (1985). The narrativization of experience in the oral style. *Journal of Education, 167*(1), 9–31.

Hahn, K. (1987). Therapeutic storytelling: Helping children learn and cope. *Pediatric Nursing, 13*(3), 175–178.

Heath, S. (1982). What no bedtime story means: Narrative skills at home and school. *Language in Society, 11,* 49–76.

Howard, G. (1991). Culture tales: A narrative approach to thinking, cross-cultural psychology, and psychotherapy. *American Psychologist, 46*(3), 187–197.

Irvin, S. (1996). Creative teaching strategies. *Journal of Continuing Education in Nursing, 27*(3), 108–114.

Klingler, A. (1997). The storyteller in heathcare settings. *Storytelling Magazine, 9*(4), 21–23.

Larkin, D., & Zahourek, R. (1988). Therapeutic storytelling and metaphors. *Holistic Nursing Practice, 2*(3), 45–53.

Livo, N., & Rietz, S. (1986). *Storytelling: Process and practice.* Littleton, CO: Libraries Unlimited.

Mayers, K. (1995). Storytelling: A method to increase discussion, familiar rapport with residents and share knowledge among long term care staff. *Journal of Continuing Education in Nursing, 26*(6), 280–282.

Mishler, E. (1986). *Research interviewing: Context and narrative.* Cambridge, MA: Harvard Press.

Moody, L., & Laurent, M. (1984). Promoting health through the use of storytelling. *Health Education, 15*(1), 8–10.

Newbern, V. (1992). Sharing the memories: The value of reminiscence as a research tool. *Journal of Gerontological Nursing, 18*(5), 13–18.

Polkinghorne, D. (1988). *Narrative knowing and the human sciences.* New York: State University of New York.

Robinson, J., & Hawpe, L. (1986). Narrative thinking and the heuristic process. In T. Sarbin (Ed.), *Narrative psychology: The storied nature of human conduct* (pp. 111–125). New York: Praeger Publishers.

Rogler, L., Malgady, R., Costantino, G., & Blumenthal, R. (1987). What do culturally sensitive mental health services mean? The case of Hispanics. *American Psychologist, 42*(6), 565–570.

Sarris, G. (1993). *Keeping Slug Woman alive: A holistic approach to American Indian texts.* Berkeley: University of California Press.

Scieska, J. (1989). *The true story of the three little pigs.* New York: Viking.

Smith, F. (1978). *Understanding reading: A psycholinguistic analysis of reading and learning to read.* New York: Holt, Rinehart, and Winston.

Wenckus, E. (1994). Storytelling: Using an ancient art to work with groups. *Journal of Psychosocial Nursing and Mental Health Services, 32*(7), 30–32.

Zurlinden, J. (1997). *Lesbian and gay nurses.* Albany, NY: Delmar.

CHAPTER 22

A Woman's Reflections on Moving Toward Wellness After a Stroke

Gerri Adreon

Creating health requires making a paradigm shift, or systems shift, to a new way of thinking about and being in relationship with our bodies, our minds, our spirits, and our connection with the universe. Very few people maintain or regain health and wholeness until they make this shift.

—Northrup, 1998, pp. 577–578

"I never want to see you again." When a woman hears these words from a man, a man she respects and admires, it is usually cause for sadness and tears. However, when my neurologist said this to me 3 years to the day after my stroke, it was music to my ears. So far, *his wish has come true*; I have not had to see this doctor since May 1997, and I hope to live to old age without ever needing his services again. I feel that perhaps my story may convince others not to wait for that wake-up call to change one's lifestyle, for it may be too late by then. I feel my story is amazing in itself, but more so because I am still here on this earth to be able to write it. Although it may be a cliche, I did truly get a second chance in life.

Before this life-threatening event happened, I never gave my health or my body a second thought. I was always a busy person, raising a son on my own, working full time, taking classes to earn a bachelor's degree at night. I enjoyed my friends, my family, my hobbies, my life. I see now that I took all of these good things for granted, especially my health. Never again! Even though I smoked (and knew I shouldn't), ate junk food and donuts (why not? my weight never varied from 110 pounds), and never exercised (too much trouble), I was rarely ill and had never been hospitalized. Every now and then a health-related article in a magazine would jump onto my radar screen from the newsstand, and I'd think, "That's a great idea. I should get my act together. I should join a health club, start swimming, jog after work," and on and on. I would say that to myself and then go along my merry way, never changing a thing.

Then, in 1994, the fates took over. God seemed to say, "I guess I'll have to scare her to death, or at least almost-to-death." I had my degree now, a stable job, had made it through the BIG 5-0 birthday, and my son had recently married a wonderful young woman. I was more secure emotionally and financially than I had ever been. I was on top of the world before my world crashed in on me. It all started very simply. I was looking out the bus window at the clear dark sky, which was filled with "billions and billions" of stars, to quote Carl Sagan. The rocking rhythm of the bus was putting me to sleep. It had been a great 3-day trip to the casinos of Atlantic City and I had even won some money, against all odds. All of a sudden, a splitting headache pierced my skull like a knife. My head pounded and I just wanted to be home in bed quickly. I did crawl into my bed that Friday night but this is where my story has a gaping hole; a black hole of nothingness for at least 24 hours. To this day I have no memory of the next day (Saturday) until I "found myself" in the emergency room (ER) of a small community hospital. The ambulance paramedics told my neighbor that I had placed the 911 call, and my neighbor informed me later that I was holding my head and screaming in pain. (I have no recollection of this at all, isn't nature wonderful?)

My actual memory of events begins again after the hospital sent me home, concluding that I had food poisoning. Heaven knows what I told the ER doctor to give her that idea; but they never did an x-ray or computed tomography (CT) scan of my head at all! The next day was Mother's Day, when I spent the entire day in bed self-diagnosed with the flu. My son was still concerned by Monday morning, and he called to see if I was feeling any better. To his amazement, I was chipper and feisty, insisting that he come home immediately to remove Bob Barker from my television set.

"What are you talking about, Mother?" he said. I replied that I hated the "Price is Right" and it would not go away. "Is the remote control broken?" he asked. "What's a remote control?" I countered. FAST FORWARD: Hospital emergency room, me on a gurney, doctors whispering to my son, me hooked up to IV tubes, beeping tones, intensive care unit (ICU), relatives one at a time with sad and frightened faces. A soft-spoken doctor, holding and patting my hand, was talking, saying to me, "I believe you had a stroke maybe 2 days ago. You have been bleeding for some time into your brain." I know he told me more, but I quit hearing, or seeing, or even comprehending where I was. A few days later, I was moved from the ICU to a regular room. Not one neu-rosurgeon or neurologist could tell me what caused this stroke be-cause, in their words, "we cannot do magnetic resonance imaging (MRI) for at least 2 months. There is so much blood on your brain that the CT scan could not allow us to see the arteries and vessels clearly. The blood will reabsorb eventually and then we will know." It was like someone telling me I was a product of Dr. Frankenstein and that his experiment went haywire. Blood was pouring into, and lying on, my brain for 2 days? How could this happen and I still be alive and men-tally functioning? Nature and the human spirit are truly amazing. The bad news was that I lost the peripheral vision in my right eye, but the doctor said it "may" return (it never did).

After 10 days, I left the hospital with a "bad attitude." I was feeling sorry for myself every day, often pacing and crying, not knowing what to do about anything. I could not drive yet, or even walk without banging into walls or light poles on my right-hand side. I felt like a horse with only one eye shield, which caused a dizzy, off-kilter feeling. In addition, I could not read or write very well and I was totally bored. My loved ones kept impressing upon me that I could have died, I should be glad I was alive. I knew all this, but I was so weak, tired, and overmedicated that I could not muster the energy to be glad about anything, let alone being alive. I was in a "life stinks, pity-party" mode. Little did I know that 1 week later I would get the lesson of my life: that things could always be worse.

FAST FORWARD AGAIN: Hospital emergency room, 105 degrees temperature, packed in ice, IV tubes once again. Then freezing and shaking with four blankets on top of me. I was like a frightened turtle, with only the tip of my nose sticking out of the blankets, trying to comprehend the clicking sound of teeth rapping against one another as being my own. This time a doctor was explaining that I had pneu-monia. Day after day my temperature would not go down, I lost 15 pounds, and my usual positive outlook was drifting away like so many storm clouds outside my hospital room window. On the sixth night of this second hospitalization a nurse arrived as usual with antibiotic se-rum, which he injected into my IV tube. Something went wrong almost immediately. A lightning bolt seemed to strike me as I went into anaphylactic shock, my throat swelling and my breathing becoming labored. My mind was in full gear as I figured out that I was literally dying. It is a strange and eerie comprehension to know that your own demise is imminent. Panic set in as I screamed, "I'm dying, I'm dying. Dear God, I'll never see my son again." In the blink of an eye, my panic was replaced with a soft whooshing sound, a bright light, and total serenity. I remember thinking that dying was not so bad, after all! This moment of peace was soon interrupted by extremely bright crash-cart lights flooding the room, as a trauma team worked on my heart, oxygen mask on my face, shouting my name over and over. I can tell you now, without giving away the ending, that I did not actually die that night. Only my old self died, while the seed of a renewed way of life was sown from which a changed human being would grow bigger and stronger in the years to come.

When I finally left the hospital for the second time, one steamy day in June 1994, I weighed 96 pounds and resembled a child's drawing of a stick person. I was awe-struck by the fact that I was still alive and that most of the world, the people, the weather, the hustle-bustle had just been going on for weeks without a thought to my particular survival. Doctors' orders were to rest, gain weight, and get my strength back. This plan sounded easy enough since I was not cleared to return to work for at least 3 months. Rest and eating came easy; the actual fight to reclaim my life and my strength was more difficult. I was so physically and mentally drained that I felt like a rag doll left out in the rain. I also felt as if I was in prison, or at least solitary confinement. Everyone else was driving here and there, going to work, having a life. I, on the other hand, was confined to my house. The heat wave of 1994 made it too oppressive to even sit outside. Friends and family became my personal chauffeurs, driving me to grocery stores, doctors' appointments, and pharmacies. No beaches or amusement parks that summer! My proud self-reliance was in shambles, and the days were spent napping, eating, and becoming addicted to Court TV (does the name O.J. Simpson sound familiar?).

The months rolled by, and I began to feel much better. I was adjusting to my loss of right-side peripheral vision, had gained weight, and started back to my job that September. Although my body was healing, my emotional self was precarious and unprepared for the work stresses and other tragedies yet unforeseen. Within a year, my beloved boss had died, a younger sister committed suicide, and one of my closest friends died of ovarian cancer at the age of 53. At this critical juncture of my own life, when I needed so much support, my sister and good friend were taken away forever. My depression grew deep. I was unable to handle the pressures of my workplace, and loneliness became a gnawing sensation in my heart. I began isolating myself from others. I felt like a rubber band, pulled tight and ready to snap. One day, I stood before the mirror looking closely at myself, and burst into tears. I declared, "You're not acting like yourself, you're a mess!" This was a turning point when I admitted my need for help from my family and friends whom I had been pushing away. I talked, I cried, I wrote daily in my private diary. Slowly my spirit began to emerge from its dormant state to begin again in a new direction: UP! But how? Where to start? What to do? The only thing I knew for sure was that I was stressed out to the maximum limits of my human capacity and was feeling quite frail. I believe that stress is the precursor to many illnesses, and that one's response to stress can eventually trigger some type of physical ailment. Stress is sneaky, like a thief in the night, quietly breaking down your immune system little by little. Stress has a cumulative effect, like a farmer whittling on a piece of wood, chipping, chipping away in silence. I have learned that you must be ever vigilant; you must know and read your own body's warning signs. Take the time to listen to your body, then take action to get back on the track to healthy living. I knew it was time to set goals and go for it. So I did exactly that.

Goal #1—Stop smoking. I realized I already had a head start on this aspect of my health program because I had not had a cigarette since my stroke, and no cravings either. The cold-turkey experience that was forced on me while in the intensive care unit was something I had been unable to accomplish for years on my own. To my surprise, it was easier to quit than I ever imagined. I often wonder if I had resolved to stop smoking years ago, would I have averted this stroke? Now I can breathe; I don't smell like a steel mill; I'm saving money; food actually tastes like something other than cardboard; employees are being forced into 20-degree weather to smoke a cigarette while I stay in my warm office; my son has stopped nagging me; and, it feels great to speak about myself as a "nonsmoker." At last!

Goals #2—Walk for one-half hour five times per week minimum. Goal #2 was less subtle. While I was sitting in the lunchroom not long after I returned to work, I became aware that most people's conversations centered around their jobs, and mostly complaints. I chomped on my Hostess Ho Ho's, nodded my head in sympathy, and threw a few complaints of my own into the mix. After the lunch hour, I felt sort of weary (after such a negative conversation, I cannot imagine why!) and walked to the building next door on an errand. Just then, a jogger with a Walkman ran by me, and a light bulb went on in my head. I can jog! Immediately common sense prevailed and I realized that jogging is not for me. However, walking was something I already knew how to do that was also good for breathing and working the heart muscle. I spend my working hours on a beautiful university campus that contains a running track and an entire football field for employees' use. It takes one-half hour to eat, then I could go on to fresh air, music in my ears, walking off the calories for 30 minutes a day. Every weekday. Sounded like a plan to me. I even invited my co-workers to walk with me, but no takers. Feeling like a lone maverick I started walking in the summer, fall, winter (inside a bubble-type dome over the field), spring. Done that, been there for 3 years. It's simple to do, it's invigorating, it breaks up the workday. I would recommend walking as a good start for anyone who does not want to put a lot of time or money into an exercise regimen. Anyone can do it; bring a friend, or go it alone. Listen to tapes: music, books, learn a new language. Erasing the mind of all thoughts and just enjoying the scenery along the walk is also a choice. That's the best part of a walking plan—there are no set rules, only whatever one's own imagination decides. After a year or two of walking during lunchtime, I even persuaded a fellow worker to join me, so I did reach at least one convert.

Some of my friends and family were astonished. They thought that I turned into a "health nut" because I quit smoking and began walking every day. This small step for womankind was not even close to being a "nut," but I sure was doing more about taking charge of my own health than ever before. At this point I was actually yearning for more to do. I read *Prevention* magazine, took notes, and was looking for another project to tackle. Aerobics videos were in all the stores, so I bought one. I even used it. However, after a few months, the aerobics guru and I were meeting in my game room less and less. Aerobics was becoming boring. Since I did not have to leave my home, I was becoming lazy and had no incentive to do the aerobics. Not only was I skipping aerobics for weeks at a time, I was beginning to hate it completely. I have learned from this mistake that exercise is a very personal thing. The premise is very simple: if you do not like to jog, you will not jog; if you do not like aerobics, you will not do aerobics. End of story.

I kept an open mind, vowing to try any and all avenues of nutrition and exercise until I found the right one(s). If I became enthusiastic and excited, then I would know I had hit the right note. The catalog of classes being offered at the community college arrived in the mail, and I turned to the index to find "Fitness and Health." A class entitled Yoga for Stress Reduction sounded just like the ticket for me. No jumping up and down to disco tunes, but a more subtle and simple approach. I wondered if the other participants were already able to put their legs behind their necks and stay that way for hours. If so, I'd be out of my league, for sure. Just stretching in my own bed as I wake up caused noise: a lot of snap, crackles, and pops from my bones. To my surprise, both men and women of every body shape imaginable were in the class, and I was more flexible than some and less flexible than others. I liked being in this middle-average range because then I would be learning something new with every lesson, and I could only become better and better. As this new adventure progressed, I soon discovered that yoga is not an exercise, it is a way of life. My instructor was vigorous, joyful, and an afficionado on this subject. Her enthusiasm was contagious and her embrace of the yoga philosophy was intriguing. Soon I was breathing, stretching, and meditating like a pro, and feeling completely at ease with the process. Currently, I do yoga every morning for 20 minutes, and it has turned into a ritual that I cannot do without.

Goal #3—Yoga as a way of life has become a reality for me. It is a perfect way to begin the day. When circumstances cause me to miss a morning yoga session, my reactions for the rest of the day are usually too quick and impulsive and lead to trouble at times. If I have not "mellowed out" before I leave the house to meet the rest of the world, it shows. However, after a little yoga/meditation in the morning, rush-hour traffic, road rage, snow and ice, voice-mail, and e-mail waiting on my computer do not have the same negative impact as they used to have. Now, all these normally nerve-wracking things are just "there." Part of the yoga philosophy is to put no judgments upon persons and circumstances, but to realize that they are just "there" and accept and move on. I know this sounds too simplistic, and it is to an extent. It takes many years of training and practice to become proficient in meditation and in "being there." However, as an amateur, I transformed this new-found practice into a more concrete and practical philosophy for myself. It is quite difficult to stop a lifetime habit of reacting, of labeling people, places, and situations as good or bad. Difficult, but not impossible. An example of applying this kind of thinking to a situation is when you are given a project at work that would take a normal human being 3 working days; you are told by your superior that he or she wants a completed product in 2 days. An immediate response might be "no can do." What happens next is what you allow to happen. Panic, anger, frustration usually rule the day. However, if you clear your mind, breathe deeply with eyes closed, you realize that problems and challenges are usually solvable. The thought process is then free to come up with possible solutions, rather than remain in a panic state. In this scenario, for instance, assistance can be requested, the deadline can be negotiated, logical reasons why this can't be done in 2 days can be pointed out. If and when all your solutions fail, you then do your best and leave it at that. The human condition has limits, and there is nothing more you can do other than your personal best. If that is not acceptable to others, it must be acceptable to yourself or else your body will rebel, become tired, sick, "burned out." When you've hit your burnout level, performing at your personal best can no longer be achieved. It is very easy to forget the fact that you are in charge; take care of yourself, or you will *not* be able to handle life in a positive and healthy manner.

Every one of us gets subtle, and not so subtle, warning signs from our bodies. Gritting teeth, inability to sleep, snapping at friends as well as foes, are all triggers that warn you: STOP! No one can take care of a problem if that person does not admit, or even see, that it *is* a problem. To quiet the mind and acquire more awareness, I would recommend any type of meditation or yoga. It doesn't matter the type, it matters in the doing. Yoga and/or meditation do not require chanting, joining a cloister, or wearing long robes. Like walking, this is another area where it is a totally personal activity. You can do it any time of the day, anywhere you choose, for as long or short a time as you desire. The place you choose can be absolutely quiet or soft music can be playing. The practice of yoga is not a one-size-fits-all, which is one of the many reasons that convinced me to embrace yoga as a step toward healthy living.

By the fall of 1997, I had come a long way in my personal quest for health. I was proud of myself, and had learned to manage many new things at the workplace: new boss, new computer program, new projects. Not one puff of a cigarette had crossed my lips; my walking regimen was down pat, I was taking vitamins and eating nutritious foods (most of the time). I looked good, felt good, and was outstretching my younger counterparts with catlike yoga moves. Despite all of this, my weight was still 15 to 20 pounds heavier than I had ever been. I was not pleased. I had heard that once you quit smoking, you inevitably gain weight; when you turn 50 years old, you gain weight; fill in the blank, you gain weight. (Get the picture? More excuses.) One evening, I was discussing my weight problem with my grown son and he jokingly said to me, "Why don't you take karate like I do? That will get you in shape!" Excuse me? Karate? Boxing gloves? Kicking? Sparring with actual people? Getting hurt? Breaking boards and concrete with body extremities? Really, the suggestion was ludicrous, so I quietly assured my loving son that he had lost his mind to even suggest such a crazy idea. However, once again a little seed was sown. Every day I drove by a local Tang Soo Do karate school on my way home from work. Every day for a month, I almost stopped. This crazy karate idea kept creeping into my consciousness. I needed to consult with Chuck Norris or Jackie Chan, but I did not think they would return my calls. My second option was to call my quasi-consultant son and ask that he accompany me on a visit, even though Tang Soo Do was a different style of karate than he was taking. He agreed. I had no idea what to expect as we stepped into an inviting, well-lighted reception area. The walls were covered with pictures of students, trophies shined from shelves, and signs were posted stating, "Please remove your shoes." An office door opened, and a young, rather petite woman smiled and asked if she could be of help. She was the instructor (Kyo Sa Nim), and she wore a white karate uniform (do-bok) with a black belt (dee) around her waist. She gave me a tour of the training room (dojang) and invited me to stay to watch a class in progress. I was fascinated, but not yet hooked. For a minimal fee, I was offered four introductory, private lessons so that I could test the waters before making any final decision to become a member of the school. After these introductory lessons, I was just about hooked.

Two weeks later, I took the plunge and signed up for an 18-month commitment. I was quite nervous and excited when I arrived for my first group class. There were 20 to 25 strangers of both sexes and all ages. I did not know it at the time, but I was the oldest one! At the beginning of class the instructor began the warm-up stretches, which I did very well because of my yoga training. Just when I mistakenly thought that karate training might be tamer than I anticipated, the following orders were shouted in a loud and stern voice by the instructor: "100 jumping jacks, 30 squat thrusts, 30 sit-ups. Begin!" At that moment I was thunderstruck. I thought I had made a terrible mistake, that I had signed up for the Marine Corps, that I was not going to make it through the next hour and still be alive. Today I can laugh about all these feelings, because I have progressed through eight promotions, having earned a red belt in Tang Soo Do Karate. I intend to stay with this program in order to earn my black belt in another 18 months.

Broken boards, belts, and certificates of achievement cover the walls of my game room at home. I have muscles in my arms and legs that I never knew existed. Incidentally, I did lose those first 10 pounds and I am still working on the next 10. The commitment and camaraderie among my fellow students is unprecedented. New and inspiring people from the karate community have become my friends. This is exactly what I needed to fill some of the gaps from the deaths of my sister and best friend. I feel so much more like a whole and complete person again, not just physically, but spiritually and emotionally as well.

The Tang Soo Do philosophy encompasses much more than physical fitness and stamina; it is a way ("the way of the worthy hand" literally) of living to your fullest potential. The overall purpose for Tang Soo Do karate training is the enhancement of the mental and physical self. It has sharpened my awareness of the connection between the mind and body; it has helped me to clear my mind of clutter; it has built stamina and strength of my physical body. This mind/body connection is a most important concept to embrace and understand. The evidence of this fact is apparent when breaking boards. The mind alone can never split a board in half, but without training, physical force alone cannot easily break a board either. It takes the mind and body working in concert to accomplish this feat. The first time I was required to break a board was during the promotion test from yellow to orange belt; it required breaking with the side of the hand (knife hand). I was very fearful of breaking a bone or severely bruising my hand. I set the fear aside, and called upon everything I had learned over the past 6 months. I psyched myself to believe I could do it—with proper breathing, concentration, focus, and balance. When my name was called, I stepped forward, bowed to the Grand Master, and said, "Permission to break, sir." All eyes were upon me as I walked toward the men in black belts holding an inch-thick square piece of wood. I approached the break station, lifted my arm, and much to my shock and amazement, my hand went crashing through the wood, splitting it cleanly in half. The guests and other students began applauding as I bowed to the Grand Master, pieces of board tucked under my arm, smiling like a Cheshire cat. There is no greater feeling than to accomplish something that you thought to be unreachable or impossible. Although I had 40 years on the young boy in *The Karate Kid* movie, I was just as jubilant and wide-eyed as he appeared in that film.

Because I am not a health professional, I felt privileged to be asked to share my personal journey from illness to health with others through the writing of this chapter. My memories of this time, both fearful and pleasant, are there to remind me of the past and to help me with the future. My health is much better than ever; but more important, I have made a promise to myself to do everything I can to get better and better every day. Results are not always quick enough, and it is very tempting to give up striving toward good health. Believe me, there are times when my mind is begging me to snuggle up on the living couch, saying over and over, "you don't have to go to karate tonight, it's snowing," These are the times that try men's souls. You just have to ignore the inner pleadings, get up, get dressed, get in the car, and go. Really, it's as simple as that!

REFERENCE

Northrup, C. (1998). *Women's bodies, women's wisdom: Creating physical and emotional health and healing* (2nd ed.). New York: Bantam Books.

CHAPTER 23

Summary/Conclusions

Ellen Olshansky

This book has presented an overview of current health issues and concerns for women, with a particular focus on the various and complex contexts in which women live and experience their health and health care. In keeping with an integrated, holistic approach to women's health, these multiple influencing factors were emphasized, in addition to the physical aspects of women's health. These health issues and concerns are included in Part I. In addition, Part III highlights some specific contextual issues that may influence women's health and well-being and provides some anecdotal/experiential perspectives.

Goals for women's wellness were delineated based on this integrated and holistic framework. The goals serve as a guideline for the variety of health care strategies and approaches included in Part II of the book. To reiterate a major intent of the book, these strategies are presented in an effort to provide the reader with an overview of both traditional and complementary approaches to women's wellness. Consistent with a true holistic perspective, a combination of approaches is included, without endorsing one particular approach over another. It is hoped that clinicians may find particular approaches or combinations of approaches useful for their particular patients.

As more attention and more scientific research are directed toward these various approaches to health care, clinicians will be better able to devise, in conjunction with their patients, a truly comprehensive plan of care, which includes a strong focus on health promotion and illness prevention. Perhaps combinations of approaches can optimize the outcome for a specific person.

As society continues the knowledge and technology explosion that is in full force, it is imperative that we maintain a human connection to our patients. A holistic and integrated approach to care will emphasize such a connection.

Index